Pulmonary Pearls

STEVEN A. SAHN, M.D.

Professor of Medicine
Director, Division of Pulmonary
  and Critical Care Medicine
Medical University of South Carolina
Charleston, South Carolina

JOHN E. HEFFNER, M.D.

Associate Professor of Medicine
Division of Pulmonary
  and Critical Care Medicine
Medical University of South Carolina
Charleston, South Carolina

HANLEY & BELFUS, INC.,/Philadelphia
THE C.V. MOSBY COMPANY/St. Louis • Toronto • London

Publisher: HANLEY & BELFUS, INC.
                    210 S. 13th Street
                    Philadelphia, PA 19107

North American and worldwide sales and distribution:
                    THE C.V. MOSBY COMPANY
                    11830 Westline Industrial Drive
                    St. Louis, MO 63146

In Canada: THE C.V. MOSBY COMPANY
                    120 Melford Drive
                    Scarborough, Canada M1B 2X5

PULMONARY PEARLS   ISBN 0-932883-16-8

Library of Congress catalog card number 88-081283

Last digit is the print number: 9 8 7 6 5 4 3 2 1

To our wives and children —

Ellie, Karen, Stacey, Jimmy, Mike, and Rachel Sahn

Ann, John, and James Heffner

CONTENTS

FOREWORD

Among the most exciting features of the field of pulmonary medicine are the innumerable diagnostic challenges faced by the clinician. The history and physical examination are aided by a variety of images, physiological measurements, and other laboratory tests that help the physician to perceive the salient facts about the nature of the symptoms and signs presented by the patient. The goal is to develop a concept that will result in an effective working diagnosis, which, in turn, will later either be confirmed or abandoned in favor of a better hypothesis. In the end, we seek a microbial or histologic diagnosis or both in most cases, or at least the necessary criteria to diagnose an entity that may not have a defined etiology, such as in some of the immunologically mediated disease states. And we sometimes are enlightened by certain unique features, often called "pearls," which become important clues to a diagnosis.

Steven Sahn and John Heffner have captured the essence of the diagnostic challenge in pulmonary medicine. In this book they have intertwined their diagnostic approaches with succinct take-home messages presented as clinical pearls. No less than 100 cases are presented in Grand Rounds fashion. This format allows the reader to study each case as an "unknown" and thus test his or her diagnostic abilities. This book contains succinct reviews of interesting pulmonary cases with appropriate supporting laboratory data and images, which make extremely interesting reading.

No doubt the many pertinent pulmonary pearls will find their way into morning reports or other roundsmanship to the enlightenment of many.

THOMAS L. PETTY, M.D.

ACKNOWLEDGMENTS

We are indebted to the fellows of the Division of Pulmonary and Critical Care Medicine, Drs. Mary Lynn Allen, Michael Baumann, Michael Milam, Charlie Strange, Sally Wooten, and Cynthia Zamora, for the selection of cases and the initiation of the presentations at our conferences. We also thank Louisa Freeman, Jeanne Jaeger, and Terri Kelly for their tireless efforts in obtaining and organizing the clinical and radiographic data.

Permission to reproduce three figures is gratefully acknowledged: Figure for Patient 14 is reproduced with permission from Strange C, Heffner JE, Collins BS, Brown FM, Sahn SA. Pulmonary hemorrhage and air embolism complicating transbronchial biopsy in pulmonary amyloidosis. Chest 1987; 92:367–369. Figure for Patient 32 is reproduced with permission from Heffner JE, Milam MG. Sarcoid-like hilar and mediastinal lymphadenopathy in a patient with metastatic testicular cancer. Cancer 1987; 60:1545–1547. Figure for Patient 59 is reproduced with permission from Heffner JE. When to consider fiberoptic bronchoscopy in the ICU. J Crit Illness 1988; 3:69–82.

PREFACE

We conceived the idea for this book in our biweekly chest conference where current patients with interesting or unusual pulmonary problems from the clinical services of the three Medical University of South Carolina hospitals are presented. Pulmonary fellows are asked to interpret the patient's chest radiograph, to formulate an initial differential diagnosis derived from pertinent radiographic and clinical findings, and to provide a management plan for further diagnostic investigations and therapeutic efforts. Our pulmonary trainees are encouraged to develop a comprehensive approach to clinical problem-solving that is based on a broad knowledge in both pulmonary and internal medicine. These efforts and the lively discussions that follow typically generate a welter of clinical information, especially from the experiences and readings of the senior pulmonologists in attendance. Several clinical pearls invariably emerge as the discussions become focused.

It occurred to us that presentation of the conference discussions in a concise format would provide valuable information that is difficult to find and not readily available in standard textbooks for practicing physicians and house officers interested in the diagnosis and management of pulmonary disease. Additionally, the style of presentation in a problem-solving format is an ideal study aid for physicians preparing for internal medicine and pulmonary board examinations. The 100 case presentations are organized in the style of our clinical conference: a brief clinical vignette is presented, accompanied by a chest radiograph and other pertinent laboratory results. The reader is encouraged to consider a differential diagnosis and to formulate a plan for diagnostic and therapeutic management based on the available data. The subsequent page discloses the patient's diagnosis followed by a discussion of the salient features of pathophysiology, clinical presentation, diagnosis, and treatment. The features of this discussion that are sufficiently valuable to warrant the designation "clinical pearls" are listed at the end of the discussion.

We have attempted to capture the atmosphere of our chest conference, presenting a large amount of information concisely. Furthermore, conclusions based on anecdotal experiences have been avoided, with the major thrust of the discussion supported by the references provided. Comments on controversial topics are clearly stated in the text to be speculative.

STEVEN A. SAHN, M.D.
JOHN E. HEFFNER, M.D.

PATIENT 1

A 55-year-old man with confusion, cough, pleuritic chest pain, and hyponatremia

A 55-year-old man was admitted because of confusion, cough, and pleuritic chest pain. He had been well until 4 days earlier when he noticed malaise, anorexia, and a low-grade fever followed by the onset of a dry cough, right-sided pleuritic chest pain, and myalgias. On the day of admission, the patient developed watery diarrhea, and the family became concerned because of his increasing confusion. The patient had been a long-time smoker, but did not have pets or occupational exposure to pulmonary toxins.

Physical Examination: Pulse 95, temperature 104.2°, respirations 25, blood pressure 120/70; dullness and tubular breath sounds at the lung bases with diffuse rales; no cardiac murmur; soft abdomen; agitated and confused.

Laboratory Findings: Sodium 120 mEq/L; BUN 69 mg/dl; creatinine 6.5 mg/dl; WBC 18,000/μl with 90% PMNs; Hct 40%; phosphate 2.1 mEq/L; LDH 4,800 IU/L; CPK 95,000 IU/L; SGOT 2,000 IU/L; urine was dark brown with a normal sediment. Chest radiograph showed bilateral alveolar infiltrates with consolidation in the right middle and left lower lobes.

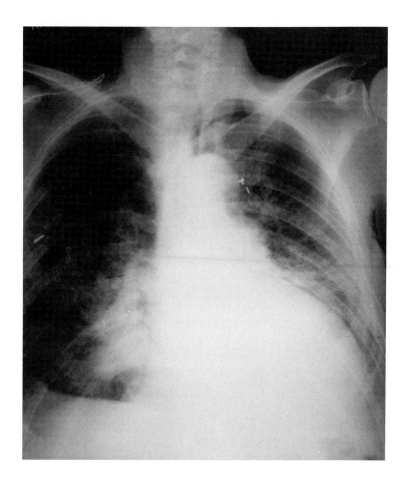

Diagnosis: Legionella pneumonia with rhabdomyolysis.

Discussion: Although Legionnaires' disease accounts for less than 10% of community-acquired pneumonias, several of the patient's clinical features suggested this diagnosis. The gradual prodrome with fever, malaise, and anorexia without accompanying upper respiratory tract symptoms is characteristic of Legionella pneumonia, as is the subsequent development of encephalopathy, relative bradycardia, watery diarrhea, and pleuritic chest pain. Although the chest radiograph demonstrating segmental or lobar consolidation is consistent with Legionnaires' disease, there are no radiographic features that distinguish the disorder from mycoplasmal or pneumococcal pneumonia. Blood chemistries do assist in this differential diagnosis, since hyponatremia, hypophosphatemia, and elevated LDH and SGOT levels are more commonly found in Legionnaires' disease than other causes of atypical pneumonia.

Once suspected, the diagnosis of Legionnaires' disease should be urgently pursued, since mortality from pneumonia increases with delay in therapy. Only 50% of patients produce sputum, which typically reveals a paucity of organisms or cellular components. Expectorated sputum may demonstrate the organism by direct immunofluorescent staining or culture on selective media. Transtracheal aspiration is an effective diagnostic technique and may have a higher yield than bronchoscopy with bronchoalveolar lavage, because growth in culture of the Legionella organism is inhibited by saline. This fact has caused some investigators to suggest that bronchoalveolar lavage should be performed with sterile water

rather than saline when Legionnaires' disease is a diagnostic possibility. A four-fold rise in acute and convalescent antibody titers is a specific test with only a 70% sensitivity, but does not assist in the initial clinical diagnosis.

Renal failure, as occurred in this patient, is an unusual finding in Legionnaires' disease. Approximately 12% of patients present with renal insufficiency, which is usually mild in degree and does not require hemodialysis. Pathologic correlations are scanty, but acute tubular necrosis or interstitial nephritis are common findings. Rare instances of irreversible rapidly progressive glomerulonephritis have been reported. Renal failure caused by associated rhabdomyolysis, as represented by the present patient, is a previously noted occurrence in Legionella pneumonia. The etiology of the muscle injury is uncertain, although it may relate to underlying metabolic disturbances such as the hypophosphatemia, acidosis, and hyponatremia that commonly accompany Legionnaires' disease. The possibility that the combined toxicity of several exotoxins from the organism plays a role has not been excluded. Muscle biopsies have not detected the presence of the organism.

The present patient could not produce sputum for evaluation, so a transtracheal aspiration was performed, demonstrating *Legionella pneumophilia* on direct immunofluorescent stains. The patient received erythromycin and rifampin, eventually recovering from the pneumonia and renal failure after a short course of hemodialysis. The sputum culture was subsequently positive for Legionella.

Clinical Pearls

1. Legionella pneumonia is occasionally associated with rhabdomyolysis-induced renal failure.

2. Use of saline during bronchoalveolar lavage may decrease the culture yield of Legionella.

REFERENCES

1. Hall SL, Wasserman M, Dall L, Schubert T. Acute renal failure secondary to myoglobinuria associated with Legionnaires' disease. Chest 1983; 84:633–635.
2. Edelstein PH, Meyer RD. Legionnaires' disease. A review. Chest 1984; 85:114–120.
3. Johnson JF, Raff MJ, Van Arsdall JA. Neurologic manifestations of Legionnaires' disease. Medicine 1984; 63:303–310.

PATIENT 2

A 40-year-old woman with arthralgias and respiratory failure

A 40-year-old woman was admitted for care of severe dyspnea and cyanosis. She had been well until one month earlier when she noted arthralgias and swelling of her fingers and wrists. Three weeks later, she developed a facial rash followed by cough, dyspnea, and bilateral pleuritic chest pain.

Physical Examination: Pulse 130; respirations 35; temperature 103°. Scattered crackles at both lung bases with tubular breath sounds, no rubs; cardiac normal; palpable splenomegaly; mild pitting edema of both ankles with redness and swelling of the distal interphalangeal joints.

Laboratory Findings: Hct 35%, WBC 7,700/μl; creatinine 1.1 mg/dl; urinalysis normal; sputum Gram stain unremarkable. ABG (room air): pH 7.54, PCO_2 27 mmHg, PO_2 48 mmHg. Chest radiograph demonstrated diffuse bilateral alveolar infiltrates with left pleural effusion.

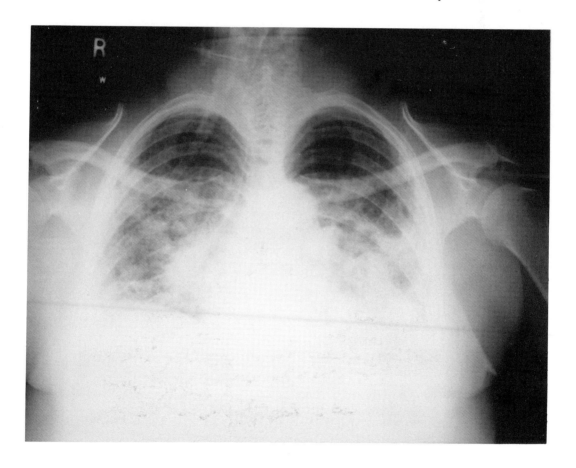

Diagnosis: Acute lupus pneumonitis.

Discussion: Systemic lupus erythematosus is a multisystem inflammatory disorder that commonly involves the lungs. The true incidence of pulmonary complications is unknown, since patients with lupus are often immunocompromised, with impaired renal and cardiovascular function causing numerous infectious and edematous respiratory conditions that may mimic lupus lung.

Lupus pneumonitis typically presents as a fulminant illness. Patients demonstrate fever and shortness of breath variably associated with pleuritic chest pain, hemoptysis, and cough. Although patients may experience pneumonitis despite mild underlying lupus, most instances occur in patients with severe systemic disease. Lupus pneumonitis, however, may be the initial manifestation of lupus, as in the present patient, and severely challenge the clinician to consider the diagnosis.

Signs and laboratory features of lupus pneumonitis are often nonspecific. Physical findings are common to other causes of respiratory insufficiency, and include fever, tachypnea, cyanosis, and basilar rales, although some patients may have coexisting skin rashes or articular findings. Blood tests are equally nonspecific, although positive ANA tests may suggest the diagnosis. The chest radiographic findings are variable, ranging from ill-defined patchy opacities to extensive bilateral alveolar infiltrates predominantly in the lower lobes commonly associated with pleural effusions. Histopathologic findings are similarly nonspecific, demonstrating interstitial edema, hyaline membranes, acute alveolitis, arteriolar thrombosis, intraalveolar hemorrhage, and alveolar cell hyperplasia.

Lupus pneumonitis is a diagnosis of exclusion. Included in the list of diagnostic possibilities are opportunistic infections, sepsis, congestive heart failure, noncardiogenic pulmonary edema, renal failure, malignancy, and multiple pulmonary emboli. If associated renal or cardiovascular conditions complicate diagnosis and the clinical setting or laboratory findings are equivocal, bronchoscopy or open lung biopsy may be indicated. Biopsy specimens are not diagnostic of lupus pneumonitis, but they may serve to exclude the presence of alternative diagnoses such as infection.

Despite early diagnosis and rapid initiation of therapy, survival in lupus pneumonitis is poor, with a 50% mortality. Up to 50% of survivors may have some degree of long-term respiratory limitation or radiographic abnormality. The remaining 25% of patients who fully recover underscore the importance of aggressive management. Ideal therapy is uncertain, but patients appear to benefit from 1 mg/kg/day of prednisone administered orally in divided doses. Although beneficial in other serious manifestations of lupus, high-dose intravenous methylprednisolone pulse therapy has not been evaluated in lupus pneumonitis. Anecdotal reports indicate benefit from azathioprine and cyclophosphamide, which should be given to patients not responding to corticosteroids.

The serum antinuclear antibody (ANA) test in the present patient was positive in a homogeneous pattern at a titer of 1:320, with decreased total hemolytic complement and positive anti-DNA. The patient was carefully evaluated for infectious etiologies, but expectorated sputums, transtracheal aspiration, and blood cultures were negative. She was treated with prednisone with a gradual improvement in her condition.

Clinical Pearls

1. The majority of patients with lupus and an abnormal chest radiograph have a secondary condition, such as heart failure or infection, causing their pulmonary condition.

2. Lupus pneumonitis is more common in patients with severe lupus but may be the initial manifestation of the underlying systemic disease.

3. Although the mortality in lupus pneumonitis is 50%, up to 25% of patients may experience complete recovery.

REFERENCES

1. Pines A, Kaplinsky N, Olchovsky D, et al. Pleuro-pulmonary manifestations of systemic lupus erythematosus: clinical features of its subgroups: prognostic and therapeutic implications. Chest 1985; 86:129–135.
2. Brasington RD, Furst DE. Pulmonary disease in systemic lupus erythematosus. Clin Exp Rheumatol 1985; 3:269–276.
3. Matthay RA, Schwarz MI, Petty TL, et al. Pulmonary manifestations of systemic lupus erythematosus: review of twelve cases of acute lupus pneumonitis. Medicine 1974; 54:397–409.

PATIENT 3

A 71-year-old woman with muscular weakness, dyspnea, and diffuse interstitial infiltrates

A 71-year-old woman developed muscular weakness, dyspnea, and a cough. She had noted arthralgias and difficulty getting out of a chair that progressed over one year.

Physical Examination: Afebrile; thin with decreased muscle mass; diffuse rales throughout all lung fields; marked proximal and distal limb muscular weakness.

Laboratory Findings: Normal CBC and electrolytes. Erythrocyte sedimentation rate 98 mm/hr. ANA positive at a titer of 1:40; rheumatoid factor negative. Creatine kinase normal at 100 IU/L; aldolase normal at 4.8 IU/ml. Chest radiograph showed bilateral diffuse interstitial infiltrates with small lung volumes. ABG (room air): pH 7.42, PO_2 76 mmHg, PCO_2 39 mmHg. Spirometry: FEV_1 0.9 L (75% of predicted), FVC 1.1 L (84% of predicted), $FEV_1/FVC\%$ 82%. An electromyogram (EMG) demonstrated nonspecific findings compatible with a myopathy.

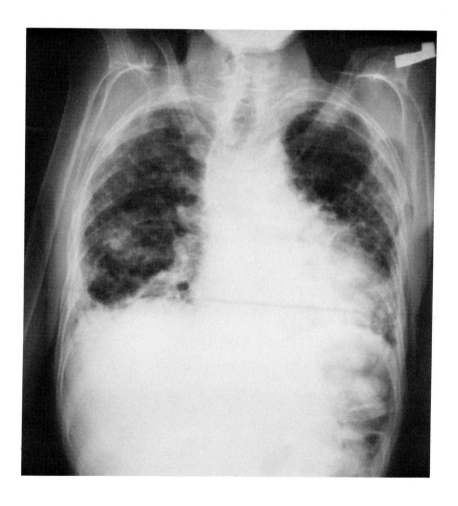

Diagnosis: Polymyositis with polymyositis-related interstitial lung disease.

Discussion: Polymyositis and dermatomyositis are inflammatory myopathies with progressive symmetric muscular weakness. The conditions are identical except for the characteristic rash associated with dermatomyositis. A definitive diagnosis of polymyositis requires the presence of progressive symmetric limb-girdle muscular weakness, biopsy evidence of myositis, elevated skeletal muscle enzymes, and EMG evidence of a myopathy. A probable diagnosis requires the presence of any three of the above criteria.

Despite active and rapidly progressive disease, this patient had normal skeletal muscle enzymes that did not become elevated during subsequent follow-up. Although this finding was initially disconcerting for the pulmonologists, the consulting rheumatologists pointed out that up to 20% of patients with polymyositis/dermatomyositis may have normal enzyme levels despite crippling disease. In fact, a normal creatine kinase level in these conditions is associated with a poor prognosis, with survival less than one year, and is usually found in patients with interstitial lung disease and underlying neoplasms.

Patients with polymyositis/dermatomyositis are subject to a multitude of pulmonary disorders. Traditional concepts limit the spectrum of pulmonary disease to interstitial lung disease, aspiration pneumonia, and ventilatory failure from muscular weakness. Recent clinicopathologic studies, however, indicate that pulmonary vasculitis, pulmonary hypertension, pulmonary edema with or without associated cardiac or renal disease, opportunistic infections after immunosuppressive therapy, and isolated diaphragmatic paresis should be considered in the evaluation of these patients.

Interstitial lung disease is a common complication reported in 10 to 40% of patients with polymyositis/dermatomyositis. The chest radiograph and histopathologic findings are nonspecific, being similar to other collagen vascular–related interstitial lung diseases. The diagnosis rests on a firm diagnosis of the underlying polymyositis, with exclusion of pulmonary processes such as congestive heart failure and infection. Lung biopsies should not be necessary. As occurred in the present patient, arthralgias are commonly present when interstitial lung disease complicates polymyositis. The development of interstitial lung disease is ominous, with mean survival less than 18 months following onset. Response to glucocorticoid therapy in this condition is variable, with a minority of patients improving.

A muscle biopsy confirmed myositis in the present patient and no other probable cause for the pulmonary abnormality existed. The patient was started on prednisone and initially improved with less muscular weakness; however, weakness recurred within six months, and the patient died of bronchopneumonia.

Clinical Pearls

1. Normal serum muscle enzyme levels do not exclude the diagnosis of polymyositis/dermatomyositis in patients with interstitial infiltrates and muscular weakness.

2. Normal serum muscle enzyme levels in polymyositis/dermatomyositis portend an unfavorable prognosis.

3. Patients with polymyositis/dermatomyositis and interstitial lung disease commonly have associated arthralgias.

REFERENCES

1. Lakhanpal S, Lie JT, Conn DL, Martin II WJ. Pulmonary disease in polymyositis/dermatomyositis: a clinicopathological analysis of 65 autopsy cases. Ann Rheum Dis 1987; 46:23–29.
2. Fudman EJ, Schnitzer TJ. Dermatomyositis without creatine kinase elevation. A poor prognostic sign. Am J Med 1986; 80:329–332.

PATIENT 4

A 27-year-old woman with mediastinal masses, a right pleural effusion, and a history of irradiated Hodgkin's disease

A 27-year-old woman was evaluated for a 2-month history of dyspnea. Eleven years earlier she underwent mantle irradiation for Hodgkin's disease that responded to therapy without known recurrence. She had smoked two packs of cigarettes a day since she was 15 years old. She denied night sweats, cough, weight loss or fever, but did note swelling in her face and hands.

Physical Examination: Breasts normal; facial edema with elevated neck veins; chest dull at the right base with decreased breath sounds and fremitus.

Laboratory Findings: CBC, liver function tests, and electrolytes normal. Chest radiograph revealed bilateral hilar and mediastinal masses extending along the right pleural surface with a right pleural effusion. Bilateral intraparenchymal masses were also present. Thoracentesis: sero-sanguinous fluid, pH 7.34, protein 5.0 g/dl, LDH 890 IU/L, glucose 76 mg/dl, leukocytes 7,900/μl with 90% lymphocytes. Cytology: atypical small "lymphocytes."

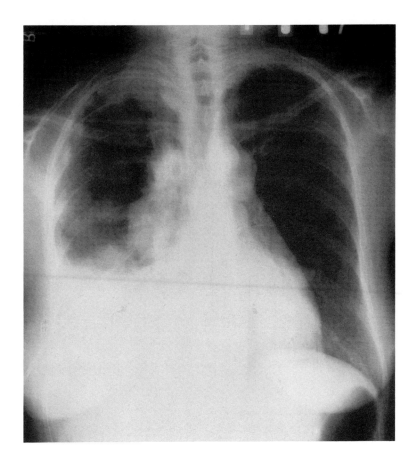

Diagnosis: Small-cell lung cancer with malignant pleural effusion and superior vena cava syndrome.

Discussion: Lung cancer is a rare disorder in young adults. The peak incidence occurs in middle age, with 70% of lung cancers diagnosed between the ages of 50 and 60 years. Several series indicate that 6% of lung cancers occur in patients younger than 39 years, with only 0.2% in patients less than 29 years of age. The profile of younger patients with lung cancer appears similar to that of patients in older age groups: the cancers tend to be advanced and unresectable when diagnosed, patients are typically smokers, and survival is poor. All cell types in young patients with lung cancer are represented, but adenocarcinoma occurs most frequently.

The patient's young age and previously treated Hodgkin's disease suggest a relationship between the thoracic irradiation and subsequent development of small-cell carcinoma. It is well established that patients with Hodgkin's disease treated with chemotherapy have a 10 to 18% incidence over 15 years of developing a second neoplasm, usually acute nonlymphoblastic leukemia. It is less well established that treated patients also are at increased risk for various solid tumors. Reported series indicate that solid tumors primarily occur in patients with Hodgkin's disease treated with radiation therapy rather than chemotherapy alone and develop after a 10-year latent period. This observation complements the general belief that radiation-induced tumors require a prolonged induction period. Squamous cell cancer of the head and neck, lung cancer, non-Hodgkin's lymphoma, and Kaposi's sarcoma represent the heterogeneous group of tumors reported to occur in 7 to 13% of patients with Hodgkin's disease treated with radiation.

Although small-cell lung cancer has a known relationship to exposure to radon daughters (e.g., uranium miners), this cell type has not been reported to occur more commonly in patients treated with radiation therapy for other malignancies. Since small-cell cancer has a close relationship to smoking, the present patient's radiation treatment combined with an unusually intense cigarette exposure for her age may have promoted this particular second neoplasm.

The clinical presentation, chest radiograph, and pleural fluid profile of the patient were compatible with a pulmonary malignancy, and a subsequent pleural biopsy was positive for small-cell cancer. A CT scan confirmed the presence of superior vena cava syndrome. The patient underwent treatment with chemotherapy for small-cell cancer, with rapid resolution of the superior vena cava syndrome and pleural effusion.

Clinical Pearls

1. Patients with treated Hodgkin's disease are at increased risk for a second malignancy. Chemotherapy predisposes to acute leukemia, and radiation therapy appears to cause solid tumors after a long induction period.

2. Young adults with lung cancer develop adenocarcinoma as the most common cell type and usually present with widespread disease and a poor prognosis.

REFERENCES

1. Coleman CN. Secondary neoplasms in patients treated for cancer: etiology and perspective. Radiation Res 1982; 92:188–200.
2. Schomberg PJ, Evans RG, Banks PM, et al. Second malignant lesions after therapy for Hodgkin's disease. Mayo Clin Proc 1984; 59:493–497.
3. Putnam JS. Lung carcinoma in young adults. JAMA 1977; 238:35-36.
4. Tucker MA, Coleman CN, Cox RS, et al. Risk of second cancers after treatment for Hodgkin's disease. N Engl J Med 1988; 318:76–80.

PATIENT 5

A 55-year-old man with ankylosing spondylitis and a unilateral lung cavity

A 55-year-old man with ankylosing spondylitis for 20 years had a routine chest radiograph. He denied pulmonary symptoms or exposure to tuberculosis. His most recent chest radiograph five years earlier showed no parenchymal abnormalities.

Physical Examination: Afebrile, thoracic kyphosis; normal chest except for dullness and decreased breath sounds over the right apex.

Laboratory Findings: CBC normal. Chest radiograph showed a right upper lobe thick-walled cavity with adjacent pleural thickening and vertebral stigmata of ankylosing spondylitis. Negative PPD with positive controls; sputum smears and cultures negative for acid-fast organisms.

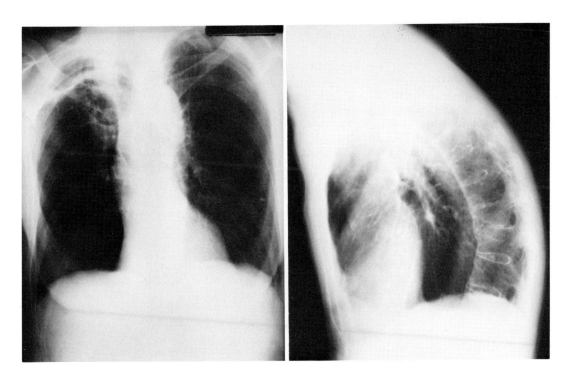

Diagnosis: Unilateral fibrobullous disease secondary to ankylosing spondylitis.

Discussion: Ankylosing spondylitis is notable for its association with several extraarticular disorders that include uveitis, ulcerative colitis, and pleuropulmonary disease. The pleuropulmonary manifestations usually develop in the seventh decade of life, 20 years after the initial diagnosis of ankylosing spondylitis, at a time when the underlying rheumatologic disorder is inactive. In evaluating patients with pulmonary complications, obvious stigmata of ankylosing spondylitis, such as thoracic spine fusion, are typically apparent.

The most common pleuropulmonary manifestations associated with ankylosing spondylitis are apical fibrobullous disease and ankylosis of costovertebral junctions, resulting in limitations of chest wall expansion. Transient exudative pleural effusions with normal glucose content and diffuse pleural thickening have been noted, but their etiologic relationship to ankylosing spondylitis has not been confirmed.

Apical fibrobullous disease is an unexplained complication of ankylosing spondylitis. Reported to occur in 10 to 30% of patients with this disorder, its true incidence is probably closer to 1 to 2%. The apical disease begins as localized peripheral fibrosis with radiographic evidence of increased interstitial markings and apical pleural thickening. Over time, the fibrotic areas break down with the formation of air spaces that may be thin-walled and cystic or thick-walled with a cavitary appearance. As notably present in this patient, the apical pleura is thickened adjacent to the cavity. The pathologic changes in the lung parenchyma may range from mild to severe in degree and, although fibrobullous disease usually begins as a unilateral process, it progresses to bilateral disease. In one series of 25 patients, however, unilateral disease in eight patients was limited to the right side in all but one patient.

Patients with fibrobullous disease are usually asymptomatic, denying cough, shortness of breath, fever, sputum or hemoptysis. The onset of these symptoms may indicate an alternative diagnosis, such as pulmonary tuberculosis, or the development of a complication of fibrobullous disease, such as aspergilloma. Aspergillus is a common saprophyte in patients with fibrobullous disease from ankylosing spondylitis and creates a risk for hemoptysis. A classic finding related to aspergillomas is pleural thickening adjacent to an apical cavity—a sign that is also noted in uncomplicated fibrobullous disease from ankylosing spondylitis. To exclude aspergillomas in these patients, tomography and serum Aspergillus precipitins are beneficial.

Patients with uncomplicated fibrobullous disease do not require therapy. Patients with aspergilloma and hemoptysis benefit from conservative management because of the morbidity of empyema and respiratory failure attached to pulmonary resection. If hemoptysis is recurrent, surgery should be considered in good operative candidates, with the remainder of patients undergoing bronchial artery embolization.

Clinical Pearls

1. Fibrobullous disease is usually an asymptomatic condition, complicating the course in 1 to 2% of patients with ankylosing spondylitis.

2. Although usually a bilateral condition, fibrobullous disease may present in a unilateral distribution.

3. Patients with fibrobullous disease related to ankylosing spondylitis with pulmonary symptoms may have underlying tuberculosis or a complicating aspergilloma.

REFERENCES
1. Rosenow EC III, Strimlan CB, Muhm JR, Ferguson RH. Pleuropulmonary manifestations of ankylosing spondylitis. Mayo Clin Proc 1977; 52:641–649.
2. Kinnear WJM, Shneerson JM. Acute pleural effusions in inactive ankylosing spondylitis. Thorax 1985; 40:150–151.
3. Davies D. Ankylosing spondylitis and lung fibrosis. Q J Med 1972; 41:395–417.

PATIENT 6

A 54-year-old man with fever, pleuritic chest pain, weight loss, and a chronic cough of 3 months' duration

A 54-year-old man with chronic alcoholism was admitted for evaluation of a chronic cough after a 3-month history of right pleuritic chest pain, fever, weight loss, and night sweats. A chest radiograph 3 months earlier showed a small right lower lobe infiltrate that was treated with an oral cephalosporin antibiotic and not reevaluated.

Physical Examination: Temperature 99°; poor dentition; decreased breath sounds; fremitus in the posterior right lower thorax.

Laboratory Findings: WBC 11,500/μl; Hct 30%; serum total protein 7.3 g/dl; serum LDH 160 IU/L; serum glucose 120 mg/dl. Chest radiograph showed scattered calcified granulomas, a right lower lobe infiltrate with air bronchograms, and a large right pleural effusion. PPD skin test was negative with positive control tests. Expectorated sputum was negative for pathogenic organisms. Thoracentesis: serous fluid; erythrocytes 130,000/μl; leukocytes 1,200/μl with 90% lymphocytes; LDH 700 IU/L; protein 5.3 g/dl; pH 7.54; amylase 40 IU/L; negative cytology; negative Gram and acid-fast stains with negative microbiologic cultures after 5 days. Fiberoptic bronchoscopy: no endobronchial lesions. Closed pleural biopsy: chronic pleural inflammation with negative microbiologic cultures and stains.

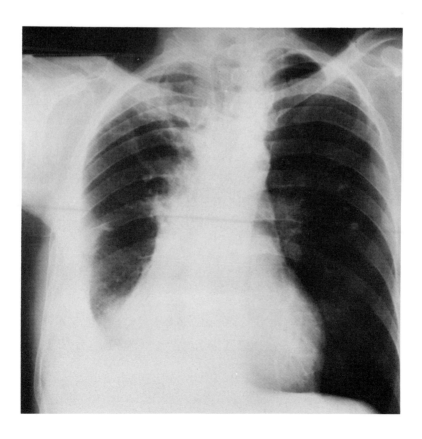

Diagnosis: Thoracic actinomycosis.

Discussion: Actinomycosis is a chronic suppurative infection caused by branching bacteria of the Actinomyces genus. *Actinomyces israelii* accounts for the vast majority of infections and is often found in association with other bacteria, as noted in this patient.

Actinomycosis is categorized into abdominal, cervicofacial, and thoracic disease. Abdominal actinomycosis is usually a complication of laparotomy and typically appears many weeks or months after surgery that characteristically involves the ileocecal region. Since these organisms often grow in the mouth and are found in abundance in patients with poor dental hygiene, cervicofacial infection is the common form of the disease. Patients present with a fluctuant mass in the lower mandible or submandibular region that may or may not be painful.

The present patient is typical of patients with thoracic actinomycosis in that the age distribution is 30 to 60 years, and males are three times as likely as females to acquire the disease. Additionally, the patient's chronic course is usual for actinomycosis, which may exist for months to years before presentation. Symptoms of cough, pleuritic chest pain, fever with night sweats, hemoptysis, superior vena cava syndrome, mild leukocytosis, and an elevated erythrocyte sedimentation rate are characteristic findings.

Thoracic actinomycosis invades the chest wall with abandon, showing little respect for anatomic barriers. Common radiographic presentations, therefore, include a chronic lower lobe infiltrate with an adjacent chest wall mass that may involve bone and pleura. In the preantibiotic era, these chest wall extensions commonly formed draining sinuses. Despite frequent involvement of the pleura, with pleural effusions in 40% of patients, large pleural effusions, as noted in the present patient, or empyemas are uncommon. Pleural fluid analysis reveals an exudate with predominantly polymorphonuclear leukocytes in the presence of pus or predominantly lymphocytes if serous fluid exists.

In the preantibiotic era, the mortality of actinomycosis approached 100%, but the advent of penicillin decreased mortality to less than 10%. Although standardization of therapy is impeded by the isolated nature of the disease, high-dose parenteral penicillin with 10 to 20 million units/day is usually successful when continued for 4 to 6 weeks. Many clinicians recommend an extended course of therapy with oral penicillin subsequently for 12 to 18 months, but recent reports indicate successful results with 2 to 3 months of treatment. The important considerations during therapy include the progression of occult foci of metastatic infection and relapse from partially treated organisms. Appropriate staging of infection by ultrasound or CT is indicated at the initiation of therapy, with consideration of gallium scans before discontinuance of antibiotics. Erythromycin, tetracycline, and clindamycin may be appropriate alternative agents for penicillin-sensitive patients.

The clinicians recommended an open lung biopsy in the present patient that demonstrated chronic inflammation with actinomycosis apparent on Gram stain. Lung specimens grew *Actinomyces israelii* and *Fusobacterium nucleatum* after 10 days. Intravenous penicillin was initiated at doses of 20 million units/day for 6 weeks. When the patient and radiograph improved, therapy was changed to oral penicillin with probenicid for an additional 3 months.

Clinical Pearls

1. A lower lobe pulmonary infiltrate with pleural or chest wall involvement in a patient with poor dentition at risk for aspiration suggests actinomycosis.
2. Large pleural effusions are unusual in thoracic actinomycosis, although pleural involvement occurs in 40% of patients.
3. Penicillin therapy for pulmonary actinomycosis is usually successful when continued for 2 to 3 months.

REFERENCES

1. Weese WB, Smith IM. A study of 57 cases of actinomycosis over a 36-year period: a diagnostic "failure" with good prognosis after treatment. Arch Intern Med 1975; 135:1562–1568.
2. Webb WR, Sagel SS. Actinomycosis involving the chest wall. AJR 1982; 139:1007–1009.

PATIENT 7

A 55-year-old man with weight loss, cough, hemoptysis, and an upper lobe cavity with a mediastinal mass

A 55-year-old man with a heavy smoking history was referred to the surgical service for evaluation of a possible pulmonary malignancy. During the previous 2 months, he had experienced a 20-pound weight loss, cough, and blood-streaked sputum. He denied prior illness but did travel extensively throughout the southeast and southwest United States.

Physical Examination: Vital signs normal; clear chest to auscultation and percussion; lymph nodes normal; no abdominal organomegaly.

Laboratory Findings: Electrolytes, renal function tests, and CBC were normal. Chest radiograph showed old calcified granulomas and a right upper lobe cavitary mass. A CT scan of the chest revealed an anterior mediastinal mass. Sputum cytology was negative but an auramine-rhodamine stain was positive for Mycobacterium.

The physicians related the right upper lobe cavity to tuberculosis but were concerned with the possible neoplastic etiology of the mediastinal mass. They subsequently elected to perform a thoracotomy for diagnosis after a percutaneous needle aspiration was nondiagnostic.

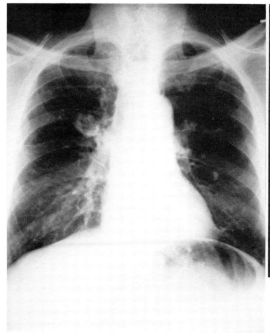 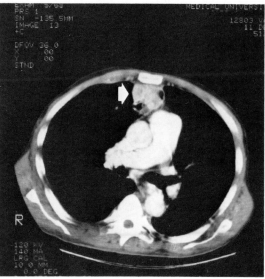

Diagnosis: Pulmonary tuberculosis with tuberculous mediastinal lymphadenitis.

Discussion: This patients's presentation was certainly suggestive of tuberculosis, although a cavitary carcinoma could have produced the same symptoms. Once the sputum smears were positive for Mycobacterium, however, greater consideration of mediastinal tuberculous lymphadenitis would have been warranted.

North American physicians are less experienced in the diagnosis of tuberculous lymphadenitis because of the low incidence of the disorder. In England, however, 40% of Asian immigrants with tuberculosis present with some form of lymphadenitis. Traditionally thought to be a childhood disease, recent series indicate that the mean age of patients presenting with tuberculous lymphadenitis is 49 years. Lymph nodes most commonly involved with tuberculosis are the intrathoracic and cervical chains, although lymphadenitis of the abdominal nodes also occurs. Within the thorax, affected nodes are most frequently paratracheal or hilar, but other mediastinal locations may be extensively involved, as occurred in this patient. Tuberculous lymphadenitis may develop during primary infection, during reactivation of a previously contained infection, or from extension of a contiguous focus.

In the setting of known pulmonary tuberculosis, enlarged mediastinal lymph nodes probably represent tuberculous lymphadenitis; however, in a middle-aged patient with a profound smoking history, major nodal enlargement could also represent a coexisting pulmonary neoplasm. This differential diagnosis is assisted by the CT appearance of the mediastinal mass. Enhancing or nonenhancing lymph nodes of uniform density do not separate tuberculous from neoplastic masses. A characteristic CT appearance of tuberculous lymph nodes is a multiloculated or multichambered mass with central lucency and thick rims of enhancement. This radiographic appearance in a patient with known tuberculosis is adequate confirmation of tuberculous lymphadenitis, obviating the need for tissue confirmation.

The present patient underwent thoracotomy with biopsy of the anterior mediastinal mass that demonstrated caseating granulomas positive for mycobacterial organisms. Subsequent culture results from the mass and sputum were positive for tuberculosis. He was treated with isoniazid and rifampin for 9 months, demonstrating resolution of the mediastinal mass over the usual time course of 4 months.

Clinical Pearls

1. Tuberculous lymphadenitis is a manifestation of primary or post-primary tuberculosis in middle-aged patients.

2. The CT appearance of involved lymph nodes can be sufficiently characteristic to confirm the diagnosis of tuberculous lymphadenitis.

REFERENCES

1. Reede DL, Bergeron RT. Cervical tuberculous adenitis: CT manifestations. Radiology 1985; 154:701–704.
2. Weir MR, Thornton GF. Extrapulmonary tuberculosis: experience of a community hospital and review of the literature. Am J Med 1985; 79:467–478.
3. Farrow PR, Jones DA, Stanley PJ, et al. Thoracic lymphadenopathy in Asians resident in the United Kingdom: role of mediastinoscopy in initial diagnosis. Thorax 1985; 40:121–124.

PATIENT 8

A 79-year-old woman with rheumatoid arthritis, hoarseness, and difficulty breathing

A 79-year-old woman with longstanding rheumatoid arthritis had a 6-month history of hoarseness and difficulty breathing. The patient was comfortable at rest but noted a "harsh noise in the windpipe" during minimal exertion such as walking across the room. The patient was in the habit of sucking on hard candy, often falling to sleep with a lozenger in her mouth, to relieve a sore and dry throat.

Physical Examination: Dry mucous membranes; scattered rales in both lung fields with inspiratory stridor localized over the larynx; normal neck examination to palpation; rheumatoid nodules with active synovitis in metacarpophalangeal joints.

Laboratory Findings: Normal CBC and electrolytes; positive rheumatoid factor. Chest radiograph showed slight increase in basilar interstitial markings. Spirometry with flow volume loop is shown below.

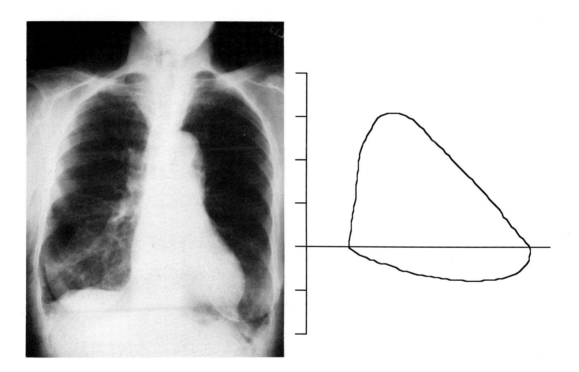

Diagnosis: Synovitis of the cricoarytenoid joint. Other possible causes of the patient's symptoms include rheumatoid nodule of the vocal cord and arteritis in the vasa nervorum of the recurrent laryngeal and vagus nerves.

Discussion: Pulmonologists are frequently reminded by their patient's problems that rheumatoid arthritis is a systemic disorder often manifested by symptoms in multiple organs. Respiratory features of the disorder include sicca syndrome with recurrent bronchitis, rheumatoid lung disease with interstitial infiltrates, necrobiotic nodules, pleural effusions, and upper airway obstruction as demonstrated by the present patient.

Upper airway obstruction in rheumatoid arthritis is related to laryngeal dysfunction that has three potential mechanisms: synovitis of the cricoarytenoid joint, rheumatoid nodules involving the vocal cords, and arteritis in the vasa nervorum of the recurrent laryngeal and vagus nerves.

Synovitis of the cricoarytenoid joint presents with variable symptoms that include hoarseness, a foreign body sensation, dyspnea, and pain radiating to the ears. Rarely, sudden occlusion of the glottis by abducted vocal cords may be a medical emergency. Indirect laryngoscopy clearly demonstrates cricoarytenoid ankylosis, which may be a finding in many patients with long-standing rheumatoid arthritis without symptoms of airway obstruction. Treatment depends on the severity of related symptoms and activity of the systemic disease. The present patient responded well to anti-inflammatory drugs, but surgical options include lateralization of the vocal cords (which may be associated with subsequent aspiration) and tracheostomy for severe airway obstruction.

Rheumatoid nodules on the vocal cords is a rare complication of rheumatoid arthritis and require resection for improvement of symptoms. Arteritis of the vasa nervorum of the recurrent laryngeal and vagus nerves causes an ischemic neuropathy, resulting in failure of vocal cord abduction. This condition is generally painless and usually occurs in association with rheumatoid vasculitis and mononeuritis multiplex.

The present patient's flow volume loop suggested upper airway obstruction with flattening of the inspiratory component. At indirect laryngoscopy, the vocal cords were observed to abduct poorly during inspiration because of fixation of the cricoarytenoid joint. She was treated with prednisone, 20 mg a day, and aspirin for 2 weeks, after which her symptoms improved. Repeat laryngoscopy demonstrated improved motion of the vocal cords, thereby confirming the diagnosis of synovitis of the cricoarytenoid joint secondary to rheumatoid arthritis.

Clinical Pearls

1. Upper airway obstruction is an extraarticular manifestation of rheumatoid arthritis and usually denotes cricoarytenoid joint synovitis.

2. Although the glottic examination may be similar in cricoarytenoid synovitis and arteritis of the vasa nervorum, the latter condition is usually painless and associated with mononeuritis multiplex.

REFERENCES

1. Lavoy MR, Hughes GRV. Laryngeal dysfunction and rheumatoid arthritis. A case report. J Rheumatol 1980; 7:759–760.
2. Lawry SV, Finerman ML, Hanafee WN, et al. Laryngeal involvement in rheumatoid arthritis. A clinical, laryngoscopic, and computerized tomographic study. Arthritis Rheum 1984; 27:873–882.

PATIENT 9

A 70-year-old man with bilateral diffuse interstitial infiltrates

A 70-year-old black male was admitted for hip surgery and was found to have an abnormal chest radiograph. The patient had been a cigarette smoker for 40 years and noted a mild chronic cough, but he denied hemoptysis, shortness of breath, or exercise limitations. He took lithium for chronic depression and worked for over 20 years blowing the dirt off of sweet potatoes after harvest with an air compressor in a barn. The patient traveled throughout the southeast United States and denied exposure to tuberculosis.

Physical Examination: Afebrile; scattered rales at both lung bases with normal respiratory excursion.

Laboratory Findings: Normal CBC and electrolytes. ANA and rheumatoid factor were positive. Chest radiograph showed bilateral, diffuse interstitial infiltrates with nodules predominantly involving the upper lung zones. PPD skin test was negative without control tests placed. ABG (room air): pH 7.42, PO_2 85 mmHg, PCO_2 38 mmHg. Spirometry: FEV_1 2.55 L (75% of predicted), FVC 3.37 L (84% of predicted), $FEV_1/FVC\%$ 76%, TLC 5.31 L (74% of predicted), RV 1.81 L (69% of predicted).

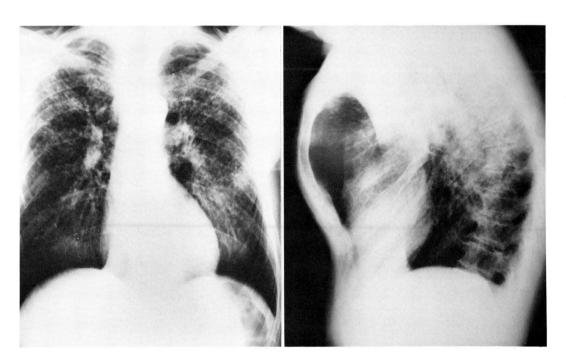

Diagnosis: Silicosis. Additional possibilities would include neoplasms, such as alveolar cell cancer, granulomatous disease, such as sarcoidosis or chronic histoplasmosis, and chronic hypersensitivity pneumonitis with pulmonary fibrosis.

Discussion: Since the import of the patient's occupational history was not immediately apparent, the patient underwent fiberoptic bronchoscopy with transbronchial biopsies to exclude neoplastic and granulomatous disorders. The biopsy specimens showed multiple silicotic nodules.

Most physicians associate silicosis with exposure to silica through mining or sandblasting occupations. Crystalline silica, however, is ubiquitous in the environment, comprising a major portion of the earth's crust. Any activity that generates 0.5 to 5.0 um silica particles capable of reaching the alveoli can cause fibrotic lung disease. After the results of lung biopsy, the clinicians more carefully interviewed the patient and learned the extent of his occupational exposure. Blowing the dirt off of harvested potatoes with a compressor in an unventilated barn resulted in clouds of dust that contained sufficient silica to cause silicosis.

Silicosis generates several clinical disorders with distinct pathologic and radiographic correlates. Chronic silicosis, as typified by this patient, develops after 20 to 40 years of occupational exposure and results in the proliferation of small discrete hyalinized nodules containing silica. The radiographic pattern of this form of silicosis comprises a reticulonodular infiltrate predominantly involving the upper lung zones and associated hilar adenopathy. The lymph nodes may calcify in an eggshell pattern that has also been noted in sarcoidosis and tuberculosis. When the silicotic nodules coalesce into masses larger than 10 mm, the disorder is termed complicated silicosis or progressive massive fibrosis. Contraction of involved lung tissue causes adjacent lung zones to undergo emphysematous changes with bleb formation.

Although 10% of patients with silicosis may have an associated connective tissue disorder, there is an additional increased incidence of antinuclear antibodies, rheumatoid factors, and circulating immune complexes that do not affect the clinical presentation or prognosis.

Accelerated silicosis may develop 5 to 15 years after initial silica exposure and causes similar pathologic and radiographic findings as chronic silicosis. The more rapid form of the disease is called acute silicosis, occurring 6 to 24 months after a particularly massive silica exposure, and may have intraalveolar deposition of proteinaceous material termed silicoproteinosis.

This patient's clinical presentation is typical of chronic silicosis with mild cough, minimal if any dyspnea, and spirometric evidence of a restrictive defect. Disabling symptoms of dyspnea usually develop after profound lung contraction has caused secondary emphysema, at which time spirometry shows an obstructive defect. The diagnosis of silicosis depends on noting the typical chest radiographic findings in the setting of a sufficient silica exposure history and should not require tissue confirmation.

Clinical Pearls

1. Exposure to dust generated through any activity can cause silicosis if sufficient quantities of free silica are present.

2. Symptoms of dyspnea in silicosis relate more closely to the presence of lung contraction with secondary emphysema and airway obstruction than with the primary restrictive defect.

REFERENCES

1. Bergen CJ, Muller NL, Vedal S, Chan-Yeung M. CT in silicosis: correlation with plain films and pulmonary function tests. AJR 1986; 146:477–483.
2. Lapp N. Lung disease secondary to inhalation of nonfibrous material. Clin Chest Med 1981; 2:219–233.

PATIENT 10

A 52-year-old man with chest trauma and a pulmonary nodule.

A 52-year-old man struck his chest and head on the steering wheel during an auto accident. During admission for observation, he was noted to have an abnormal chest radiograph. The patient smoked heavily but denied chest symptoms.

Physical Examination: Tender sternum with a forehead abrasion.

Laboratory Findings: Chest radiograph showed a 2.5 cm nodule in the right infrahilum overlying the thoracic vertebral column on the lateral view (arrows). Low-voltage spot films demonstrated a smooth-bordered lesion without apparent calcifications. A CT scan revealed the nodule to have central calcification in a lobular pattern interlaced with low density tissue. Because chest radiographs from two years earlier showed the nodule to have grown slightly, a thoracic surgeon recommended its removal.

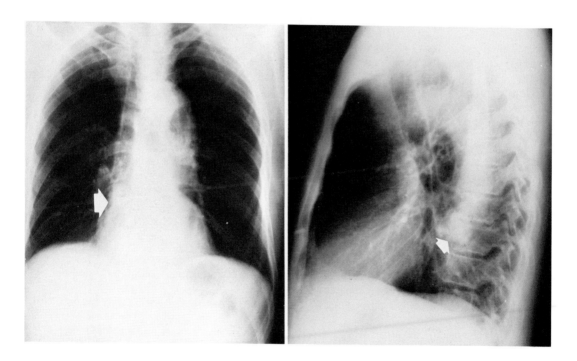

Diagnosis: Pulmonary hamartoma.

Discussion: Hamartoma derives from the Greek words for "error" and "tumor" and denotes a lesion made up of the tissues normally found in the involved organ but present in abnormal amounts, distribution, or degrees of differentiation. Previously thought to be a tumor-like developmental abnormality, pulmonary hamartomas are now considered to be benign neoplasms of mesenchymal cell origin. Cartilage, with varying degrees of calcification and ossification, is the dominant mesenchymal component, with additional fat or myxomatous tissue present. Cystic spaces and branching channels lined by respiratory epithelium are thought to be incorporated into the growing nodule from terminal bronchioles rather than being a component of the neoplastic process.

Pulmonary hamartomas are the third most common cause of pulmonary nodules, representing 6 to 8% of localized parenchymal masses requiring evaluation, and are the second commonest benign pulmonary neoplasm behind bronchial adenomas. The peak incidence of pulmonary hamartomas is in the fifth to sixth decades, with equal distribution between sexes. Most lesions present as an asymptomatic 1 to 4 cm solitary pulmonary nodule usually in the lung periphery and appear, as occurred in this patient, as an incidental finding. Ten to 15% of hamartomas, however, are endobronchial, presenting with cough, hemoptysis, pneumonia, atelectasis, or chest pain.

The diagnostic approach to hamartomas is assisted by their often distinctive radiologic appearance. They are typically well-circumscribed, solitary, and lobulated, with a diameter less than 2.5 cm. Although present in less than 5% of patients, the calcification pattern that occurred in this patient may simulate a kernel of popcorn. The detection of fat by CT scanning is a more important radiologic finding, since it occurs in up to 50% of hamartomas and indicates that the nodules are benign. Most pulmonologists would be satisfied with a diagnosis of hamartoma based on CT evidence of lobulated calcifications and fat tissue and would observe the lesion. Since hamartomas may enlarge over a 2-year period and are not considered to have malignant potential, the documented growth in this patient's lesion would not necessitate resection.

Often the radiographic evaluation of a hamartoma will be indeterminate, or a patient (or physician) may require certainty of benignity before comfortably agreeing to simple observation. In such instances, fine-needle aspiration may diagnose a hamartoma in more than 80% of instances. Evidence of cartilage fragments is diagnostic and fibromyxomatous tissue is considered suspicious for the diagnosis of hamartoma.

In our pulmonary division, this patient's CT evidence of nodule calcification intermixed with fat densities would have warranted observation, but we would perform needle aspiration if the patient requested greater diagnostic certainty.

Clinical Pearls

1. CT scan evidence of fat or popcorn calcification in a solitary pulmonary nodule are valuable clues to the presence of a hamartoma.

2. Up to 50% of hamartomas contain fat, whereas only 5% or less have popcorn calcifications.

3. Fine-needle aspiration can satisfactorily diagnose hamartoma and exclude malignancy in a solitary pulmonary nodule if cartilage is detected by cytologic or histologic methods.

REFERENCES

1. Hamper UM, Khouri NF, Stitik FP, Siegelman SS. Pulmonary hamartoma: diagnosis by transthoracic needle-aspiration biopsy. Radiology 1985; 155:15–18.
2. Siegelman SS, Khouri NF, Scott WW Jr, et al. Pulmonary hamartoma: CT findings. Radiology 1986; 160:313–317.
3. Fudge TL, Ochsner JL, Mills NL. Clinical spectrum of pulmonary hamartomas. Ann Thorac Surg 1980; 30:36–39.

PATIENT 11

A 52-year-old man with recurrent pneumonia and hilar calcifications

A 52-year-old man was evaluated for recurrent pneumonia. Despite being a long-time smoker, the patient was a vigorous exerciser until 2 years earlier when he developed cough and mild dyspnea on exertion. He discontinued smoking but noted progressive cough with occasional blood-streaked sputum. Six months before admission, he developed fever and purulent sputum with a right lower lobe infiltrate that responded to oral antibiotics. Because of two similar instances of pneumonia, he was referred for evaluation.

Physical Examination: No lymphadenopathy; low-pitched wheeze over the right mainstem bronchus; decreased breath sounds with mild crackles in the right lower lobe region.

Laboratory Findings: Normal CBC and electrolytes. Chest radiograph showed several hilar calcifications, one of which was 1 cm and near the right bronchus intermedius (arrow).

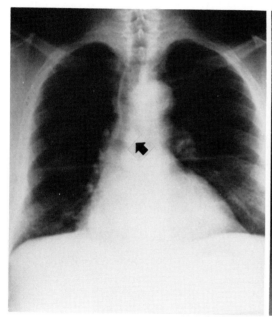 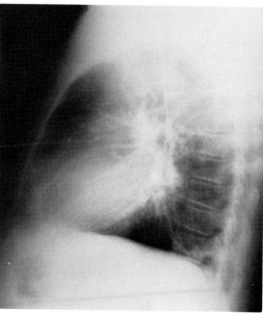

Diagnosis: Broncholith.

Discussion: The vast majority of patients presenting in this fashion would most likely have bronchogenic carcinoma. This patient's presentation, however, suggests the possibility of broncholithiasis because of the hilar calcifications and his residence in a state indigenous for histoplasmosis.

Broncholithiasis has a venerable history, with its first description dating to the Greeks in the 4th century BC. Originally defined by its most notable feature of a patient "spitting of stones," the spectrum of broncholithiasis has been extended to include any condition in which calcified material exists within an airway or hilar calcifications extrinsically compress a bronchus. The etiology of the broncholith is almost always infection in a peribronchial lymph node involved with histoplasmosis or tuberculosis, although occasional episodes result from actinomycosis, coccidioidomycosis, and cryptococcosis.

The clinical presentation of patients with broncholithiasis is similar to the present case summary. Any age group is at risk, with men and women having equal incidence. Patients typically note cough, fever, hemoptysis, bronchorrhea, recurrent pneumonia, lung abscess, and bronchiectasis, with symptom duration from months to as long as 20 years. Lithoptysis is diagnostic of the disorder but is an unusual finding. The key to suspecting broncholithiasis is close scrutiny of the patient's chest radiograph. The presence of parenchymal infiltrates or lobar atelectasis in the setting of hilar calcifications suggests broncholithiasis, and the diagnosis is even more likely if a large calcification is near a bronchus serving an area of infiltration.

Diagnosis can be made at fiberoptic bronchoscopy, since the airways are always abnormal and a characteristic white calcified node is apparent in nearly 50% of patients. A nondiagnostic bronchoscopy study can be aided by tomography or CT scanning, which detects the broncholith in nearly every patient.

Patients who are minimally symptomatic may require only observation. Most patients, however, have bothersome or severe symptoms that require broncholith removal. The fiberoptic bronchoscope may occasionally remove small broncholiths in select patients. The rigid bronchoscope, however, with its larger biopsy forcep is more effective at fracturing and removing broncholiths, although only a minority of patients are successfully treated, and hemoptysis may occur during stone manipulation. A single report indicates that a large mobile broncholith can be shattered by a YAG laser, allowing bronchoscopic removal. Most patients with serious symptoms require surgical removal with a bronchotomy, segmentectomy, lobectomy, or pneumonectomy. Because of the nonmalignant nature of the disorder, as much lung tissue as possible should be preserved.

The present patient underwent fiberoptic bronchoscopy, which demonstrated an immobile broncholith in the right lower lobe bronchus. A CT scan of the chest confirmed a single broncholith with distal bronchiectasis. The patient underwent thoracotomy with right lower lobe lobectomy without recurrence of symptoms during prolonged follow-up.

Clinical Pearls

1. Symptoms of recurrent pneumonia or lobar atelectasis suggestive of bronchogenic carcinoma warrant scrutiny of the chest radiograph for hilar calcifications that indicate the possibility of broncholithiasis.

2. If broncholithiasis is suspected after bronchoscopy, tomography or CT scanning is indicated to confirm the diagnosis.

REFERENCES

1. Cole FH, Cole FH, Khandekar A, Watson DC. Management of broncholithiasis: Is thoracotomy necessary? Ann Thorac Surg 1986; 42:255–257.
2. Dixon GF, Donnerberg RL, Schonfeld SA, Whitcomb ME. Advances in the diagnosis and treatment of broncholithiasis. Am Rev Respir Dis 1984; 129:1028–1030.
3. Miks VM, Kvale PA, Riddle JM, Lewis JW Jr. Broncholith removal using the YAG laser. Chest 1986; 90:295–297.

PATIENT 12

A 15-year-old boy with a history of Down's syndrome, diffuse pulmonary infiltrates, and respiratory failure

A 15-year-old boy with Down's syndrome was well until he noted a headache followed by a dry cough. The symptoms persisted, progressing to shortness of breath and peripheral cyanosis. The family denied that the patient had recent drug ingestion, rigors, purulent sputum, or skin rash. Other members of the family with whom the patient lived noted similar symptoms but not as severe.

Physical Examination: Physical characteristics typical of Down's syndrome; central and peripheral cyanosis without clubbing; diffuse rales across all lung fields; grade II/VI ejection murmur along the left sternal border.

Laboratory Findings: WBC 8,500/μl with 85% PMNs. ABG (room air): pH 7.55, PCO_2 28 mmHg, PO_2 40 mmHg; sputum unavailable. Chest radiograph showed diffuse alveolar infiltrates with a patchy distribution.

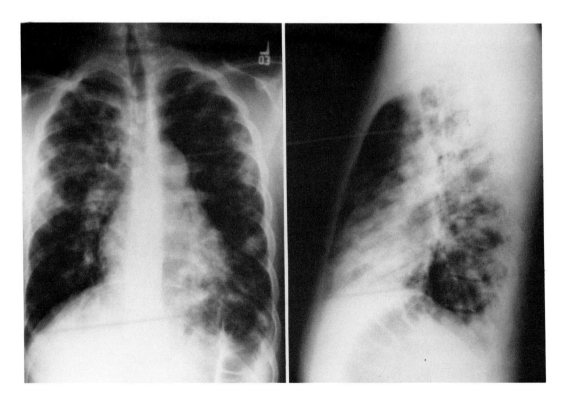

Diagnosis: Infectious pneumonia due to *Mycoplasma pneumoniae* with a right-to-left shunt through an atrial septal defect.

Discussion: Because of improvements in medical management and home and institutional care, the life expectancy of patients with Down's syndrome has increased over the last 50 years from 9 years in 1929 to over 30 years presently. As many as 25% of patients may live into their sixth decade. Despite these advances, patients with Down's syndrome still have an increased mortality rate compared to the general population and to similarly retarded persons without Down's syndrome. The reasons for this excess mortality include the occurrence in Down's syndrome of congenital heart disease, malignancies, early senility, stroke, and a high incidence of respiratory and nonrespiratory infections.

Patients with Down's syndrome have a 50- to 100-fold increased susceptibility for respiratory infections, and instances of pneumonia are more severe compared to the general population. This increased risk for pneumonia is most apparent in patients who are institutionalized and thereby exposed to a greater quantity of pathogens but also occurs in patients cared for at home. The pathogens range from viral to bacterial and include *Mycoplasma pneumoniae*, as was diagnosed in this patient on the basis of the typical clinical findings, outbreak in family members, and positive serologic studies.

The pathogenesis of lowered host defenses against infection in Down's syndrome is poorly understood, but the additional observations of an increased risk for autoimmune disorders and malignancies suggest that a defect in immunoregulation exists. Specific defects detected include abnormalities in immunoglobulin levels, bactericidal activities of phagocytic cells, and T-cell function, and indicate that multiple immunologic dysfunctions may combine to produce an increased susceptibility to infection.

Patients with Down's syndrome also have a 40-fold increased risk of congenital heart disease that includes atrioventricular communis, ventricular septal defect, tetralogy of Fallot, atrial septal defect, and patent ductus arteriosus. The present patient apparently had a small atrial septal defect that was not clinically important until he developed severe pneumonia. The attendant hypoxic vasoconstriction with increased pulmonary hypertension activated a potential right-to-left shunt that was detected on echocardiography during the acute illness. The patient was treated with high flow oxygen by mask that raised the PO_2 to 50 mmHg until he improved on erythromycin therapy.

Clinical Pearls

1. Patients with Down's syndrome are at increased risk for severe pneumonia.
2. The presence of profound hypoxia during episodes of pneumonia may result from intracardiac shunts through congenital cardiac defects.

REFERENCES

1. Breg WR. Down's syndrome: a review of recent progress in research. Pathobiol Annu 1977; 7:257–303.
2. Thase ME. Longevity and mortality in Down's syndrome. J Ment Defic Res 1982; 26:177–192.

PATIENT 13

A 20-year-old woman with wheezing, urticaria, pulmonary infiltrates, and eosinophilia

A 20-year-old woman was discharged from the hospital after normal labor and delivery. One week later she noticed low-grade fever, cough productive of clear sputum, and mild wheezing. She presented at the emergency room because of "hives." She denied medications, a smoking history, or foreign travel.

Physical Examination: Lung examination was normal except for occasional scattered rales. Skin revealed localized urticaria over the upper trunk.

Laboratory Findings: CBC was normal except for a WBC of 9,000/μl with 40% eosinophils. Chest radiograph showed bilateral patchy infiltrates.

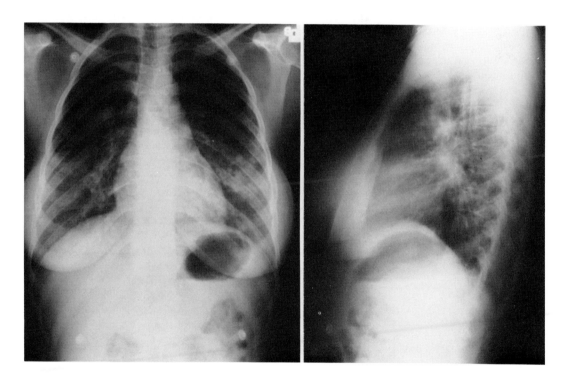

Diagnosis: Loffler's syndrome (simple pulmonary eosinophilia) from transpulmonary migration of *Ascaris lumbricoides*. Other major diagnostic considerations include other nematode ingestions and a drug reaction, despite the patient's negative medication history.

Discussion: This patient's presentation is typical of the pulmonary manifestations of ascariasis, with symptoms first occurring 1 to 3 weeks after ingestion of ascarid eggs. The ova hatch in the gastrointestinal tract where the larvae burrow through the intestinal wall, finding their way into the venous circulation. Filtered by the lung, the larvae mature in the alveoli where they increase in size over a 2-week period before migrating into the upper airway. They are subsequently swallowed, reentering the alimentary system to complete their life cycle.

During residence in the lung, ascaris larvae promote a peripheral eosinophilia that may be mild or sufficiently intense that 60% of circulating leukocytes are eosinophils. Eosinophils may also be found in the expectorated sputum of these patients. The association of peripheral eosinophilia with a pulmonary infiltrate is an important clinical condition with a wide differential diagnosis. Careful evaluation of clinical manifestations usually narrows the diagnostic possibilities.

Loffler's syndrome, or simple pulmonary eosinophilia, is noted for transient pulmonary infiltrates and usually a mild self-limited illness. Symptoms include fever, cough, nocturnal asthma, rash, and occasional urticaria. The chest radiograph usually shows patchy infiltrates that migrate and evolve rapidly but may be miliary, thereby simulating tuberculosis. Nearly 25% of patients in Loffler's original series had ascariasis, but other nematodes such as hookworm can cause the condition along with various drug reactions, including penicillin, sulfonamides, and nitrofurantoin.

Other pulmonary eosinophilic disorders differ from Loffler's syndrome on the basis of chronicity of symptoms or associated conditions. These entities include chronic eosinophilic pneumonia, pulmonary eosinophilia with asthma such as bronchopulmonary aspergillosis, and pulmonary eosinophilia associated with systemic vasculitis. Tropical eosinophilia caused by filariasis may simulate Loffler's syndrome, but its occurrence is limited to tropical endemic regions.

Pulmonary ascariasis is usually suggested by the characteristic clinical presentation and is further supported by a personal or family history of parasite infestation. Confirmation requires detection of larvae in expectorated sputum. Unfortunately, serologic tests are not helpful, and since the worms have not yet matured in the gut during the period of pulmonary symptoms, stool examinations for ova and parasites are unrevealing.

On further questioning, the present patient recalled seeing a long worm in the commode after one of her children had a bowel movement. She had believed at the time that the worm had come in through the water supply rather than from her child. She continued with mild symptoms and eosinophilia that resolved without therapy after 8 days. Occasionally, severe cough and shortness of breath may warrant corticosteroid therapy that has been anecdotally noted to improve respiratory symptoms. Definitive therapy is dibendazole. Since the drug only affects mature worms in the gut, therapy should be delayed for 3 months after the pulmonary symptoms to allow time for completion of the life cycle.

Clinical Pearls

1. Sputum examination for larvae can be diagnostic of ascariasis in pulmonary eosinophilia.

2. Pulmonary transmigration precedes gut infestation, with mature ascarid worms making stool examinations for ova and parasites negative during the phase of respiratory symptoms.

REFERENCES
1. Barrett-Connor E. Parasitic pulmonary disease. Am Rev Respir Dis 1982; 126:558–563.
2. Crofton JW, Livingstone JL, Oswald NC, Roberts ATM. Pulmonary eosinophilia. Thorax 1952; 7:1–35.

PATIENT 14

An 89-year-old man with bilateral pulmonary infiltrates and progressive dyspnea on exertion of 2 years' duration

An 89-year-old black male farmer presented with progressive exertional dyspnea of over 2 years' duration. He denied cough, fever, weight loss, hemoptysis, or use of any medication. He recently discontinued smoking because of increasing dyspnea that limited his walking to 20 feet.

Physical Examination: Normal except for diffuse rales.

Laboratory Findings: ABG (room air): pH 7.42, $PaCO_2$ 39 mmHg, PaO_2 56 mmHg; Hct 39%; WBC 4,300/μl; platelet count normal; electrolytes normal; renal and liver function tests normal. The chest radiograph demonstrated diffuse bilateral infiltrates with a mixed alveolar and reticulo-nodular pattern involving all lobes.

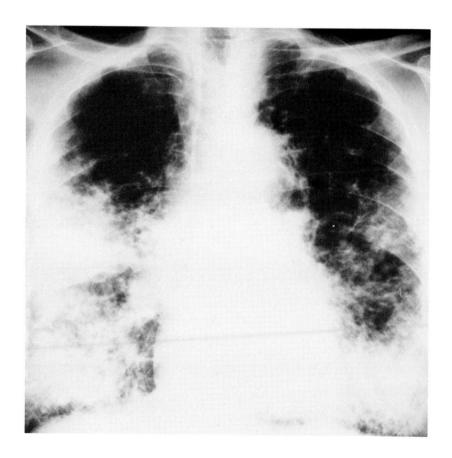

Diagnosis: Pulmonary parenchymal amyloid. Other diagnoses to consider are metastatic cancer, alveolar cell cancer, and lymphoma.

Discussion: The patient underwent flexible fiberoptic bronchoscopy with transbronchial lung biopsies. The airway examination was normal. After the third transbronchial lung biopsy, brisk uncontrollable hemorrhage developed that continued despite efforts to tamponade the hemorrhage with the bronchoscope. The patient became hypotensive and asystolic, expiring despite the initiation of cardiopulmonary resuscitation. A chest radiograph obtained immediately postmortem demonstrated air in the left ventricle and major cardiothoracic vessels.

The transbronchial biopsies and subsequent autopsy demonstrated waxy, amorphous, eosinophilic material replacing alveolar walls and infiltrating blood vessels. Congo red stains were positive for amyloid. There was no evidence of endobronchial or extrapulmonary deposition of amyloid; therefore, the final diagnosis was pulmonary parenchymal amyloidosis.

Infiltration of amyloidosis limited to the respiratory tract is a rare disorder. Localized pulmonary amyloidosis is classified into three distinct pathologic types: tracheobronchial, parenchymal nodular, and diffuse alveolar septal disease. Since most patients with pulmonary amyloid from systemic amyloidosis have coexisting myocardial amyloid deposition, the normal cardiac evaluation at autopsy excludes systemic disease.

Previous reports support the efficacy and safety of flexible fiberoptic bronchoscopy with transbronchial biopsies for the diagnosis of pulmonary amyloidosis. The present patient's complication of massive hemoptysis with air embolism indicates that bronchoscopy is not without risk in this disorder. The autopsy demonstrated profound amyloid vasculopathy, and postmortem radiocontrast studies of the lung specimen showed bidirectional patency of a bronchovenous fistula in the area from which the biopsies were obtained. These findings suggest that infiltration of vessels with amyloidosis predisposes to a loss of arterial vasoconstriction capacities, resulting in free hemorrhage and air embolism after lung biopsy, and indicate a need for caution in performing transbronchial biopsies in patients in whom pulmonary amyloidosis is suspected.

Clinical Pearls

1. Slowly progressive dyspnea without associated symptoms in an elderly patient with bilateral alveolar infiltrates suggests pulmonary amyloid.
2. Bronchoscopy with transbronchial biopsy in a patient with suspected pulmonary amyloid risks massive pulmonary hemorrhage and air embolism because of amyloid vasculopathy.

REFERENCES
1. Hui AN, Koss MN, Hochholzer L, Wehunt WD. Amyloid presenting in the lower respiratory tract. Arch Pathol Lab Med 1986; 110:212–218.
2. Celli BR, Rubinow MD, Cohen AS, Brody JS. Patterns of pulmonary involvement in systemic amyloidosis. Chest 1978; 74:543–547.
3. Yood RA, Skinner M, Rubinow A, et al. Bleeding manifestations in 100 patients with amyloidosis. JAMA 1983; 249:1322–1324.

PATIENT 15

A 34-year-old man with a history of Down's syndrome and an anterior mediastinal mass

A 34-year-old asymptomatic man with Down's syndrome was evaluated for an abnormal chest radiograph.

Physical Examination: Normal.

Laboratory Findings: CBC and electrolytes normal. Chest radiograph showed an anterior mediastinal mass that was most apparent on the lateral view. The mass was confirmed on CT scan and shown to be solid without calcifications.

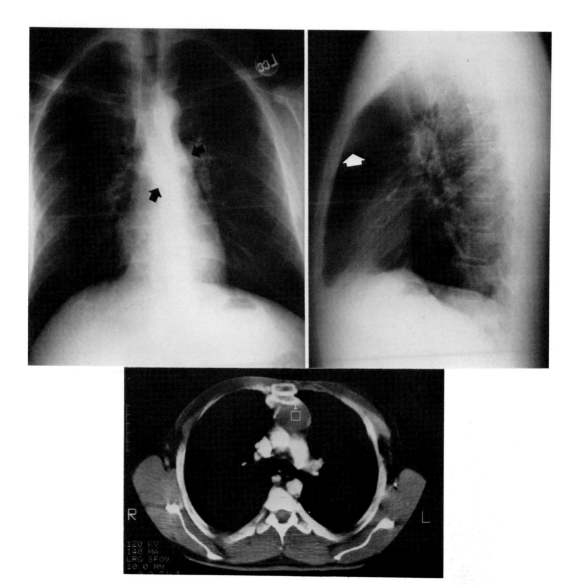

Diagnosis: Thymic cyst. Other likely possibilities include thymoma, lymphoma, and dermoid cyst. A substernal thyroid goiter is unlikely because of the absence of tracheal deviation or a palpable goiter.

Discussion: An impressive aspect of this patient's presentation is the subtle radiographic findings on plain chest views in contrast to the large size of the mediastinal mass demonstrated on CT scan. This lack of chest radiographic sensitivity is characteristic of thymic masses that may appear (1) well-defined, (2) indistinct, as they blend into normal structures, or (3) undetectable on routine films. Up to 35% of thymomas detected by CT scan are not apparent on chest radiographs. Subsequently, the chest CT scan is paramount in the evaluation of a suspected thymic mass, since it not only confirms their existence but also clearly defines their location, degree of infiltration, and tissue density. In this instance, the CT scan demonstrated that the solid mass completely obscured normal thymus morphology, thereby strongly suggesting a thymic origin.

Solid thymic masses are usually thymomas, since these neoplasms account for 15% of all mediastinal tumors. Usually occurring in the fifth decade of life, 50% of these tumors are asymptomatic; incidental findings in the other 50% include paraneoplastic syndromes such as myasthenia gravis, red cell aplasia, or hypogammaglobulinemia. Thymomas may be benign or malignant, although the two forms differ only in degree of local infiltration and not in histologic appearance or probability of calcification. Other less likely possibilities for a solid thymic mass include germ cell tumors, thymolipomas, thymic carcinoid tumors, malignant lymphomas of the thymus, and, rarely, metastatic carcinoma.

The approach to a thymic mass after CT confirmation is surgical resection, since percutaneous needle aspirations or mediastinoscopy biopsies do not adequately exclude malignant disease. At median sternotomy, the present patient was found to have a multiloculated cystic mass containing thick brown material characteristic of a thymic cyst. Thymic cysts are rare, accounting for approximately 1% of all mediastinal masses. They are usually developmental abnormalities, and may occur anywhere along the embryologic descent of the thymus from the neck to anterior mediastinum. Cervical thymic cysts can cause tracheal or esophageal obstruction; however, mediastinal cysts are usually asymptomatic, although they have been reported to occur with aplastic anemia or subsequent to radiation therapy of Hodgkin's disease. As exemplified by this patient, despite their cystic nature, they may appear solid on CT scan, possibly because of consolidation of cystic hemorrhage.

Clinical Pearls

1. Up to 35% of thymic masses noted on CT scan may be inapparent on routine chest radiographs.

2. The radiographic evidence of calcification or histopathologic examination of biopsy specimens may not separate benign from malignant thymomas.

3. Thymic cysts may appear solid on CT scan examination.

REFERENCES

1. Graeber GM, Thompson LD, Cohen DJ, et al. Cystic lesions of the thymus. An occasionally malignant cervical and/or anterior mediastinal mass. J Thorac Cardiovasc Surg 1984; 87:295–300.
2. Day DL, Gedgaudas E. The thymus. Radiol Clin North Am 1984; 22:519–538.

PATIENT 16

A 51-year-old woman with chronic myelogenous leukemia with the acute onset of nausea, vomiting, dyspnea, and left upper quadrant and anterior chest pain

A 51-year-old black woman with chronic myelogenous leukemia diagnosed 18 months previously was admitted to the hospital with the acute onset of dyspnea, nausea, vomiting, and left upper quadrant and left anterior chest pain. The pain was constant, "stabbing," and had a pleuritic component. She had been treated with hydroxyurea for the past several months. A low-grade fever for the past several days was attributed to an upper respiratory tract infection.

Physical Examination: Temperature 99°; pulse 88; respirations 26. Obese female in minimal distress due to upper abdominal and lower chest pain; tenderness on palpation in the epigastrium, left upper quadrant and left anterior rib cage; tender splenomegaly.

Laboratory Findings: WBC 21,000/μl, 53% PMNs, 27% lymphocytes, 7% basophils, 6% myelocytes. Hct 37%; platelet count 996,000/μl. Urinalysis unremarkable; liver function tests normal; serum amylase 72 IU/L. Chest radiograph: moderate left pleural effusion with contralateral mediastinal shift. Abdominal ultrasound: normal biliary system, enlarged spleen with echogenic focus. An abdominal CT was ordered.

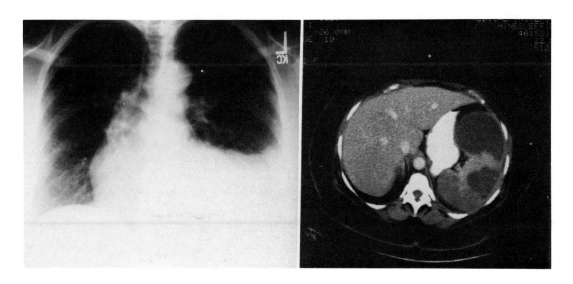

Diagnosis: Splenic infarction with pleural effusion.

Discussion: Thrombocythemia, the autonomous production of platelets, is a feature of the myeloproliferative syndromes. Either thrombosis or hemorrhage can occur as a result of the elevated platelet count in addition to abnormalities of platelet function.

Splenic infarction can occur with vasoocclusion because the arteries of the spleen are "end arteries" without collateral circulation and may occur in the setting of massive splenomegaly due to a myeloproliferative disorder. Vascular occlusive phenomena tend to be associated with the hemoglobinopathies, such as SS, SA, and SC disease. Splenic infarcts also can occur from bland emboli from valvular vegetations. These infarcts frequently become secondarily infected with abscess formation.

Patients with splenic infarction may be asymptomatic or may present with the acute onset of severe left upper quadrant pain, which may or may not radiate to the shoulder, depending upon the location of the diaphragmatic inflammation. On physical examination, the patient may be splinting the left hemithorax, have abdominal guarding, and, at times, have a friction rub over the spleen which is frequently palpable. There may be evidence of a left pleural effusion.

The chest radiograph is usually abnormal and shows an elevated left hemidiaphragm, atelectasis, a small left pleural effusion, and evidence of splenomegaly.

A pleural effusion may occur secondary to splenic infarction if the infarct causes diaphragmatic inflammation. The effusion is a nonspecific exudate with a modest number of leukocytes and a predominance of PMNs. If splenic abscess or subdiaphragmatic abscess secondary to splenic rupture develops, the effusion may increase in size and contain a larger percentage of PMNs, though remaining sterile.

The diagnosis is based on clinical and radiographic findings with the aid of noninvasive imaging. Technetium scanning and ultrasound may be helpful but CT scanning probably is the most useful. By nuclear medicine scanning, the infarct resolves over 2-3 weeks with or without volume loss. Control of underlying initiating factor and symptomatic therapy is all that is usually necessary.

The CT scan of the present patient showed a markedly enlarged spleen with multiple low density areas compatible with splenic infarction. She was treated with bedrest, analgesia, and busulfan in an attempt to reduce the platelet count. Symptoms abated over several days and the left pleural effusion resolved by 2 weeks.

Clinical Pearls

1. Splenic infarction may occur in the setting of chronic myelogenous leukemia due to massive splenomegaly or an elevated platelet count and platelet abnormalities.

2. Splenic infarction can cause a left pleural effusion secondary to diaphragmatic inflammation.

3. The pleural fluid is a nonspecific sterile exudate with a modest number of leukocytes and a predominance of PMNs.

REFERENCES

1. Sears DA, Udden MM. Splenic infarction, splenic sequestration, and functional hyposplenism in hemoglobin S-C disease. Am J Hematol 1985; 18:261–268.
2. Cardamone JM, Edson JR, McArthur JR, Jacob HS. Abnormalities of platelet function in the myeloproliferative disorders. JAMA 1972; 221:270–273.
3. Spencer RP. "Healing" of a splenic infarct. J Nucl Med 1974; 15:303–304.

PATIENT 17

A 22-year-old man with a history of pulmonary tuberculosis, and a right pleural effusion

A 22-year-old man was evaluated for shortness of breath. He began monitored therapy four months earlier for pulmonary tuberculosis with isoniazid and rifampin, and tolerated therapy well. During the preceding two weeks, however, he noted the onset of dyspnea with a heavy feeling in his chest.

Physical Examination: Afebrile; no lymphadenopathy. Chest examination: dullness at the right base with egophony and decreased fremitus. Cardiac and abdominal examinations normal.

Laboratory Findings: CBC and electrolytes normal; serum albumin 3.8 g/dl. Chest radiograph showed normal lung fields with a right-sided pleural effusion. Thoracentesis: milky fluid; glucose 130 mg/dl; protein 5.2 g/dl; triglycerides 538 mg/dl; cholesterol 78 mg/dl; leukocytes 1,200/μl with 98% lymphocytes; erythrocytes 2,200/μl. Negative smears for Mycobacteria and other organisms. A chest CT scan was normal except for the pleural effusion.

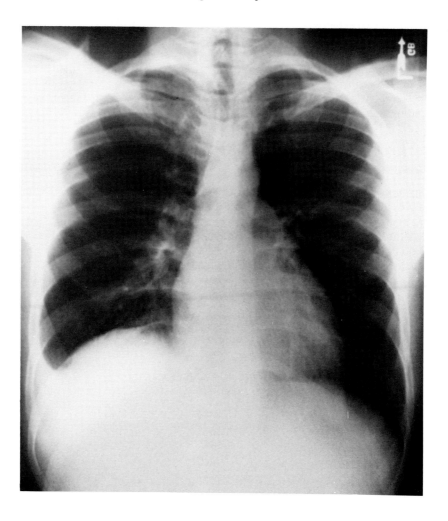

Diagnosis: Chylous effusion during resolution of pulmonary tuberculosis.

Discussion: Although chylous and pseudochylous effusions both share a characteristic milky appearance, they differ in their chemical makeup and diagnostic implications. Chylous effusions have fat globules accounting for their opalescent appearance and subsequently contain chylomicrons and triglyceride levels above 110 mg/dl. The presence of chylomicrons produces a creamy layer in a tube of the fluid that is allowed to stand. The addition of ethyl ether clears the opaqueness of the fluid. In contrast, pseudochylous effusions contain cholesterol and/or lecithin-globulin complexes that impart the milky appearance. No creamy layer forms with standing, the turbidity does not clear with ethyl ether, and triglyceride levels are usually normal.

The clinical conditions associated with chylous or pseudochylous effusions differ. Pseudochylous effusions develop in the setting of chronic inflammatory pleural effusions such as those resulting from tuberculosis or rheumatoid arthritis. Inflammatory cells are sequestered in the pleural space and over time release cholesterol that may be present in levels greater than 1,000 mg/dl. In contrast, the formation of a chylothorax is dependent on injury to the thoracic duct with spillage of chyle into the pleural space. Since the thoracic duct delivers 1 to 2 liters of fluid a day into the venous circulation, its interruption can result in massive effusions.

A wide range of clinical conditions result in chylothorax, including malignancy, trauma, surgery, and miscellaneous disorders such as aortic aneurysms, lymphangiomyomatosis, and sarcoidosis. As many as 15% of adult chylothoraces are idiopathic and may result from minor trauma such as coughing or stretching. Although tuberculosis is included in medical reviews as a cause of chylothorax, this association is not well documented. Only one case report in the English literature notes the occurrence of chylothorax in a patient with tuberculosis. In this instance, a large paravertebral lymph node obstructed the thoracic duct and was confirmed to be of tuberculous origin after surgical removal. Considering the prevalence of tuberculosis with mediastinal lymphadenopathy, the association with chylothorax must be rare.

The present patient was evaluated with a CT scan to exclude the possibility of lymphoma or other malignancy as a cause of the chylothorax. He refused a lymphangiogram, which may have defined the site of leak or suggested an etiology. With continuation of antituberculous therapy, the effusion gradually resolved over the ensuing 6 months.

Clinical Pearls

1. Chylous and pseudochylous effusions can be differentiated by their cholesterol and triglyceride content; clearing of turbidity with the addition of ethyl ether is a quick bedside test for chylothorax.

2. Chylothorax has been reported to result from mediastinal tuberculous adenitis and thoracic duct obstruction, but the association is exceedingly rare.

REFERENCES
1. Vennera MC, Moreno R, Cot J, Marin A, et al. Chylothorax and tuberculosis. Thorax 1983; 38:694–695.
2. Hughes RL, Mintzer RA, Hidvegi DF, et al. The management of chylothorax. Chest 1979; 76:212–218.

PATIENT 18

A 33-year-old woman with a 3-week history of intermittent fevers, productive cough, and myalgias followed by right upper quadrant pain

A 33-year-old woman was admitted to the hospital for evaluation for tuberculosis. She had a 3-week history of productive cough, intermittent fever, myalgias, fatigue, and right upper lobe consolidation on chest radiograph. There was a 1-week history of right upper quadrant pain. There was no history of alcohol abuse. She had received a week of erythromycin therapy.

Physical Examination: Temperature 98.8°; pulse 86; respirations 20; no acute distress; rhonchi without consolidation in the right upper lung zone; minimal hepatomegaly and tenderness on palpation of the liver.

Laboratory Findings: WBC 8,300/μl, 55% PMNs, 42% lymphocytes; Hct 41%; LDH 197 IU/L, SGOT 262 IU/L, SGPT 220 IU/L. Chest radiograph: resolving right upper lobe infiltrate and minimal right hilar adenopathy. PPD and controls negative. Sputum smear for AFB: negative; sputum Gram stain: many PMNs and no predominant organism; sputum culture: oral flora.

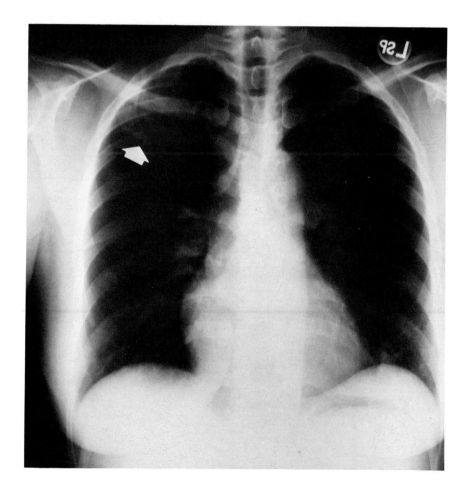

Diagnosis: Mycoplasma pneumoniae pneumonia with hepatitis.

Discussion: Mycoplasma produces an illness that ranges from a mild upper respiratory tract infection to severe bronchitis and pneumonia. This smallest free-living organism is transmitted from man to man by means of aerosols and requires prolonged close contact; therefore, it is seen frequently in families, on college campuses, and in the military. It occurs most commonly in the 5 to 25 year age group. Pneumonia develops in from 5 to 40% of those infected with *M. pneumoniae.* Pneumonia is unusual in young children and tends to be more common in older children and adults. With pneumonia, fever, chills, nonproductive cough, headache, and fatigue are usual findings. Sputum may be purulent but hemoptysis is unusual. Patients may complain of nonpleuritic chest pain, and gastrointestinal symptoms may occur.

Chest examination usually shows rhonchi and rales without consolidation. Symptoms tend to be more impressive than physical findings. Sputum Gram stain usually reveals PMNs without a predominant organism. Chest radiograph characteristically shows a unilateral bronchopneumonia in a lower lobe. Upper lobe involvement is seen in about 25% of patients and may mimic tuberculosis. Bilateral infiltrates and hilar adenopathy have been reported; hilar adenopathy is most common in children. The clinical course of pneumonia is usually self-limited but, on occasion, may be life-threatening. Erythromycin and tetracycline reduce the duration of symptoms and hasten chest radiograph resolution but do not appear to eradicate the organism from the respiratory tract.

Extrapulmonary manifestations are infrequent and include hemolytic anemia, arthralgias and arthritis, Stevens-Johnson syndrome, meningoencephalitis, and myocarditis. Up to 45% of patients with *M. pneumoniae* pneumonia develop gastrointestinal symptoms of anorexia, nausea, vomiting, and diarrhea. Incidental liver function abnormalities have been noted in isolated case reports and were noted in 9 of 42 (21%) patients with Mycoplasma pneumonia hospitalized at a community hospital. The hepatitis appears to be self-limited and tends to parallel the course of the pneumonia. Of interest is a report of the association of *M. pneumoniae* infections and chronic hepatitis.

The present patient responded to erythromycin therapy with a resolution of symptoms, clearing of chest radiograph, and resolution of liver function abnormalities. Cold agglutinins were positive at a titer of 1:256 on admission and showed a four-fold rise at three weeks. Acute and convalescent serum for complement fixation antibody titers showed a four-fold rise. Studies for viral hepatitis were negative.

Clinical Pearls

1. *Mycoplasma pneumoniae* pneumonia may present as an isolated right upper lobe infiltrate mimicking tuberculosis.

2. Liver enzymes may be elevated (up to 20% of patients) in *Mycoplasma pneumoniae* pneumonia and should be considered an extrapulmonic manifestation that does not necessarily require an extensive evaluation for another etiology.

3. When hepatitis is associated with pneumonia, Mycoplasma should be considered as an etiologic agent.

REFERENCES
1. Murray HW, Masur H, Senterfit LB, Roberts RB. The protean manifestations of *Mycoplasma pneumoniae* infection in adults. Am J Med 1975; 58:229–242.
2. Jansson E, Wegelius R, Visakorpi JK. Chronic active hepatitis and concomitant Mycoplasma infection. Lancet 1972; 1:1395.
3. Dean NL. Mycoplasmal pneumonias in the community hospital. Clin Chest Med 1981; 2:121–131.

PATIENT 19

A 32-year-old man with a history of nephrotic syndrome and shortness of breath

A 32-year-old man was admitted with shortness of breath. One year earlier, he had developed nephrotic syndrome from biopsy-proven membranous glomerulonephritis. He did well until three days before admission when he noted slowly progressive dyspnea despite a stable weight. His only medication was furosemide.

Physical Examination: Pulse 100; respirations 20; temperature 98°. Scattered crackles at both lung bases; cardiac normal; abdomen normal; moderate pitting edema of both ankles.

Laboratory Findings: Hct 35%, WBC 8,700/µl; creatinine 2.5 mg/dl; 4+ proteinuria. Chest radiograph demonstrated bibasilar atelectasis.

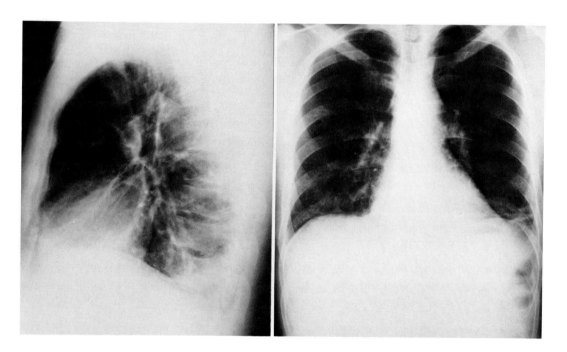

Diagnosis: Pulmonary emboli from nephrosis-induced renal vein thrombosis.

Discussion: Renal vein thrombosis with thromboembolic disease is a common and serious complication of nephrotic syndrome. Occurring more frequently in membranous and membrano-proliferative glomerulonephritis compared to lupus, diabetic, amyloid, sarcoid or sickle cell nephropathy, the true incidence of renal vein thrombosis is uncertain but probably occurs in 30 to 40% of nephrotic patients. The pulmonologist's interest in renal vein thrombosis is stimulated by the 8% frequency of pulmonary thromboemboli in nephrosis and the 50% frequency in patients with renal vein thrombosis, which may be the first manifestation of nephropathy. Isolated thromboses also occur in the deep venous systems and arterial circulation in 20 to 40% of patients with nephrosis. These occurrences make nephrosis the biggest risk factor for thromboembolic disease in medicine.

Renal vein thrombosis is a result of nephrosis rather than the cause, as evidenced by patients with primary renal vein thrombosis without accompanying renal insufficiency. The exact pathogenic mechanisms underlying vascular thrombosis in nephrosis are uncertain but urinary loss of clotting inhibitors, hemoconcentration due to an edematogenic state and diuretics, increased platelet aggregation, and heightened hepatic synthesis of fibrinogen and other clotting substances probably combine to cause a hypercoagulability state. Furthermore, immunologic injury of the glomeruli may initiate the clotting cascade through effects on the Hageman factor. This mechanism is supported by the observation that circulating immune complexes are more commonly found in patients with nephrosis and renal vein thrombosis compared to those with nephrosis alone.

Diagnosis of renal vein thrombosis is complicated by the two clinical presentations of the disease. An acute presentation comprises flank pain, hematuria, and unexplained rapid deterioration of renal function often associated with pleuritic chest pain or dyspnea, as occurred in the present patient. Evaluation of these patients has classically involved renal venography to confirm the presence of renal vein thrombosis. The asymptomatic chronic form is difficult to detect and may be the more common presentation. One prospective study screened 155 nephrotic patients with renal venography, finding renal vein thrombosis in 33 patients, of whom 30 were asymptomatic. Although the decision to periodically evaluate patients with nephrosis for asymptomatic renal vein thrombosis is controversial, most agree that the presence of undetected thrombosis is a considerable risk factor for thromboembolic disease. Due to the invasiveness and cost of renal venography and the insensitivity of intravenous pyelography, renal ultrasound and CT have been employed as screening examinations.

Heparin with subsequent coumadin anticoagulation is the treatment for patients with renal vein thrombosis with or without thromboembolic disease. Systemic anticoagulation improves symptoms of acute disease and may occasionally resolve the renal vein clot, thereby improving renal function. Anticoagulation is usually continued until the patient is no longer nephrotic, since the prognosis in untreated renal vein thrombosis is poor, being largely determined by the occurrence of thromboembolic disease.

The present patient underwent a lung scan that was highly probable for pulmonary emboli. He received intravenous heparin with improvement of symptoms. A subsequent abdominal CT scan documented the presence of renal vein thrombosis.

Clinical Pearls

1. Renal vein thrombosis eventually occurs in 30 to 40% of patients with nephrotic syndrome.

2. Pulmonary thromboemboli complicate the course of 8% of patients with nephrotic syndrome and 50% of patients with renal vein thrombosis.

3. The majority of patients with nephrosis and renal vein thrombosis are asymptomatic but are still at risk for thromboembolic disease.

REFERENCES

1. Gatewood OMB, Fishman EK, Burrow CR, et al. Renal vein thrombosis in patients with nephrotic syndrome: CT diagnosis. Radiology 1986; 159:117–122.
2. Llach F. Hypercoagulability, renal vein thrombosis, and other thrombotic complications of nephrotic syndrome. Kidney Int 1985; 28:429–439.

PATIENT 20

A 50-year-old man with alcoholism, dyspnea, and a large right pleural effusion

A 50-year-old man with alcoholism was admitted with dyspnea on exertion. He had a history of several bouts of acute pancreatitis, the most recent being three months prior to admission.

Physical Examination: Thin, in no acute distress; flat percussion note; decreased fremitus and decreased breath sounds in the right chest.

Laboratory Findings: Normal WBC and differential; Hct 33%; serum amylase 581 IU/L. Chest radiograph: large right pleural effusion. Thoracentesis: serosanguinous fluid; 1500 nucleated cells/μl, 5% PMNs, 47% macrophages, 29% lymphocytes, amylase 25,000 IU/L, protein 4.0 g/dl, LDH 221 IU/L, glucose 119 mg/dl, pH 7.35. Three days following the thoracentesis, the pleural fluid had reaccumulated.

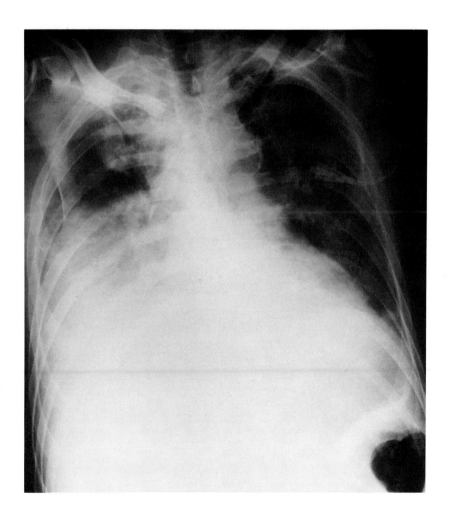

Diagnosis: Pancreaticopleural fistula.

Discussion: Pleural effusions from chronic pancreatitis are less frequent and present differently from those associated with acute pancreatitis. Patients with large or massive pleural effusions from chronic pancreatitis usually manifest only respiratory symptoms with dyspnea, chest pain, or cough. The effusions tend to recur rapidly following thoracentesis. Left pleural effusions are slightly more common than right and bilateral effusions may occur. Patients presenting with large pancreatic pleural effusions frequently do not have a history of pancreatic disease, although the majority are alcoholics. Due to the paucity of abdominal symptoms, the patient with a chronic pancreatic pleural effusion may not be diagnosed unless the pleural fluid amylase is measured. In contrast to acute pancreatitis, the amylase in the chronic state is always elevated and may reach levels greater than 100,000 IU/L. The serum amylase frequently is elevated due to back-diffusion, although it may be normal.

The treatment of chronic pancreatic pleural effusion has not been standardized. A reasonable approach is initially to manage the patient conservatively with drainage of the pleural space, usually with tube thoracostomy, bowel rest to decrease flow of pancreatic secretions, and nutritional support via hyperalimentation. The conservative approach is successful in about half of patients. Surgery is indicated for effusions that are refractory to conservative treatment. The fistulous tract needs to be identified preoperatively, if possible, to plan the optimal surgical approach. Endoscopic retrograde pancreatography has been useful for this purpose and, in addition, delineates the pancreatic duct. CT has been reported to be useful in identifying the fistulous tract. If the fistula cannot be identified, intraoperative pancreatography should be performed.

The patient failed with conservative treatment and underwent a surgical procedure with resolution of the pleural effusion by eight days.

Clinical Pearls

1. Patients with chronic pancreatic pleural effusions present with predominantly respiratory symptoms of dyspnea and chest pain and do not have concurrent abdominal symptoms.

2. The pleural fluid may be bloody, probably due to the high concentration of amylase in the fluid.

3. Other causes of high amylase pleural effusions include acute pancreatitis, esophageal rupture (amylase salivary in origin), neoplasm (<10%), ruptured ectopic pregnancy, and pneumonia (rare).

REFERENCES

1. Anderson WJ, Skinner DB, Zuidema GD, Cameron JL. Chronic pancreatic pleural effusions. Surg Gynecol Obstet 1973; 137:827–830.
2. Cameron JL. Chronic pancreatic ascites and pancreatic pleural effusions. Gastroenterology 1978; 74:134–140.
3. Pottmeyer EW III, Frey CF, Matusuno S. Pancreaticopleural fistulas. Arch Surg 1987; 122:648–654.

PATIENT 21

A 24-year-old woman with a history of Noonan's syndrome presenting with dyspnea on exertion and a left pleural effusion

A 24-year-old woman with Noonan's syndrome noted progressive dyspnea on exertion without associated symptoms. The patient underwent pulmonary valve replacement with a porcine prosthesis for congenital pulmonary stenosis 10 years earlier. She had no exposure to tuberculosis and her only medications comprised progesterone and estrogen replacement therapy.

Physical Examination: Typical body habitus of Noonan's syndrome with webbed neck and shield chest; no lymphadenopathy; chest dull at left base with decreased breath sounds and fremitus; grade II/VI SEM at left sternal border; mild mental retardation.

Laboratory Findings: CBC, liver function tests, and electrolytes normal. Chest radiograph revealed moderate left pleural effusion, scoliosis, and wire sutures and stent from previous cardiac surgery. Thoracentesis: serous fluid, pH 7.44, protein 3.5 g/dl, LDH 203 IU/L, glucose 76 mg/dl, leukocytes 1,400/μl with 78% lymphocytes. Cytology, Gram stain, and smears for Mycobacterium were negative.

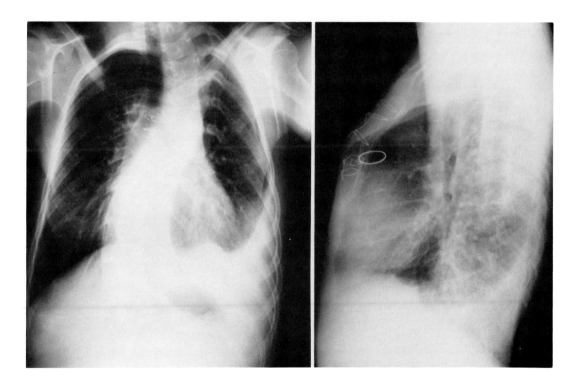

Diagnosis: Chylothorax from congenital lymphangiectasia.

Discussion: Noonan's syndrome shares many of the phenotypic features of Turner's syndrome, such as short stature, webbed neck, shield chest, and mental retardation. It is distinguished from Turner's syndrome by a normal karotype and frequent associated cardiovascular anomalies such as pulmonary stenosis, atrial septal defect, and eccentric left ventricular hypertrophy. An additional shared feature of these two conditions is a predilection for anomalies of the lymphatic system. As many as 20 to 35% of patients with either syndrome have peripheral lymphedema ascribed to hypoplasia or aplasia of the superficial lymphatics.

Patients with Noonan's syndrome also develop abnormalities of the intestinal and pulmonary lymphatics. Intestinal lymphangiectasia in this condition presents with protein-losing enteropathy and lymphopenia with decreased circulating T-cells. Pulmonary lymphangiectasia typically presents with chylothorax and lymphangiographic evidence of abnormally dilated and tortuous thoracic lymphatics with occasional absence of the thoracic duct. It was subsequently learned that surgeons first noted absence of the thoracic duct in the present patient during median sternotomy for pulmonic valve replacement. Her subsequent postoperative course was complicated by a chylothorax, and a postoperative lymphangiogram was consistent with congenital pulmonary lymphangiectasia showing characteristic dilated lymphatics.

This patient's presentation demonstrates that pleural fluid in chylothorax is not necessarily milky in appearance and may be serous or serosanguinous in greater than 50% of patients. The diagnosis is confirmed by the presence of elevated pleural fluid triglyceride content above 110 mg/dl. Her fluid triglyceride concentration was 1,100 mg/dl with a normal cholesterol level, confirming the clinical suspicion of chylothorax. Tuberculous pleurisy was an additional diagnostic possibility, but other causes of a pleural effusion in a young patient, such as collagen vascular disease or pulmonary emboli, seemed unlikely because of the absence of associated symptoms. The patient was placed on a low-fat diet supplemented by medium-chain triglycerides and had a gradual resolution of the chylothorax over the next 3 months.

Clinical Pearls

1. Patients with Noonan's syndrome have a predilection for lymphatic abnormalities that may present as a chylothorax.

2. The gross appearance of pleural fluid in chylothoraces may be serous or serosanguinous rather than milky.

REFERENCES

1. Baltaxe HA, Lee JG, Ehlers KH, Engle MA. Pulmonary lymphangiectasia demonstrated by lymphangiography in 2 patients with Noonan's syndrome. Radiology 1975; 115:149–153.
2. Fisher E, Weiss EB, Michals K, et al. Spontaneous chylothorax in Noonan's syndrome. Eur J Pediatr 1982; 138:282–284.

PATIENT 22

A 20-year-old man with a 3-month history of right upper quadrant and back pain with intermittent fevers

A 20-year-old white man presented with a 3-month history of right upper quadrant and back pain and intermittent fevers.

Physical Examination: Afebrile; chest examination unremarkable; minimal, right upper quadrant tenderness; normal liver scan; pain elicited on percussion over the lumbar region.

Laboratory Findings: Alkaline phosphatase 640 IU/L; SGOT 107 IU/L; LDH 453 IU/L. Chest radiograph: reticulonodular interstitial lung disease with right pneumothorax. Lumbar spine films: lytic lesion of Ll. FVC 4.03 liters (76% of predicted); FEV_1 3.20 liters (73% of predicted); FEV_1/FVC ratio 79%; DL/VA 4.95; TLC, FRC, RV all minimally reduced. ABG (room air): pH 7.41, PCO_2 41 mmHg, PO_2 96 mmHg.

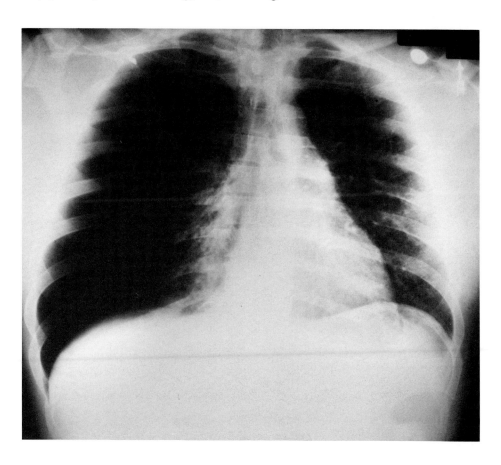

Diagnosis: Histiocytosis X involving lung, liver, and bone.

Discussion: In the early 1950s, Lichtenstein introduced the term histiocytosis X (HX) to include eosinophilic granuloma of bone, Hand-Schuller-Christian disease, and Letterer-Siwe disease. These diseases are typified by proliferation of morphologically characteristic histiocytes, often accompanied by eosinophils. Pulmonary involvement occurs in all forms of the disease but may be the sole manifestation in primary pulmonary HX. Although primary pulmonary HX can occur in the extremes of age, it most commonly affects young white adults and tends to have a male predominance. The disease may be discovered by routine chest radiograph or patients may present with respiratory symptoms (dyspnea, cough or pneumothorax), constitutional symptoms, or less commonly with extrapulmonary disease. Approximately 60% of patients at the time of diagnosis are cigarette smokers. Physical examination of the chest may be unremarkable early in the disease. Routine laboratory examination is nonspecific, with blood eosinophilia not being reported. The chest radiograph initially shows small, nodular and reticular bilateral and diffuse opacities, but larger nodules, cysts, or "honeycomb lung" may be seen. Pulmonary function tests may be within normal limits in up to 15% of patients but usually show a reduced FVC and an increased RV/TLC ratio. Poor prognostic features include extremes of age, recurrent pneumothorax, extrapulmonic disease, prolonged symptoms, extensive initial pulmonary involvement with cyst formation, and a low diffusing capacity. Pathologically, the lesions consist of a focal interstitial infiltrate of histiocytes, macrophages laden with pigment, lymphocytes, and eosinophils that are centered on airways. Initial lesions tend to be cellular and mitotically active. As the disease progresses stellate fibrotic scars, cystic changes, and bronchiolectasis ensue. When difficulty arises in differentiating HX cells from macrophages by light microscopy, the dilemma usually can be resolved by electron microscopy. HX cells are smaller and contain granules, pentalaminar structures of constant width (40 to 45 nm) scattered throughout the cytoplasm. The presence of these ultrastructural granules in HX cells, also called the Birbeck or Langerhans cell granules or HX bodies, confirms the diagnosis. S-100 protein, documented by an immunoperoxidase technique, in the HX cell also is confirmatory.

In the present patient the transbronchial lung biopsy was compatible with the diagnosis of HX; this was confirmed by ultrastructural studies, which demonstrated the HX cells and granules in both tissue and BAL fluid. S-100 protein also was demonstrated in the lung tissue and BAL fluid.

The patient was treated with radiation therapy to the lumbar spine, and prednisone, cyclophosphamide, and vincristine for 1 year because of extrapulmonary disease in the liver and bone. During this time, the patient's back and upper abdominal pain resolved, liver functions returned to normal, and pulmonary function and chest radiograph remained stable.

Clinical Pearls

1. The histologic lesions of pulmonary HX, which are characteristic and specific, are an infrequent finding in transbronchial biopsy specimens.

2. The majority of adults with histiocytosis X have a good prognosis but those with multisystem disease have the worst outcome.

3. Electron microscopy of BAL specimens demonstrate HX cells; this is one of the few examples of a definitive diagnostic role for BAL in noninfectious pulmonary disease.

4. In progressive pulmonary disease or extrapulmonary involvement, a therapeutic trial of vinca alkaloids, alkylating agents, and antimetabolites in conjunction with corticosteroids appears justified.

REFERENCES

1. Basset F, Corrin B, Spencer H, et al. Pulmonary histiocytosis X. Am Rev Respir Dis 1978; 118:811–820.
2. Colby TV, Lombard C. Histiocytosis X in the lung. Hum Pathol 1983; 14:847–856.
3. Flint A, Lloyd RV, Colby TV, Wilson BW. Pulmonary histiocytosis X: immunoperoxidase staining for HLA-DR antigen and S-100 protein. Arch Pathol Lab Med 1986; 110:990–993.

PATIENT 23

A 35-year-old man with a history of epilepsy and mediastinal lymphadenopathy

A 35-year-old man with a history of epilepsy was referred for pulmonary evaluation because of an abnormal chest radiograph. He felt well, specifically denying pulmonary problems, and his most recent seizure was 5 years earlier. He was a nonsmoker, and his only medications were diphenylhydantoin and phenobarbital.

Physical Examination: Normal except for mild gingival hyperplasia.

Laboratory Findings: CBC normal. Chest radiograph revealed mediastinal adenopathy.

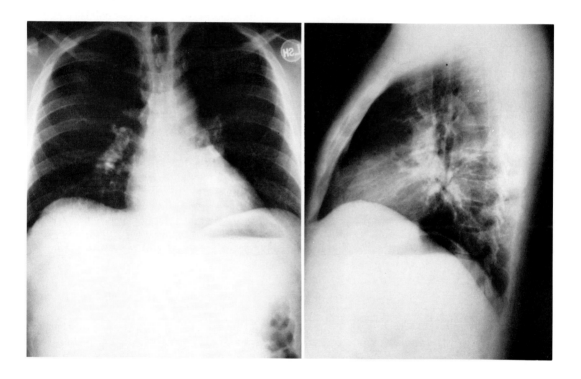

Diagnosis: Diphenylhydantoin-induced hilar adenopathy.

Discussion: Reactions to pharmacologic agents generate varied signs and symptoms that often present diagnostic difficulties when they simulate the manifestations of specific diseases. Since 3 to 5% of drug reactions affect the lung, the pulmonologist is often challenged with their evaluation.

Diphenylhydantoin was introduced 50 years ago as the first nonsedating antiepileptic. Although an effective and usually well-tolerated drug, it has an unusually broad spectrum of adverse reactions. Diphenylhydantoin is a particularly interesting agent because of its potential to generate several disparate pulmonary reactions that include drug-induced lupus syndromes, hypersensitivity reactions, and hilar adenopathy with a pseudolymphoma presentation.

Of the more than 20 drugs that can induce a lupus syndrome with positive antinuclear antibodies (ANA), procainamide and diphenylhydantoin are the most common. More than 50% of patients will have some pulmonary manifestation, which may be pleural effusion, pleuritic pain, atelectasis, or diffuse interstitial infiltrates. Commonly associated symptoms include arthralgias and skin lesions. Patients with diphenylhydantoin-induced lupus syndrome are older (sixth decade) compared to patients with systemic lupus erythematosus (third decade), and notably lack renal or central nervous system involvement. Patients may require 2 months to recover after discontinuation of the drug, but symptoms may recur in the absence of drug rechallenge after several years in some patients.

Hypersensitivity pulmonary reactions have been documented with diphenylhydantoin usage. Patients present with cough, dyspnea, and fever within 3 to 6 weeks of initiation of the drug. A maculopapular rash, generalized lymphadenopathy, liver function test abnormalities, or eosinophilia may be associated findings. The chest radiograph demonstrates bilateral reticular, nodular, and alveolar infiltrates with or without hilar or mediastinal adenopathy. Most patients recover upon discontinuation of the drug.

A presentation with hilar adenopathy (pseudolymphoma), as demonstrated by the present patient, is a rare manifestation of diphenylhydantoin toxicity. Radiographic abnormalities simulate Hodgkin's disease and malignant lymphoma and have been associated with reduced levels of immunoglobulin A. The adenopathy usually develops within the first few months of drug use but may remain undetected for prolonged periods if the patient is asymptomatic. If symptoms occur, they are related to a hypersensitivity reaction. The key to management is to suspect the etiology of the adenopathy in patients on diphenylhydantoin and to discontinue therapy. Patients typically improve, with normalization of chest radiographs within 2 to 3 weeks.

The abnormal chest radiograph in the present patient was attributed to a drug reaction, although alternative diagnoses such as lymphoma or sarcoidosis could not be excluded. After diphenylhydantoin was withdrawn, the hilar adenopathy regressed after 2 weeks of observation, obviating further evaluation.

Clinical Pearls

1. Diphenylhydantoin is one of the most common causes of drug-induced lupus syndrome, which usually resolves after discontinuance of therapy but may recur later.

2. Hypersensitivity reactions with pulmonary infiltrates, eosinophilia, and high fever are associated with diphenylhydantoin therapy.

3. Hilar adenopathy is a rare manifestation of diphenylhydantoin toxicity that may be associated with decreased IgA levels.

REFERENCES

1. Sorrell TC, Forbes IJ, Burness FR, Rischbieth RHC. Depression of immunologic function in patients treated with phenytoin sodium (sodium diphenylhydantoin). Lancet 1971; 2:1233–1235.
2. Cooper JAD, White DA, Matthay RA. Drug-induced pulmonary disease. Part 2: Noncytotoxic drugs. Am Rev Respir Dis 1986; 133:488–505.
3. Alacon-Segovia D. Drug-induced lupus syndrome. Mayo Clin Proc 1969; 44:664–681.

PATIENT 24

A 59-year-old man with a 20-year history of sarcoidosis presenting with massive hemoptysis

A 59-year-old black man who was ventilator dependent was transferred to our hospital with a tracheostomy in place. He was status post cardiac arrest, which occurred during bronchoscopy for evaluation of hemoptysis. The patient had a history of intermittent minimal hemoptysis for the previous several months. Sarcoidosis was diagnosed approximately 20 years prior by mediastinoscopy. There was a history of chronic steroid therapy.

Physical Examination: Blood pressure 110/70; triggering ventilator at 16 breaths/min; unresponsive to verbal stimuli but responsive to pain; moved all extremities; diffuse rhonchi and basilar rales.

Laboratory Findings: WBC 19,200/μl, 83% PMNs, 15% lymphocytes; Hct 34%; platelet count 241,000/μl; PT 14 sec, PTT 32 sec. Chest radiograph: bilateral hilar adenopathy with calcification of hilar and mediastinal lymph nodes and right supraclavicular lymph nodes, diffuse nodular opacities throughout both lung fields. PFTs: FVC 1.2 L, FEV$_1$ 0.71 L.

On the second hospital day, acute massive bleeding from the tracheostomy tube occurred. The patient was not an operative candidate. It was decided that bronchial artery embolization would not be offered to this patient with postanoxic encephalopathy who had been comatose for the preceding two weeks. The pulmonary hemorrhage continued; the patient could not be oxygenated or ventilated adequately and shortly thereafter had a cardiac arrest.

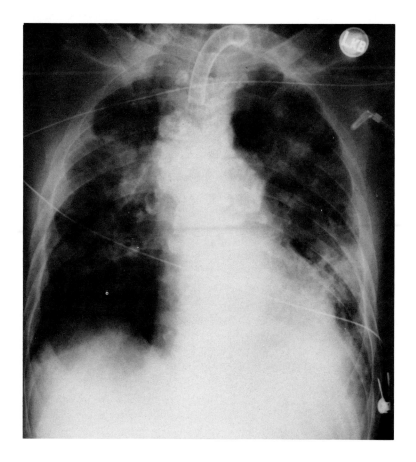

Diagnosis: Sarcoidosis with massive hemoptysis due to erosion of a broncholith into a pulmonary artery.

Discussion: The most common causes of mediastinal calcification are generally considered to be tuberculosis and histoplasmosis, but other infectious agents such as coccidioides, cryptococcus, and actinomyces have been noted. Silicosis also is a documented cause of hilar and mediastinal lymph node calcification. It was believed that sarcoidosis was a rare cause of hilar and mediastinal lymph node calcification; however, if patients with a diagnosis of sarcoidosis for >10 years are considered, more than 20% will have mediastinal lymph node calcification. This phenomenon appears to be more common in patients with stage II disease; the calcifications tend to become more dense and larger over time. Whether calcium deposition in lymph nodes involved with sarcoidosis results from necrosis or hyalinized fibrosis is unclear.

In the majority of instances, calcified mediastinal nodes are of no clinical consequence; however, at times, calcified peribronchial lymph nodes can erode the airway and lung parenchyma. The most common symptoms associated with a broncholithiasis are cough, hemoptysis, and bronchial obstruction; lithoptysis is an uncommon late finding. Hemoptysis due to broncholithiasis most commonly is minor and may be chronic and intermittent. Massive hemoptysis is rare and usually is a late complication resulting from erosion of the broncholith into the lung parenchyma, causing rupture of a pulmonary or bronchial artery or from an aortotracheal fistula. Massive or submassive hemoptysis resulting from sarcoidosis most commonly is seen with complicating aspergilloma or with fibrocystic sarcoidosis and is rare with broncholithiasis.

Radiographic manifestations of broncholithiasis include disappearance of a calcified focus on serial radiographs, changing positions of a calcified focus, and evidence of bronchial obstruction, either lobar or segmental atelectasis or partial obstruction with air trapping; right middle lobe atelectasis is the most common obstructive manifestation. After the diagnosis is confirmed by fiberoptic bronchoscopy, tomography and CT scan, management depends on the size of the stone, its location, and its complications. Observation probably is warranted in the absence of clinically important symptoms or complications. Surgical intervention is indicated for recurrent or massive hemoptysis, repeated pneumonia, and fistulas (see Patient 11).

Postmortem examination in the present patient demonstrated erosion of a right peribronchial lymph node into the lung parenchyma, resulting in rupture of a branch of the pulmonary artery. Even if more aggressive therapy had been attempted, bronchial artery embolization would not have been effective.

Clinical Pearls

1. Sarcoidosis is a cause of mediastinal lymph node calcification and is most commonly found in patients with stage II sarcoidosis who have had the disease for greater than 10 years.

2. Broncholithiasis can cause massive hemoptysis by erosion into the lung parenchyma; it is usually a late complication and is preceded by episodes of minor hemoptysis.

3. Sarcoidosis can cause massive hemoptysis when it is associated with aspergilloma, is of the fibrocystic variety, and when complicated by broncholithiasis.

REFERENCES

1. Bollengier WE, Guernsey JM. Broncholithiasis with aortotracheal fistula. J Thorac Cardiovasc Surg 1974; 68:588–591.
2. Israel HL, Lenchner G, Steiner RM. Late development of mediastinal calcification in sarcoidosis. Am Rev Respir Dis 1981; 124:302–305.
3. Lin C-S, Decker WH. Broncholith as a cause of fatal hemoptysis. JAMA 1978; 239:2153.
4. Shin MS, Kiang-Jey H. Broncholithiasis: detection by computed tomography in patients with recurrent hemoptysis of unknown etiology. J Comput Tomogr 1983; 7:189–193.

PATIENT 25

A 78-year-old woman with rheumatoid arthritis presenting with bilateral pleural effusions and pulmonary nodules

A 78-year-old white woman was referred for evaluation of bilateral pleural effusions and pulmonary nodules. She had a long-standing history of rheumatoid arthritis, with the articular manifestations being minimal and controlled with aspirin. Over the preceding several weeks, the patient had noted increased dyspnea with exertion and fatigue. She did not drink alcohol and was not a cigarette smoker. She denied cough, sputum production, fever, or hemoptysis. There was no history of a prior malignancy.

Physical Examination: Temperature 98.9°; pulse 100, irregularly irregular; respirations 24. Thin, chronically ill-appearing female in no acute distress; symmetrical joint involvement with active synovitis and subcutaneous nodules over extensor surfaces of forearms; evidence of small to moderate bilateral pleural effusions; breast and pelvic examination normal.

Laboratory Findings: WBC 8700/μl with normal differential; Hct 35%; ESR 32 mm/h. Serum rheumatoid factor 1:128. Chest radiograph: bilateral pleural effusions and multiple nodules throughout both lung fields. Right thoracentesis: yellow, turbid, nucleated cells 5600/μl, 65% lymphocytes, 20% PMNs, 10% monocytes, total protein 4.8 g/dl, glucose 60 mg/dl, pH 7.32, LDH 480 IU/L. Gram and AFB stains negative; cytology negative. Left thoracentesis: yellowish-green, turbid fluid, nucleated cells 6800/μl, 55% lymphocytes, 35% PMNs, total protein 5.2 g/dl, glucose 53 mg/dl, pH 7.30, LDH 500 IU/L. Gram and AFB stains negative; cytology negative. A diagnostic procedure was performed.

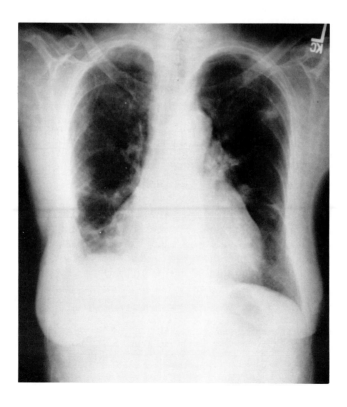

Diagnosis: Pulmonary rheumatoid nodules and rheumatoid pleural effusions.

Discussion: Nodular lesions in the lungs and pleurae in patients with rheumatoid arthritis were described at autopsy 40 years ago and were similar to the subcutaneous rheumatoid nodule described 10 years previously. The parenchymal nodules can occur at any time during the course of rheumatoid disease and may precede the articular manifestations. They appear to be more common in men (1.5:1), but not with the predilection seen with rheumatoid pleurisy. The nodules vary in size from a few millimeters up to 7 cm in diameter and generally result in no respiratory symptoms unless they are large and undergo necrosis with cavitation, which may be responsible for cough and hemoptysis. The nodules often are discovered on a routine chest radiograph or when a radiograph is obtained because the patient has symptoms of concomitant pleurisy. Pleural effusion or pleural thickening is seen in about 35% of patients with rheumatoid pulmonary nodules with a tendency to occur more frequently when the nodules are multiple rather than single lesions; nodules are more commonly multiple than single and cavitation is present more commonly with multiple lesions. Rheumatoid nodules may be subradiographic and discovered only at postmortem examination.

Subcutaneous nodules are identified in most patients (80%) with rheumatoid pulmonary nodules. Other systemic manifestations, especially cardiac lesions, are found commonly in patients with rheumatoid nodules; pericardial, myocardial, and endocardial lesions have been documented at postmortem examination.

Rheumatoid nodules are characterized by a central area of necrosis surrounded by palisading histiocytes and epithelial cells and an outer zone of chronic inflammatory cells, including multinucleated giant cells and macrophages. The history of these lesions is variable; some have increased in size and number under observation and others have resolved either spontaneously or in association with corticosteroid therapy. Depending upon the availability of serial radiographs spanning months to years, a histologic diagnosis of the nodules may be necessary at the time the patient is evaluated. Metastatic carcinoma, granulomatous diseases of the lung (including tuberculosis and fungal infections), and Wegener's and lymphomatoid granulomatosis need to be excluded. Special stains and culture help to eliminate the infectious granulomatoses, but careful histologic examination is necessary to exclude Wegener's and lymphomatoid granulomatosis on the basis of lack of destructive vascular lesions.

Approximately 15% of patients with rheumatoid pleurisy have normal pH, normal glucose, and low LDH pleural effusions; this usually occurs in the individual who has minimal pleural fibrosis that allows glucose entry and hydrogen ion efflux from the pleural space and limits the degree of pleural fluid acidosis.

In the present patient, transthoracic needle aspiration of one of the nodules showed necrosis, histiocytes, and multinucleated giant cells; AFB and KOH stains were negative as were cultures. The patient's clinical course and chest radiograph have been stable over the past 11 months without treatment.

Clinical Pearls

1. Rheumatoid pulmonary nodules are a relatively uncommon manifestation of rheumatoid lung disease and usually present as multiple (1–7 cm) round densities that may cavitate and are often accompanied by rheumatoid pleural effusions or pleural thickening; nodules are more common in males.

2. Nodules rarely produce symptoms except when they are large and cavitate, resulting in hemoptysis. The diagnosis usually is suspected on routine radiograph or when patients present with symptoms of rheumatoid pleurisy.

REFERENCES
1. Walker WC, Wright D. Pulmonary lesions and rheumatoid arthritis. Medicine 1968; 47:501–519.
2. Walters MN-I, Ojeda VJ. Pleuropulmonary necrobiotic rheumatoid nodules. Med J Aust 1986; 144:648–651.
3. Kaye VR, Kaye RL, Bobrobe A. Rheumatoid nodules. Review of the spectrum of associated conditions and a proposal of a new classification; with a report of 4 seronegative cases. Am J Med 1984; 76:279–292.

PATIENT 26

A 75-year-old man with fatigue, weight loss, fever, low back pain, and a pulmonary nodule

A 75-year-old black farmer was admitted with weight loss, fatigue, occasional fevers, and low back pain of several months duration. He denied loss of sensation or weakness in the legs. The patient denied cough, hemoptysis, dyspnea, or night sweats.

Physical Examination: Temperature 98.8°; respirations 16; cachectic but in no distress; no lymphadenopathy; examination of lungs was normal; no pain elicited with flexion or extension of the spine; no tenderness to palpation over the vertebrae; neurologic examination was intact.

Laboratory Findings: WBC 2400/μl, 51% PMNs, 7% bands, 29% lymphocytes, 9% monocytes; Hct 32%. Chest radiograph: a 1-cm nodule in the right upper lobe posteriorly. Lumbosacral spine films: destruction of the end plate of the inferior margin of L3 with associated partial collapse of the vertebral body, evidence of loss of disc space. PPD skin test positive.

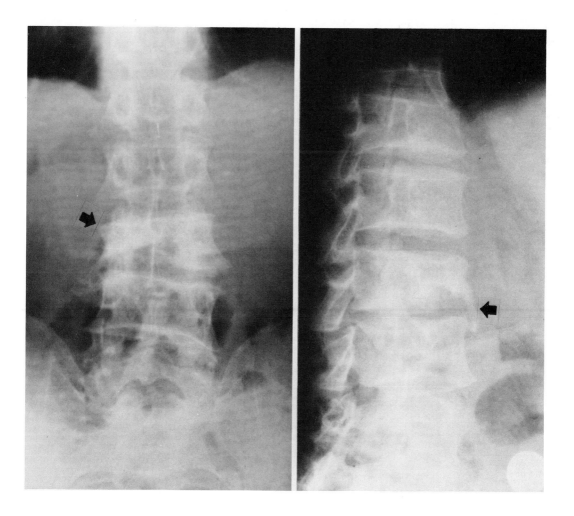

Diagnosis: Pulmonary and vertebral tuberculosis (Pott's disease).

Discussion: Skeletal tuberculosis represents less than 1% of cases of tuberculosis and less than 10% of cases of extrapulmonary tuberculosis. It usually is the consequence of reactivation of a focus that was initiated during hematogenous seeding but may also occur from contiguous spread from a caseating lymph node or from lymphatic spread from the lung or kidney. The age of patients with skeletal tuberculosis appears to be increasing, with the majority presenting between the fifth and seventh decades. Pain over the affected vertebrae of several weeks' to years' duration, with or without limitation of motion, is the most common presenting symptom. The pain is often associated with weight loss, fatigue, and fever. Vertebral collapse or subluxation with pressure on the spinal cord or nerve roots produces a variety of neurologic symptoms.

Approximately half the patients with skeletal tuberculosis have radiographic evidence of active or inactive pulmonary tuberculosis. Early skeletal changes include radiolucency of the vertebral body and loss of bony cortex with later vertebral collapse, producing the characteristic "anterior wedging." The disc space becomes destroyed and, when infection spreads along the anterior and longitudinal ligaments, it can produce vertebral body scalloping. Paravertebral abscesses, which are commonly associated, may be missed on plain film but are identified easily on CT scan. The differential diagnosis of back pain and vertebral collapse in the elderly is osteoporosis, malignancy, and infection. In osteoporosis, there is preservation of the bony cortex; in infection, the disc space is destroyed; and in malignancy, the vertebral pedicles are lost. Paravertebral soft tissue shadows and calcification, uncommon in malignant disease of the spine, suggest infection. Radioisotope scans are nondiagnostic except if they show increased areas of uptake throughout the skeleton, suggesting malignancy. The diagnosis of skeletal tuberculosis is easily established by bone biopsy, either by histology or culture. Chemotherapy is the mainstay of treatment, with surgery being reserved for those patients who fail to respond to chemotherapy alone and selected cases with neurologic complications. The optimal duration of therapy for bone tuberculosis is unknown, but probably 12 months of isoniazid and rifampin therapy is adequate.

The present patient underwent needle aspiration of the L1 vertebra that showed granulomatous inflammation, which subsequently cultured *M. tuberculosis*. On chemotherapy consisting of isoniazid, rifampin and pyrazinimide for 2 months and isoniazid and rifampin for an additional 10 months, the patient's symptoms abated, the pulmonary nodule resolved, and the lumbar spine lesion underwent further sclerosis without progression.

Clinical Pearls

1. Tuberculosis of the spine should be considered in the differential diagnosis of back pain and vertebral collapse in the elderly.

2. Tuberculosis destroys the disc space, whereas malignant disease involving the vertebral bodies results in loss of the pedicles.

3. The diagnosis of tuberculosis of the spine is best established by culture or histology of the bony or paravertebral lesion.

REFERENCES

1. Alvarez S, McCabe WR. Extrapulmonary tuberculosis revisited: a review of experience at Boston City and other hospitals. Medicine 1984; 63:25–85.
2. Mann JS, Cole RB. Tuberculous spondylitis in the elderly. A potential diagnostic pitfall. Br Med J 1987; 294:1149–1150.
3. Davidson PT, Horwitz I. Skeletal tuberculosis. Am J Med 1984; 48:77–84.

PATIENT 27

A 54-year-old man with a several-month history of bilateral chest pain, dyspnea on exertion, and a pulmonary nodule

A 54-year-old man presented with bilateral, aching, diffuse chest pain and dyspnea on exertion for several months. He had a 20 pack/year history of cigarette smoking and had quit 8 years prior. As a boiler repairman, he had heavy exposure to asbestos for 4 years, 32 years prior.

Physical Examination: Atrial fibrillation with slow ventricular response; respirations 16; decreased bilateral expansion; slight diminution in breath sounds without adventitious sounds; clubbing absent.

Laboratory Findings: FVC 2.91 L (55% of predicted); FEV$_1$ 2.17 L (84% of predicted); FEV$_1$/FVC ratio 93%; DL/VA 5.44. ABG (room air): pH 7.37, PCO$_2$ 42 mmHg, PO$_2$ 79 mmHg. Chest radiograph: bilateral pleural thickening, diaphragmatic calcified pleural plaques and interstitial lung disease; a 4 × 3 cm lesion in the left mid-lung zone.

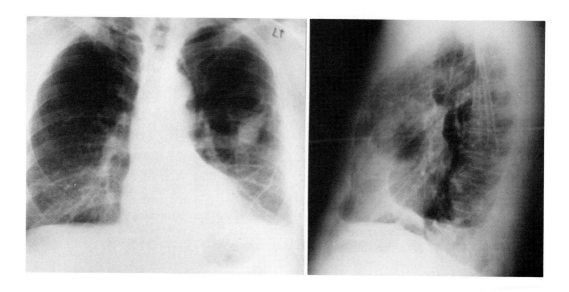

Diagnosis: Rounded atelectasis due to asbestos-induced pleural disease.

Discussion: The entity "rounded atelectasis" (shrinking pleuritis with atelectasis, pseudotumor) was first described in the European literature in the 1950s and 60s. Patients had a thoracotomy because of suspected pulmonary neoplasm. At operation, no tumor was found but a thick, fibrous membrane covering part of the lung was noted; the underlying parenchyma was atelectatic. Following decortication, the lung expanded and appeared normal. Silica, blunt chest trauma, mitral disease, and post-cardiac injury syndrome all have been implicated in the pathogenesis of shrinking pleuritis with atelectasis, but asbestos exposure remains the major cause.

Rounded atelectasis probably develops due to the following sequence of events. (1) Asbestos-induced pleural effusion results in atelectasis within an area of the lobe compressed by the effusion. A cleft forms between the atelectatic lung and the aerated parts of the lobe. (2) The lobe tilts at the cleft and becomes fixed in a new position by the progressive fibrinous exudate on the lung surface, especially at the cleft. (3) The pleural fluid is reabsorbed and normal lung expands toward the chest wall; however, the atelectatic segment becomes engulfed within the visceral pleura of the remainder of the reexpanded lobe.

The pulmonary lesion tends to have a curved outline but may not be strictly round. It may be oval, lobulated, or irregular in shape. The margins may be sharp or poorly defined. Often the proximal inferior border is blurred by vessels and bronchi entering the lesion. The diameter of the lesion ranges from 2.5 to 5.0 cm, is most commonly located along the posterior surface of a lower lobe medially or laterally, and is almost always separated from the diaphragm by lung tissue. The lung adjacent to the lesion has features essentially pathognomonic for rounded atelectasis. The blood vessels adjacent to the mass often are crowded together in a curved fashion as they approach the lesion. Initial direction of the vessels is toward the base of the lung before sweeping caudad like the "tail of a comet" as they enter the lower part of the lesion. The "comet tail" (composed of vessels and bronchi) cannot be seen in all projections but usually can be visualized by tomography. Chronic pleural thickening is almost always present in rounded atelectasis, and free pleural effusion is almost never seen at the time the lesion is diagnosed. Pleural thickening is usually localized over the affected lobe or, at minimum, more striking than elsewhere in the pleural space. The lesion is virtually always in contact with the thickened pleura and forms an acute angle with it, indicating an intrapulmonic rather than pleural or extrapleural location. There usually is no evidence of volume loss, since rounded atelectasis seldom involves a large part of the lobe. The lesion usually does not change over time but, on occasion, there has been spontaneous reduction or disappearance. When the typical radiographic features are present in a patient with a history of asbestos exposure, the diagnosis can be made with confidence. Obviously, if a series of films are available showing a static lesion, the diagnostic impression is strengthened. CT scan usually is not additive to tomography. In the patient without characteristic findings on previous chest radiographs, transthoracic needle aspiration probably is the procedure of choice. The lesion in the present patient has been unchanged radiographically for 3 years.

Clinical Pearls

1. Rounded atelectasis is an unusual form of peripheral lobar collapse most commonly caused by asbestos-induced pleural disease.

2. It has distinctive radiographic features, so that in the presence of chronic pleural thickening from asbestos exposure, the findings are highly suggestive of the diagnosis.

3. CT scan usually is not additive to tomography in confirming the characteristic features of rounded atelectasis.

REFERENCES

1. Schneider HJ, Felson B, Gonzalez LL. Rounded atelectasis. AJR 1980; 134:225–232.
2. Mintzer RA, Gore RM, Vogelzang RL, Holz S. Rounded atelectasis and its association with asbestos-induced pleural disease. Radiology 1981; 139:567–570.
3. Dernevik L, Gatzinsky T, Hultman E, et al. Shrinking pleuritis with atelectasis. Thorax 1982; 37:252–258.

PATIENT 28

A 59-year-old man with a history of acute myelogenous leukemia presenting with acute shortness of breath and bilateral pulmonary infiltrates

A 59-year-old man developed the sudden onset of shortness of breath during hospitalization for chemotherapeutic management of acute myeloid leukemia. His symptoms developed several hours after receiving the twelfth dose of high-dose cytosine arabinoside (ARA-C). He had previously received Adriamycin during an earlier hospitalization.

Physical Examination. Temperature 99°; respirations 32; pulse 120; blood pressure 108/67. Patient appeared in moderate respiratory distress; diffuse rales; crisp heart sounds with a brisk point of maximal cardiac impulse; abdomen normal.

Laboratory Findings: Hct 26%, WBC 800/μl with 50% neutrophils; platelets 50,000/μl. ABG (100% O_2 nonrebreathing face mask): pH 7.45, $PaCO_2$ 30 mmHg, PaO_2 65 mmHg. Chest radiograph showed bilateral alveolar infiltrates with a normal sized heart.

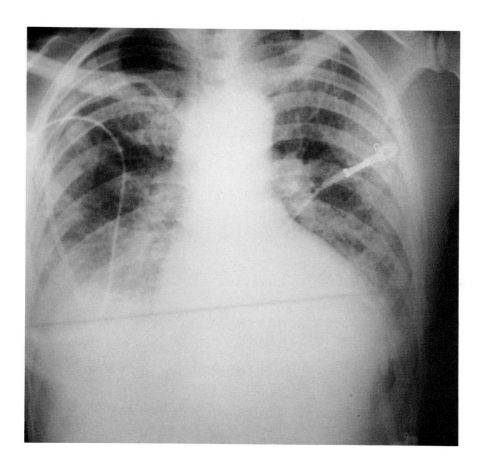

Diagnosis: ARA-C-induced pulmonary edema. Other considerations include pulmonary hemorrhage, pulmonary infection, and cardiogenic pulmonary edema, possibly related to Adriamycin-induced cardiotoxicity.

Discussion: Cytotoxic chemotherapeutic agents have been increasingly recognized as important causes of pulmonary dysfunction. Although these drugs are considered under the single general category of "cytotoxic agents," their chemical structures and modes of action vary widely, which explains the diverseness of the pulmonary reactions they generate. Depending on the particular drug, manifestations of pulmonary toxicity may range from chronic pneumonitis with fibrosis to more acute disorders, such as hypersensitivity pneumonitis and noncardiogenic pulmonary edema. Mechanisms of lung injury are equally varied and include idiosyncratic and immunologic reactions, modulation of fibroblast replication, and oxidant lung injury.

Diagnosis of cytotoxic drug-induced pulmonary dysfunction is complicated not only by the diverse clinical presentations, but also by the patient's medical condition. Underlying pulmonary neoplasm, high inspired oxygen concentrations, previous gamma irradiation, and multiple drug regimens with agents having potential pulmonary toxicity often contribute to lung dysfunction, thereby obscuring the role of any one particular cytotoxic drug.

ARA-C is one of the most important drugs for the treatment of acute myeloid leukemia in the adult. Its major adverse reactions are profound myelosuppression, mucositis, and hypoproteinemia resulting from gastrointestinal protein loss. Although the literature is not extensive, ARA-C is also recognized as a cause of pulmonary toxicity. Manifestations of the sudden onset of respiratory distress attributable to pulmonary edema. Although cardiomegaly may be radiographically apparent, the pulmonary edema is noncardiogenic with normal left ventricular ejection fractions. Pulmonary edema may occur after the first dose of ARA-C or three weeks after the initiation of therapy. Most patients recover from the drug-induced pulmonary edema, but corticosteroids are anecdotally noted to accelerate resolution. The incidence of ARA-C pulmonary toxicity can be decreased if patients are pretreated with corticosteroids before receiving chemotherapy.

The present patient received corticosteroids with the presumptive diagnosis of ARA-C induced pulmonary edema. Adriamycin cardiotoxicity was excluded by an echocardiogram that demonstrated adequate left ventricular function. Alternative diagnoses such as pulmonary hemorrhage and pulmonary infection could not be immediately excluded, but the characteristic onset of pulmonary edema subsequent to initiation of ARA-C made these diagnoses less likely. After 24 hours, the patient progressively improved, clearing the radiographic infiltrates and normalizing oxygenation.

Clinical Pearls

1. ARA-C causes pulmonary toxicity that is characterized by a rapid onset of respiratory distress with noncardiogenic pulmonary edema.

2. Most patients survive ARA-C lung toxicity, and corticosteroids may accelerate the rate of symptom resolution.

REFERENCES

1. Hewlett RI, Wilson AF. Adult respiratory distress syndrome (ARDS) following aggressive management of extensive acute lymphoblastic leukemia. Cancer 1977; 39:2422–2425.
2. Andersson BS, Cogan BM, Keating MJ, et al. Subacute pulmonary failure complicating therapy with high-dose ARA-C in acute leukemia. Cancer 1985; 56:2181–2184.

PATIENT 29

A 67-year-old man with cough, hemoptysis, weight loss, and upper lobe pulmonary infiltrates

A 67-year-old man was evaluated for cough, hemoptysis, and weight loss. He related a smoking history but denied previous pulmonary disease, rheumatologic problems, or exposure to tuberculosis. He was in the Navy 20 years earlier and subsequently worked in outdoor jobs ranging from construction to landscaping throughout the midwestern and southeastern United States.

Physical Examination: No skin abnormalities or lymphadenopathy; chest apical rales; no clubbing.

Laboratory Findings: CBC normal; liver function tests normal; PPD and controls negative. Sputum for fungus and acid fast organisms negative on smear and culture. Chest radiograph showed bilateral apical dense infiltrates.

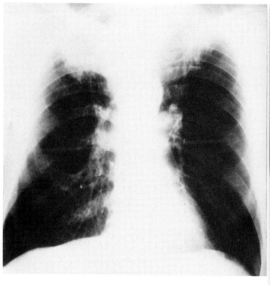 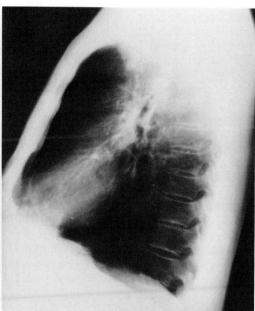

Diagnosis: Primary pulmonary sporotrichosis. Other diagnostic possibilities include tuberculosis and other fungal infections such as chronic histoplasmosis.

Discussion: Sporothrix schenckii is a dimorphic fungus with low virulence that is a rare cause of primary pulmonary infection. Widespread in nature, the organism typically causes cutaneous infection after scratches from thorny bushes or plants. Inhalation or aspiration of organisms also occurs, however, allowing penetration of the 2 to 3 μm spores to the alveolus, establishing a focus of pulmonary infection.

Pulmonary infection is chronic and insidious in onset. Symptoms are nonspecific and include cough, blood-streaked sputum, fever, chest pain, weight loss, anorexia, and night sweats—a constellation that is compatible with pulmonary tuberculosis. Men are more commonly infected than women and the average age at presentation is 45 years. Although distributed worldwide, 73% of sporotrichosis cases in this country occur within the Missouri and Mississippi River valleys.

Clinical features suggesting the diagnosis include an occupation or hobby that increases the patient's exposure to fungal spores. Particularly suspicious activities include greenhouse operations, landscaping, and construction work. Virtually any outdoor activity, however, has been associated with sporotrichosis, and 35% of patients with pulmonary infection do not have an exposure history. Patients may present with characteristic cutaneous findings; however, 90% of patients with pulmonary involvement have primary disease without extrapulmonary manifestations. More than half of patients have an underlying impairment of host defenses such as diabetes mellitus, alcoholism, or renal insufficiency—a finding similar to other infectious causes of chronic upper lobe infiltrates.

The radiographic manifestations of sporotrichosis mimic tuberculosis, cancer, anaerobic lung infections, and other chronic fungal disorders in the upper lobe predominance. The infiltrates range from linear streaking to fibronodular densities with or without cavities that are typically thin-walled and irregular. One-third of patients have bilateral disease, and hilar adenopathy or pleural effusions occur rarely.

The diagnosis of sporotrichosis requires demonstration of the organism in tissue or culture. Serologic studies are not commonly employed, although a tube agglutination test in titers of 1:80 or greater suggests the diagnosis. The organism is rarely seen in sputum, but its detection can be enhanced by using a direct fluorescent antibody stain. Sputum cultures may be positive in 80% of patients, with growth occurring rapidly in 3 to 5 days. Some colonies may never become pigmented, and cultures may be discarded as overgrown with "yeast." The organisms may be difficult to detect in specifically stained pathologic specimens unless nonfungal polysaccharides are first dissolved.

The best therapy for pulmonary sporotrichosis is poorly defined. Localized cavitary disease in a good operative candidate warrants consideration of surgical removal after preoperative therapy with amphotericin B or SSKI. Multifocal or extensive unresectable pulmonary disease should be managed with systemic amphotericin B. Infiltrative pulmonary disease without cavities may be treated with SSKI alone, but if the infiltrates do not improve, resection or amphotericin B should be considered.

The present patient underwent a nondiagnostic fiberoptic bronchoscopy followed by an open lung biopsy that revealed chronic inflammation on pathologic examination and *Sporothrix schenckii* on culture. He was treated with 2 gm of amphotericin B with regression of the infiltrates and improvement of symptoms.

Clinical Pearls

1. A suggestive exposure history is found in only 65% of patients with pulmonary sporotrichosis.

2. The organism may be difficult to detect in pathologic specimens even with appropriate stains unless the nonfungal polysaccharides are dissolved.

3. Expectorated sputums are positive in up to 80% of patients with pulmonary sporotrichosis.

REFERENCES

1. Sarosi GA, Armstrong D, Davies SF, et al. Laboratory diagnosis of mycotic and specific fungal infections. Am Rev Respir Dis 1985; 132:1373–1379.
2. Rohatgi FK. Pulmonary sporotrichosis. South Med J 1980; 73:1611–1617.
3. Pluss JL, Opal SM. Pulmonary sporotrichosis: review of treatment and outcome. Medicine 1986; 65:143–153.

PATIENT 30

An 82-year-old woman with a history of congestive heart failure presenting with weight loss, shortness of breath, and diffuse pulmonary infiltrates

An 82-year-old black woman was admitted from a nursing home because of weight loss, anorexia, and shortness of breath over the previous two months. She had had several similar episodes in the previous two years ascribed to chronic congestive heart failure, but the present symptoms did not improve with increased diuresis. One year earlier she had received a transvenous pacemaker for persistent bradycardia. The patient denied smoking, recent travel, fever, or cough.

Physical Examination: Temperature 98°; pulse 70; blood pressure 110/79. Chest normal; regular cardiac rhythm; hepatosplenomegaly.

Laboratory Findings: Hct 30%, WBC 6,700/μl; serum sodium 128 mEq/L; slightly elevated BUN and creatinine. Chest radiograph revealed massive cardiomegaly with a transvenous pacemaker in place. The lung fields were abnormal, with a diffuse reticulonodular infiltrate interpreted as congestive heart failure.

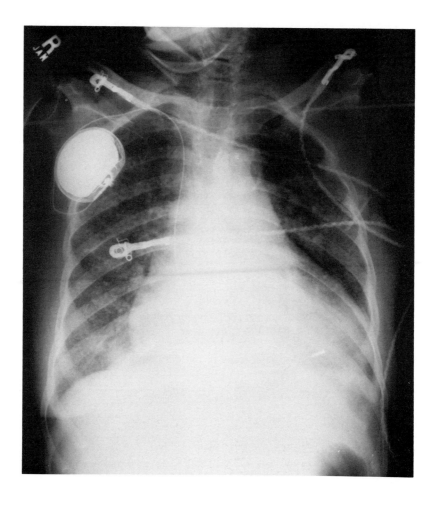

Diagnosis: Miliary tuberculosis.

Discussion: Two major trends in the epidemiology of tuberculosis in the last 30 years have an important impact on the diagnosis of the disease. First, the incidence of pulmonary tuberculosis has decreased annually, while the incidence of extrapulmonary tuberculosis has remained stable. Subsequently, a greater proportion (15%) of patients with tuberculosis present with extrapulmonary disease that may be initially occult and difficult to diagnose. Second, tuberculosis in the United States has become primarily a disease of the elderly. Tuberculosis rates are three times higher in patients older than 65 years of age, and 30% of all tuberculosis occurs in this elderly age group. Considering that our general population is becoming older and that 40% of the elderly in urban areas already have positive PPD skin tests, the importance of engendering a strong clinical suspicion for tuberculosis in clinicians caring for elderly patients is paramount.

A recently realized result of the "aging" of tuberculosis in this country is the increasing prevalence of tuberculosis transmission among residents in nursing homes. As many as 35% of nursing home residents have either a previous exposure to tuberculosis or a positive PPD. When these sources of infection are combined with the large number of elderly residents who were not exposed to tuberculosis during childhood, the nursing home's closed living conditions becomes an ideal environment for transmitting progressive primary tuberculosis. Recent studies indicate that the rate of conversion of PPD skin tests among new residents of nursing homes ranges between 5 and 10% and that these new converters have a 5%

probability of developing active tuberculosis within the first year of conversion.

Miliary tuberculosis may be particularly difficult to diagnose in the elderly population where the disease has a high mortality. As many as 50% of these patients have underlying medical problems such as diabetes mellitus, renal insufficiency, or cardiovascular disease, as demonstrated by the present patient. These medical disorders, combined with the often indolent and nonspecific symptoms of miliary tuberculosis, obscure the correct diagnosis. In this setting, the miliary pattern on the chest radiograph may be misinterpreted and attributed to coexisting problems such as pneumonia or congestive heart failure.

A high index of suspicion and recognition of the characteristic clinical features of miliary tuberculosis are requisite in caring for elderly patients: patients typically have malaise, fever, weight loss, and fatigue, although these symptoms may be absent in 30% of patients. Symptoms may be indolent or develop rapidly, but the average duration of symptoms before diagnosis is 16 weeks. Blacks are at particular risk because of the 2 to 1 ratio of tuberculosis in black compared to white patients. Hyponatremia and anemia are common, but any combination of hematologic abnormalities is possible.

The combination of an indolent illness unresponsive to diuretics with diffuse nodular infiltrates in an elderly patient from a nursing home suggested the possibility of tuberculosis in the present patient. Sputum specimens were unremarkable, but gastric aspirates were positive on smear and culture for *Mycobacterium tuberculosis*.

Clinical Pearls

1. Despite improvements in public health and a declining incidence of pulmonary tuberculosis, extrapulmonary tuberculosis has not decreased in frequency and now accounts for 15% of all instances of tuberculosis.

2. Up to 35% of nursing home residents are potential sources of tuberculous infection, accounting for the 5 to 10% annual conversion rate of skin tests in previously unexposed residents.

3. The average duration of symptoms in patients with miliary tuberculosis before diagnosis is 16 weeks.

REFERENCES

1. Alvarez S, McCabe WR. Extrapulmonary tuberculosis revisited: A review of experience at Boston City and other hospitals. Medicine 1984; 63:25–55.
2. Weir MR, Thornton GF. Extrapulmonary tuberculosis. Experience of a community hospital and review of the literature. Am J Med 1985; 79:467–478.
3. Welty C, Burstin S, Muspratt S, Tager IB. Epidemiology of tuberculous infection in a chronic care population. Am Rev Respir Dis 1985; 132:133–136.

PATIENT 31

A 26-year-old man with tuberculous pleurisy and an intrapleural foreign body after thoracentesis

A 26-year-old man was admitted with a 6-week history of fatigue, fever, weight loss, productive cough, and progressive dyspnea on exertion. He was a construction worker and had not been able to perform his job adequately over the preceding few weeks. He had a 10 pack/year history of cigarette smoking, occasional alcohol use, and no previous tuberculosis skin tests.

Physical Examination: Temperature 100.6°; pulse 100; respirations 24. In no acute distress; flat percussion note, decreased fremitus and absent breath sounds over entire left hemithorax; heart sounds heard best over midline and to right of sternum; absence of clubbing.

Laboratory Findings: WBC 9300/µl, 70% PMNs, 25% lymphocytes, 5% monocytes; Hct 32%. Liver function tests normal; PPD 15 mm. Chest radiograph: large left pleural effusion with contralateral mediastinal shift, right upper lobe cavitary infiltrate. Sputum Gram stain: few PMNs, no predominant organism; sputum culture: normal flora; sputum AFB smear negative; sputum culture for TB and fungus: plated. Thoracentesis: serous, nucleated cells 4500/µl, 80% lymphocytes, 15% PMNs, 4% macrophages, total protein 5.1 g/dl, LDH 250 IU/L, pH 7.33, glucose 65 mg/dl, amylase 40 IU/L. Cytology negative; AFB smear negative; TB and fungal culture pending; pleural biopsy: caseating granuloma.

1000 ml of pleural fluid was removed, with relief of dyspnea. Post-thoracentesis chest radiograph: diminished volume of pleural fluid, air-fluid level, and evidence of radiopaque foreign body in left pleural space.

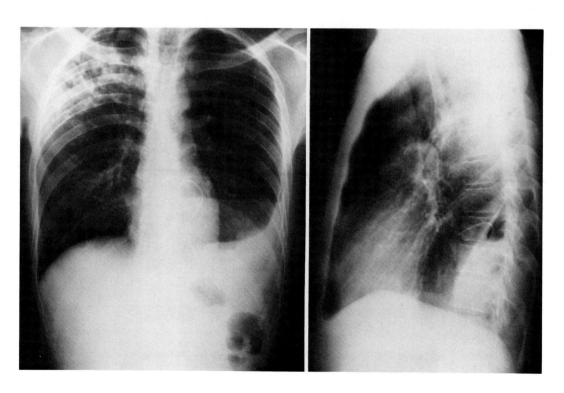

Diagnosis: Intrapleural foreign body (polyethylene catheter). Removal from pleural space using thoracoscopy under local anesthesia.

Discussion: Thoracoscopy was originally introduced more than 70 years ago by Jacobaeus to investigate idiopathic pleurisy; he also was the first individual to use the instrument therapeutically to guide lysis of pleural space adhesions that were preventing collapse therapy for pulmonary tuberculosis. Thorascopic pneumolysis became unnecessary as tuberculosis declined and chemotherapy developed, and the enthusiasm for thoracoscopy diminished. Recently, however, an increased resurgence in its use for diagnostic purposes has emerged. The introduction of a rigid scope with a cold light source has allowed a thorough exploration of the entire hemithorax, including the mediastinum, and has improved on the sensitivity of closed needle biopsy in the diagnosis and staging of malignant disease of the lungs or pleura.

Several therapeutic uses of the thoracoscope have emerged recently: removal of intrapleural foreign bodies, chemical pleurodesis, and debridement of post-pneumonectomy empyema cavities. There have been isolated reports of removal of an intrapleural foreign body with the thoracoscope using general anesthesia; no complications were noted.

Although the presence of a small piece of sterile tubing in the pleural space may not be associated with adverse effects, removal may be warranted in some individuals with predisposing conditions. For example, in the immunosuppressed patient or the patient with a prosthetic device, the risk of sepsis could be devastating. Furthermore, there always is the possibility of extrapleural migration of the foreign body into the vascular space. There are no absolute indications for removal of these sterile, inert foreign bodies, usually the result of a sheered catheter. However, the patient may insist upon removal or there may be medical indications for extraction. If the foreign body can be removed by thoracostomy, a formal thoracotomy with its morbidity, potential mortality, and economic burden can be avoided.

Thoracoscopy, in addition to confirming a malignant pleural process, can be used for directed chemical pleurodesis. Tetracycline can be instilled directly or talc can be insufflated into the pleural space. Thoracoscopy also has been used for the evaluation and treatment of inadequately drained, postpneumonectomy empyema cavities. This procedure may be of value in selected patients with empyema, as it may allow better aspiration of debris with assurance of optimal positioning of chest tubes. Other potential therapeutic indications for thoracoscopy may be in the setting of chest trauma, where the bleeding source can be identified and possibly stopped by electrocautery.

The patient had rigid thoracoscopy under local anesthesia with preoperative morphine (3 mg) and midazolam (1 mg) intravenously with removal of a 2-cm polyethylene catheter within 5 minutes upon entering the pleural space. He tolerated the procedure well and was returned to his room within 30 minutes. There were no complications from the procedure and the patient had no pleural space sequelae over the ensuing 4 months. *M. tuberculosis* was cultured from the sputum and pleural tissue; he was was treated with antituberculosis chemotherapy.

Clinical Pearls

1. Therapeutic indications for thoracoscopy are removal of an intrapleural foreign body, chemical pleurodesis, and debridement of empyemas that have been drained inadequately.

2. There are no absolute indications for removal of a sterile, intrapleural foreign body; however, in the immunocompromised patient or the patient with a prosthetic device where sepsis may be devastating, removal probably is indicated.

3. An intrapleural foreign body may be removed rapidly and easily by thoracoscopy under local anesthesia.

REFERENCES

1. Brodsky JB, Weltil RS, Mark JBD. Thoracoscopy for retrieval of intrathoracic foreign bodies. Anesthesiology 1981; 54:91–92.
2. Oakes DD, Sherck JP, Brodsky JB, Mark JBD. Therapeutic thoracoscopy. J Thorac Cardiovasc Surg 1984; 87:269–273.
3. Moore JP, Fendley SA, Rodning CB. Extraction of an intrapleural foreign body with a flexible endoscope. J Thorac Cardiovasc Surg 1986; 91:929–936.

PATIENT 32

A 23-year-old man with a history of testes cancer presenting with mediastinal adenopathy and pulmonary nodules

A 23-year-old white male was evaluated for an enlarged left testis.

Physical Examination: Normal except for a firm, nontender left testis.

Laboratory Findings: CBC, liver function tests, and indices of renal function normal; α-fetoprotein and β human chorionic gonadotropin levels normal. Chest radiograph was normal (not shown). Abdominal CT scan was unremarkable without enlarged abdominal lymph nodes.

Orchiectomy was performed revealing an embryonal cell cancer. Three months later, the patient was asymptomatic, but a chest radiograph demonstrated hilar and paratracheal lymphadenopathy with several 1 to 2 cm nodules in both lung fields. The physical examination was normal and serum markers of tumor activity were again nonelevated. Sputum specimen smears obtained for acid-fast and fungal pathogens were negative. A chest and abdominal CT scan confirmed the mediastinal lymphadenopathy and defined the pulmonary nodules, but there was no evidence of abdominal lymphadenopathy or hepatic masses. A bone scan was normal.

The patient underwent mediastinoscopy and biopsy of a right paratracheal lymph node that demonstrated noncaseating granulomas consistent with sarcoidosis. Oncology consultants presented recent medical reports, stating an association between sarcoid-like mediastinal lymphadenopathy and testes cancer that develops after curative resection and does not necessarily indicate recurrent disease.

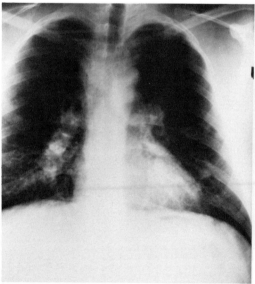
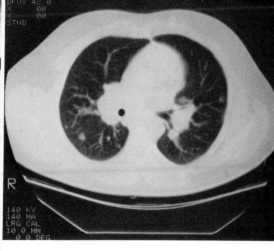

Diagnosis: Metastatic embryonal cell cancer with a sarcoid-like reaction.

Discussion: Sarcoidosis is characterized by diffuse epithelial granulomas in several organ systems and usually presents with a distinctive clinical pattern. Many neoplasms such as cancer of the lung, uterus, and stomach may produce local sarcoid-like reactions but do not generate the generalized systemic features of sarcoidosis. These local tissue reactions are not difficult to distinguish from true sarcoidosis because of their regional association with the primary neoplasm. Several reports, however, demonstrate that patients with resected testicular cancers without known tumor recurrence may develop mediastinal lymphadenopathy with pathologic features of granulomatous inflammation indistinguishable from sarcoidosis. The etiology of these local sarcoid-like reactions and their relationship to sarcoidosis are uncertain, but their occurrence may present considerable difficulty in excluding metastatic tumor recurrence.

The present patient underwent mediastinoscopy, confirming the benign granulomatous reaction in mediastinal lymph nodes. However, the pulmonary nodules could not be considered manifestations of nodular sarcoidosis without tissue confirmation. Therefore, the patient underwent needle aspiration of one of the nodules demonstrating metastatic disease. Since the cure rate in metastatic cancer of the testes is directly related to the bulk of metastatic disease, recurrent malignant disease must be aggressively evaluated. If needle aspiration of the lung nodule in the present patient had been nondiagnostic or cytologically consistent with granulomatous inflammation, a repeat needle aspiration or an open lung biopsy would have been necessary.

The patient was started on chemotherapy that included VP-16, cisplatin, and bleomycin but no corticosteroids. Four weeks later, a repeat chest radiograph was normal, showing complete resolution of the pulmonary nodules and mediastinal lymphadenopathy.

Clinical Pearls

1. A sarcoid-like reaction with mediastinal granulomatous lymphadenopathy can occur after curative resection of testes cancer and does not necessarily denote tumor recurrence.

2. Pulmonary nodules may be the only manifestation of metastatic disease in testes cancer and can develop concurrently with a mediastinal sarcoid-like reaction.

REFERENCES

1. Fossa SD, Abeler V, Marton PF, et al. Sarcoid reaction of hilar and paratracheal lymph nodes in patients treated for testicular cancer. Cancer 1985; 56:2212–2216.
2. Dhakhwa RB, Harmon E, Safirstein BH. Sarcoidosis presenting as multiple pulmonary nodules. JAMA 1976; 236: 2529–2530.
3. James DG, Jones-Williams W. Sarcoidosis and Other Granulomatous Disorders. Philadelphia, W.B. Saunders, 1985.

PATIENT 33

A 15-year-old boy with a 1-month history of abdominal pain and ascites

A 15-year-old black male was in good health until 4 weeks prior to admission when he developed intermittent abdominal discomfort. He was placed on antacids by his local physician but returned 1 week later because of continued pain and abdominal swelling. There was no history of fever or chills. The patient denied TB exposure.

Physical Examination: Temperature 98.1°; pulse 84; respirations 16. No acute distress; protuberant abdomen with bulging flanks and a fluid wave; decreased bilateral expansion, diminished breath sounds in the bases; no masses or hepatosplenomegaly; no lymphadenopathy.

Laboratory Findings: WBC 5700/μl, 62% PMNs, 31% lymphocytes, 4% eosinophils; Hct 43%. Urinalysis normal; PPD skin test negative; controls positive. Chest radiograph: slightly reduced lung volumes, parenchyma normal. CT scan of the abdomen: ascites, normal liver and spleen; no masses or lymphadenopathy. Paracentesis: serosanguinous fluid, nucleated cells 1600/μl, 59% lymphocytes, 27% macrophages, 13% PMNs, RBC 10,500/μl (87% fresh); total protein 5.9 g/dl, glucose 95 mg/dl, amylase 46 IU/L. Gram stain: no organisms; aerobic and anaerobic cultures negative; AFB smear negative; TB and fungus culture pending; cytology negative. A laparoscopy was performed.

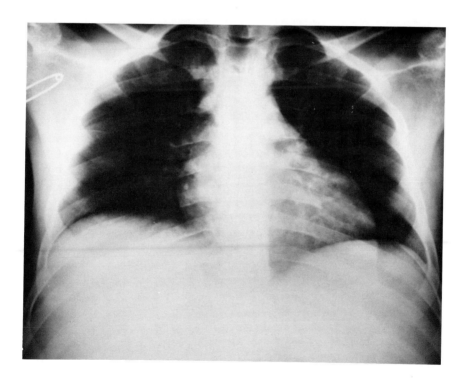

Diagnosis: Sarcoidosis with ascites due to peritoneal involvement.

Discussion: Patients with sarcoidosis who develop ascites usually have either severe liver disease with portal hypertension and hypoalbuminemia or marked pulmonary fibrosis with hypoxemia and hypercapnia with cor pulmonale and systemic venous hypertension. Peritoneal involvement with ascites secondary to sarcoidosis is an extremely rare occurrence, with only a few patients previously reported in the literature. In only one patient was the peritoneum the only organ involved with noncaseating granulomas. The pleura and pericardium are involved infrequently with noncaseating granuloma but the peritoneum appears to be affected rarely. The production of ascites due to peritoneal involvement with sarcoidosis appears to be due to increased capillary permeability similar to that postulated for the development of sarcoid pleural effusions.

The ascitic fluid in sarcoid peritonitis may be serous, serosanguinous, or bloody, and has been reported to have a total protein concentration greater than 5.5 g/dl. There generally is a small number of lymphoctyes. The etiology of the hemorrhage in sarcoid ascites is unclear. The prognosis of patients with ascites due to peritoneal sarcoidosis appears to be good, with resolution of the ascites within several weeks with or without steroid therapy. This is in contrast to patients with ascites from hepatic sarcoidosis, in whom the risk of esophageal variceal bleeding is high and a common cause of death. Furthermore, patients who develop right heart failure from severe pulmonary sarcoid disease also have a poor prognosis; respiratory failure represents the major cause of death in sarcoidosis.

Patients with sarcoid of the peritoneum may present with abdominal pain, dyspnea on exertion, or increased abdominal girth. At laparoscopy, the operator may visualize diffuse nodular lesions in the peritoneum, bowel wall, and mesentery. The diagnostic impression may be malignancy when the peritoneal lesions are accompanied by enlarged retroperitoneal lymph nodes and nodules in the liver. Peritoneal sarcoidosis should be considered in the appropriate clinical setting. Biopsy shows typical noncaseating granulomas that are negative on stain and culture.

At laparoscopy, the present patient had diffuse nodular lesions on the bowel wall, mesentery, and peritoneum, with the bowel fused together in the left upper quadrant. Histology showed noncaseating granulomas containing numerous multinucleated giant cells. Stains and cultures for tuberculosis and fungi were negative. A transbronchial lung biopsy demonstrated noncaseating granulomas with negative stains and cultures. The patient was treated with prednisone 40 mg daily, with resolution of the ascites by 1 month. He continues asymptomatic on low-dose, alternate-day steroids 4 months following initiation of treatment.

Clinical Pearls

1. Ascites due to sarcoidosis most commonly occurs in the setting of portal hypertension or cor pulmonale.

2. Sarcoid involvement of the peritoneum with ascites is rare but may be a presenting manifestation or part of multisystem involvement.

3. Peritoneal sarcoidosis may result in hemorrhagic ascites and at laparoscopy may simulate malignancy.

REFERENCES
1. Papowitz AJ, Li JKH. Abdominal sarcoidosis with ascites. Chest 1971; 59:692–695.
2. Wheeler JE, Rosenthal AS. Bloody ascites in sarcoidosis. Chest 1985; 88:917–918.
3. Becker WF, Coleman WO. Surgical significance of abdominal sarcoidosis. Ann Surg 1961; 153:987–995.

PATIENT 34

A 66-year-old man with carcinoma of the colon, left hydronephrosis, and left pleural effusion

A 66-year-old man with recurrent carcinoma of the colon presented with pulmonary edema secondary to acute renal failure. Following emergency hemodialysis and stabilization, abdominal ultrasound demonstrated bilateral hydronephrosis and retrograde pyelograms bilateral ureteral obstruction secondary to extrinsic depression. Bilateral nephrostomy tubes were placed; however, the left nephrostomy tube became dislodged shortly following placement and a left renal stent was placed by cystoscopy. At the time of cystoscopy, dye injection demonstrated extravasation of contrast into the left perirenal space.

Physical Examination: Following dialysis, nephrostomy tube and stent placement, the patient was relatively asymptomatic.

Laboratory Findings: Chest radiograph 2 days following stent placement: left pleural effusion. Thoracentesis: clear yellow fluid; total protein 0.7 g/dl, LDH 58 IU/L, WBC 230/μl, RBC 15,000/μl, glucose 172 mg/dl, pH 7.20, PF/S creatinine > 1.0. Simultaneous urinalysis from the left renal stent: pH = 5.0. CT scan of abdomen: perirenal collection of fluid and left hydronephrosis.

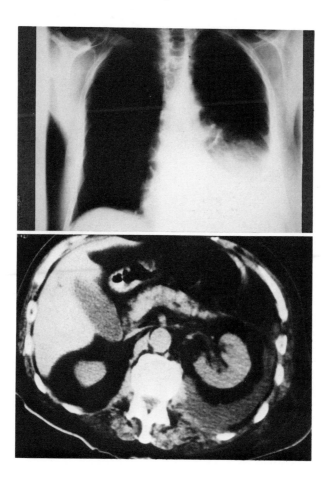

Diagnosis: Urinothorax.

Discussion: Pleural effusions associated with renal disease occur with nephrotic syndrome, salt and water excess leading to congestive heart failure, uremic pleurisy, peritoneal dialysis, and urinary tract obstruction. Effusions secondary to obstructive uropathy have a unique pathogenesis and are termed urinothorax. With rare exception, hydronephrosis with extravasation of fluid into the perirenal space appears to be a prerequisite for the development of a urinothorax. Causes of urinothorax reported in the literature include bladder and prostate cancer, posterior urethral valves, renal cysts, nephrolithiasis, surgical ureteral manipulation, blunt kidney trauma, renal transplant, and ileal conduit with ureteral obstruction. Obstructive uropathy leads to perirenal fluid accumulation and ipsilateral pleural effusion. Removal of the obstructing lesion generally results in rapid resolution (days) of the effusion.

Depending on the size of the pleural effusion and the underlying pulmonary status, the patient may present with dyspnea or be asymptomatic. The diagnosis should be suspected in the setting of obstructive uropathy and can be confirmed by thoracentesis if the pleural fluid to serum creatinine ratio is greater than 1.0. The ratio of pleural fluid to serum creatinine appears to be specific for the diagnosis, especially if measured within the first few days of pleural fluid formation. Other clues to the diagnosis on thoracentesis are the finding of a low pH transudate. This is a unique combination as all other low pH effusions (pH < 7.30) have been associated with exudates (empyema, esophageal rupture, carcinoma, rheumatoid pleurisy, tuberculosis, and lupus pleuritis).

The pathogenesis of the low pH transudate is not clearly established, although it is most likely related to the low pH of the extravasated urine with some back-diffusion of hydrogen ions as the fluid passes from the retroperitoneal into the pleural space. Obviously, an alkaline urine at the time of extravasation would result in a normal pH effusion.

In the present patient, the pleural effusion resolved over 4 days, following improved drainage from the nephrostomy.

Clinical Pearls

1. A pleural effusion (urinothorax) can develop following obstructive uropathy ipsilateral to the obstructed kidney.
2. Diagnosis of urinothorax is established by finding a pleural fluid to creatinine ratio of >1.0, and is most specific in the first 2 or 3 days following pleural fluid formation.
3. Urinothorax is the only cause of a low pH transudate.

REFERENCES
1. Stark BD, Schanes JG, Baron RL, Koch DD. Biochemical features of urinothorax. Arch Intern Med 1982; 142:1509–1511.
2. Carcillo J, Salcedo JR. Urinothorax as the manifestation of nondialated obstructed uropathy following renal transplantation. Am J Kid Dis 1985; 5:211–213.
3. Leung FW, Williams AJ, Oill PA. Pleural effusion associated with urinary tract obstruction: support for a hypothesis. Thorax 1981; 36:682–683.

PATIENT 35

A 32-year-old woman resuscitated from near-drowning

A 32-year-old woman was admitted after being resuscitated from a near-drowning incident at the ocean.

Physical Examination: Respirations 21; pulse 120; blood pressure 108/69. Lethargic, arousable woman with an oral endotracheal tube; diffuse rhonchi.

Laboratory Findings: CBC and electrolytes normal. ABG (60% O_2): pH 7.53, $PaCO_2$ 29 mmHg, PaO_2 68 mmHg. Chest radiograph was normal with adequate placement of the endotracheal tube.

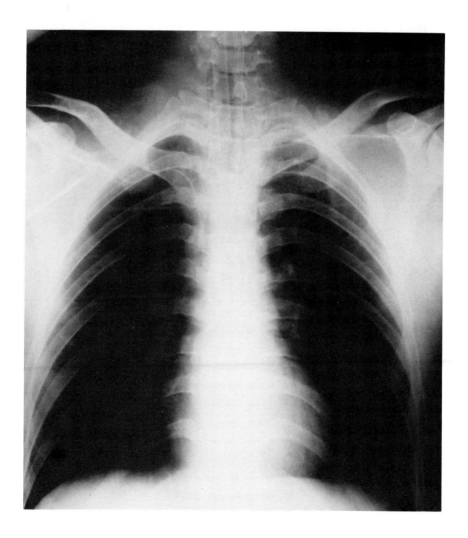

Diagnosis: Near-drowning.

Discussion: The course of victims of near-drowning varies depending on the duration of submersion, the degree of water aspiration, and the severity of resultant hypoxemia. Recent patient series no longer support the traditional wisdoms that major serum electrolyte changes underlie the pathophysiology of near-drowning or that the pattern of electrolyte alterations depends on the salinity of the aspirated fluid. Since most patients aspirate less than 10 ml/kg, resultant fluxes in serum electrolyte concentrations are negligible and do not by themselves aggravate pulmonary, cardiovascular, or neurologic function.

The etiology of hypoxia in near-drowning varies depending on the type and quantity of aspirated fluid. Up to 12% of patients develop laryngospasm, which prevents significant aspiration, and experience hypoxia by simple asphyxiation. The remaining 80-85% of patients undergo varying degrees of aspiration. If the aspirated fluid is ocean water, the irritative effects of hypertonicity and accompanying organic and particulate debris may generate exudative flooding of the alveoli with resultant ventilation perfusion mismatch and shunt. Aspiration of fresh water removes alveolar surfactant causing hypoxia from alveolar collapse. Both types of aspiration may initiate noncardiogenic pulmonary edema, progressing to the adult respiratory distress syndrome that may be first manifest after 24 hours of observation.

Patients present with altered mental status that ranges from confusion to profound coma, depending on the severity and duration of cerebral anoxia. The prognosis for recovery is varied, being modified by the temperature of the submersion, age of the victim, and presence of comorbid medical conditions. The course of the pulmonary manifestations of near-drowning similarly vary. Patients with brief submersions experiencing laryngospasm may have no respiratory sequelae. Conversely, patients with extensive aspiration and alveolar damage may develop prolonged respiratory failure, requiring mechanical ventilation. Their subsequent course may then be further complicated by pneumonia and other complications of mechanical ventilation.

Management of near-drowning victims is largely supportive. Hypothermia is slowly reversed, and patients with respiratory failure are intubated, mechanically ventilated, and managed with positive end-expiratory pressure if profoundly hypoxic. There are no benefits in using hypotonic or hypertonic intravenous solutions dictated by the type of fluid submersion, since electrolyte shifts are clinically unimportant. Prophylactic corticosteroids or antibiotics are of no benefit, and recent data do not support the use of corticosteroids for the management of the adult respiratory distress syndrome.

The present patient improved with resolution of hypoxia, allowing extubation several hours after admission. She progressively became more alert without neurologic sequelae.

Clinical Pearls

1. Serum electrolyte abnormalities dependent on the salinity of the aspirated fluid are negligible and do not contribute to the pathophysiology of near-drowning.

2. As many as 12% of near-drowning victims experience laryngospasm and develop hypoxia from simple asphyxia.

3. Patients seldom aspirate more than 10 ml/kg of fluid during a near-drowning episode.

REFERENCES

1. Modell J, Graves S, Ketover A. Clinical course of 91 consecutive near-drowning victims. Chest 1976; 70:231–238.
2. Fine N, Myerson DA, Myerson PJ, Pagliaro JJ. Near-drowning presenting as the ARDS. Chest 1974; 65:347–349.

PATIENT 36

A 64-year-old man with COPD presenting with increased cough, purulent sputum, fever, and dyspnea

A 64-year-old man with a long history of symptomatic COPD was seen with the chief complaints of increased cough, purulent sputum production, intermittent fevers, and dyspnea. He was currently smoking cigarettes. He was seen by an emergency room physician 7 days prior and was started on ampicillin without change in symptoms.

Physical Examination: Temperature 101°; pulse 110; respirations 24; minimal respiratory distress; basilar rales without evidence of consolidation.

Laboratory Findings: WBC 12,500/μl, 80% PMNs, 2% bands. Sputum Gram stain: many PMNs with intracellular and extracellular gram-negative diplococci. Sputum culture: a predominance of *Branhamella catarrhalis* with a few colonies of other normal respiratory tract flora. Chest radiograph: minimal bilateral lower lobe and retrocardiac infiltrates.

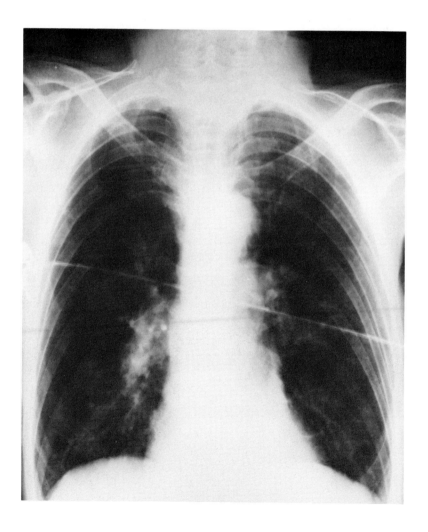

Diagnosis: Branhamella catarrhalis pneumonia.

Discussion: Branhamella catarrhalis, a commensal of the oropharynx, is now recognized as a pathogen in the lower respiratory tract in patients with chronic bronchitis, bronchiectasis, asthma, pneumoconiosis, and immunosuppression.

These patients, usually with a history of chronic lung disease, have cough, increased sputum, and dyspnea, similar to the presentation of many patients with an exacerbation of COPD. The chest radiograph frequently shows transient patches of bronchopneumonia in contrast to the unchanged radiograph in the usual COPD patient with exacerbation. Sputum gram stain shows an abundance of PMNs and gram-negative diplococci, which may be the predominant organism. Herein lies the problem, as these organisms, in the majority of cases, are commensals of the upper respiratory tract. A Gram stain showing Branhamella as the predominant organism, especially when intracellular, and being the predominant organism on culture, strongly suggests the diagnosis. Isolation of *B. catarrhalis* from the sputum in a concentration $> 10^7$ cfu/ml strengthens the diagnosis.

Establishing the etiologic diagnosis is important in relation to therapy, as *B. catarrhalis* produces beta-lactamase of the penicillinase type in a large percentage of cases, often exceeding 50%. Therefore, penicillins and first- and second-generation cephalosporins generally demonstrate weak activity against *B. catarrhalis*. The tetracyclines, third-generation cephalosporins, erythromycin, and trimethoprim-sulfamethoxazole usually are effective agents.

The present patient was treated with erythromycin in conjunction with inhaled beta agonists and chest physiotherapy, with a good response.

Clinical Pearls

1. *Branhamella catarrhalis* pneumonia or purulent bronchitis is a cause of exacerbation of COPD.

2. Sputum Gram stain showing an abundance of PMNs and gram-negative intracellular and extracellular diplococci suggests the diagnosis. Isolation of predominantly pure cultures of this organism from the sputum and quantitative bacteriology demonstrating greater than 10^7 cfu/ml of the organism appear to be diagnostic.

3. Since the majority of these organisms are beta-lactamase-producing, penicillins and first- and second-generations cephalosporins are frequently not effective. The patient should be treated with erythromycin, tetracycline, or trimethoprim-sulfamethoxazole.

REFERENCES

1. McNeely DJ, Kitchens CS, Kluge RM. The fatal neisseria *(Branhamella catarrhalis)* pneumonia in an immunodeficient host. Am Rev Respir Dis 1976; 114:399–402.
2. Ninane G, Joly J, Kraytman M. Bronchopulmonary infection due to *Branhamella catarrhalis*: 11 cases assessed by transtracheal puncture. Br Med J 1978; 1:276–278.
3. Slevin NJ, Aitken J, Thornley PE. Clinical and microbiological features of *Branhamella catarrhalis* bronchopulmonary infection. Lancet 1984; 1:782–783.

PATIENT 37

A 71-year-old woman with respiratory failure and a several-week history of cough, fever, shortness of breath, and malaise

A 71-year-old nonsmoking black woman was brought to the emergency room with cough, fever, and shortness of breath. She noted weakness and anorexia six weeks earlier that resulted in a 20 lb weight loss. A bothersome cough with purulent sputum had been present for two weeks. Difficulty with breathing began the evening before admission.

Physical Examination: Chronically ill appearing elderly patient with severe dyspnea. Edentulous without lymphadenopathy; right basilar consolidation with rales.

Laboratory Findings: WBC 12,000/μl, 90% PMNs; Hct 29%; serum albumin 2.1 g/dl. ABG (room air): pH 7.40, PCO_2 30 mmHg, PO_2 49 mmHg.

The patient was intubated in the emergency room and the chest radiograph showed bilateral alveolar infiltrates worse on the right with bilateral pleural effusions. Gram stain of suctioned sputum showed leukocytes with mixed flora.

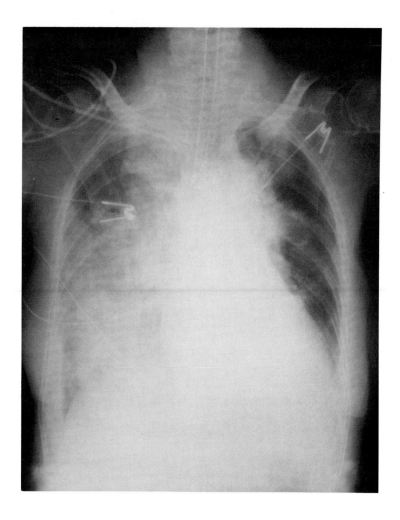

Diagnosis: Tuberculous pneumonia with respiratory failure.

Discussion: Tuberculosis is a chronic infection that typically evolves in an indolent manner. On occasion, however, patients may present with acute hypoxic respiratory failure after an antecedent subacute illness. Miliary tuberculosis is the most notable form of the disease associated with respiratory insufficiency, and multiple reports indicate that the adult respiratory distress syndrome may be the initial presentation of the disease.

It is less widely recognized that pulmonary tuberculosis can also promote respiratory failure. Previous angiographic studies had indicated that this form of tuberculosis would not be expected to cause severe hypoxia, since alveoli and adjacent alveolar capillaries are obliterated in unison, thereby preserving matching of ventilation with perfusion. Subsequently, however, several reports have clearly substantiated the association between pulmonary tuberculosis and respiratory failure, which may be the patient's initial clinical manifestation of infection. Additional autopsy studies indicate that the presence of respiratory failure may be a major cause of the clinician's failure to diagnose pulmonary tuberculosis in many patients antemortem.

The present patient demonstrated several clinical features that suggested the possibility of tuberculous pneumonia. The patient's advanced age coincides with the increasing occurrence of tuberculosis in the elderly. Furthermore, the patient's history indicated a 2-month illness documented by weight loss; most patients with tuberculosis note deteriorating health for several weeks before the onset of respiratory failure, in contradistinction to acute respiratory failure from bacterial pneumonia. And finally, the presence of anemia and hypoalbuminemia should prompt a search for an underlying chronic disorder, since these findings occur regularly in patients with tuberculosis and respiratory failure.

The majority of patients with tuberculous pneumonia and respiratory failure have positive sputum smears for tuberculosis. An elderly patient with marked dyspnea, however, may be unable to provide an adequate specimen and will benefit from the physician's commitment to urgently pursue the diagnosis rather than ascribe the respiratory failure to nontuberculous bacterial pneumonia. Patients can survive respiratory failure from tuberculosis if they receive prompt initiation of antituberculous therapy, consideration of possible adrenal insufficiency, and general critical care support.

Auramine-rhodamine stains of suctioned sputum from the present patient were packed with acid-fast organisms that subsequently grew *Mycobacterium tuberculosis.* Pleural fluid was also positive for tuberculosis. The patient was started on antituberculous therapy but died 7 days later with respiratory failure and renal failure.

Clinical Pearls

1. Noncavitary alveolar infiltrates with respiratory failure in an elderly patient with a preceding illness lasting longer than 1 week should suggest tuberculosis.
2. Patients with respiratory failure from pulmonary tuberculosis almost always have anemia and hypoalbuminemia.

REFERENCES
1. Dyer RA, Chappel WA, Potgieter PO. Adult respiratory distress syndrome associated with miliary tuberculosis. Crit Care Med 1985; 13:12–15.
2. Agarwal MK, Muthuswamy PP, Banner AS, et al. Respiratory failure in pulmonary tuberculosis. Chest 1977; 72:605–609.

PATIENT 38

A 28-year-old woman with substernal chest discomfort, dysphagia, and a mediastinal mass

A 28-year-old woman was referred to our hospital when she entered a local hospital for surgery on a ganglion cyst and was found to have a "mediastinal mass" on chest radiograph. She stated that for the previous year she had experienced midsternal chest pain described as a "pulling inward sensation"; the discomfort was episodic and resolved spontaneously. She also admitted to occasional dysphagia. This was the first time that she was told she had an abnormal chest radiograph, even though she had had previous films.

Physical Examination: Vital signs normal; no acute distress; lungs normal; remainder of physical examination: normal.

Laboratory Findings: CBC and chemistries normal. Chest radiograph: posterior mediastinal mass just below the level of the carina. Esophagram: large impression on the right lateral wall of the esophagus, displacing it toward the left and slightly anterior to the mediastinal mass, which was at T7. CT scan: posterior mediastinal mass. The patient had a right thoracotomy.

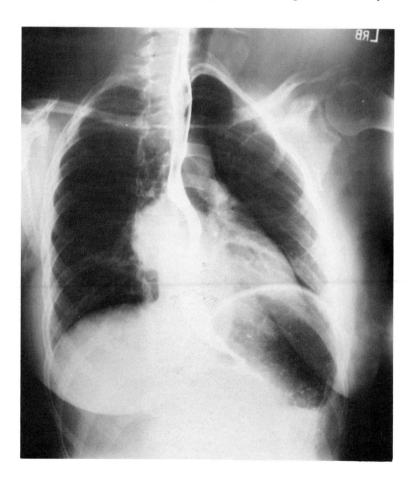

Diagnosis: Mediastinal bronchogenic cyst.

Discussion: Bronchogenic cysts are unusual congenital abnormalities that result from improper budding of the tracheobronchial tree during development. Bronchogenic cysts occur in both the parenchyma and mediastinum with an incidence of about 2:1, respectively. These thin-walled cysts are lined by respiratory epithelium and generally contain a mucoid substance. The cyst walls often contain elastic fibers, smooth muscle, mucous glands, and cartilage. Bronchial communication is rare unless infection develops that may be detected radiographically by the development of an air-fluid level. Most mediastinal bronchogenic cysts are located near the carina, commonly connected by a stalk to a major airway. In a series of 14 pathologically proven cases of mediastinal bronchogenic cysts, 7 were in the posterior mediastinum, 5 in the middle mediastinum, and 2 in the superior mediastinum.

Pressure symptoms may occur with an enlarging cyst, particularly in a subcarinal location. These include substernal chest pain, exertional dyspnea, cough, stridor or dysphagia. Depending on its location, a mediastinal bronchogenic cyst may become large, with the patient remaining asymptomatic and the lesion being discovered on a routine chest radiograph.

Radiographically, the cysts are seen as a homogeneous mass with a clearly defined border inferior to the carina, and a predilection for the right hemithorax, often overlaying the right hilum. The configuration is usually spherical or oval; the cyst may change in configuration during fluoroscopy or with an inspiratory and expiratory radiograph. These solitary lesions may displace the esophagus, usually to the left. CT scan will verify the location of the cyst and may show either a fluid or solid density, the latter at times being confused with a malignant process. Surgery usually is recommended either for diagnostic purposes or relief of symptoms. Recently, diagnosis and therapy have been recommended using transbronchial needle aspiration through the fiberoptic bronchoscope for a bronchogenic mediastinal cyst adjacent to a central airway.

The present patient had a right thoracotomy and excision of a 4.5 cm diameter cyst from the posterior mediastinum in the subcarinal area. Upon sectioning of the cyst, the pathologist noted a greenish-gold, viscous fluid; the anterior surface of the cyst wall showed occasional fibrous strands and thickening. The cyst was lined with respiratory epithelium and surrounded by chronic inflammatory infiltrate.

Clinical Pearls

1. Bronchogenic cysts are congenital abnormalities that are more commonly found in the lung parenchyma than the mediastinum.

2. Most mediastinal bronchogenic cysts are situated near the carina and, therefore, may cause symptoms such as chest pain, cough, or exertional dyspnea due to pressure on surrounding structures. Bronchogenic cysts should be considered in the differential diagnosis in patients with symptoms of major upper airway obstruction.

3. The characteristic radiographic features of a mediastinal bronchogenic cyst are a well-defined homogeneous density inferior to the carina, protrusion to the right of the midline, and overlay of the right hilum.

REFERENCES
1. Maier HC. Bronchogenic cysts of the mediastinum. Ann Surg 1948; 127:476–502.
2. Davis JG, Somonton JH. Mediastinal carinal bronchogenic cysts. Radiology 1956; 67:391–395.
3. Rogers LF, Osmer JC. Bronchogenic cysts: review of 46 cases. AJR 1964; 91:273–283.
4. Schwartz AR, Fishman EK, Wang KP. Diagnosis and treatment of bronchogenic cysts using transbronchial needle aspiration. Thorax 1986; 41:326–327.

PATIENT 39

A 34-year-old woman with a history of treated pulmonary tuberculosis presenting with chronic cough and poor exercise tolerance

A 34-year-old woman sought evaluation for a chronic cough and poor exercise tolerance. She was a nonsmoker and denied asthma or rhinitis symptoms. Her past medical history was notable for pulmonary tuberculosis successfully treated with isoniazid and rifampin one year earlier.

Physical Examination: Normal vital signs; clear chest to auscultation and percussion; cardiac examination normal.

Laboratory Findings: CBC and electrolytes normal; sputum smear for fungus and acid-fast organisms negative. Chest radiograph showed several calcified granulomas and a poorly visualized left mainstem bronchus, appearing narrowed on a right anterior oblique view. Tomograms demonstrated left bronchostenosis. Spirometry was normal except for a decreased FEV_3.

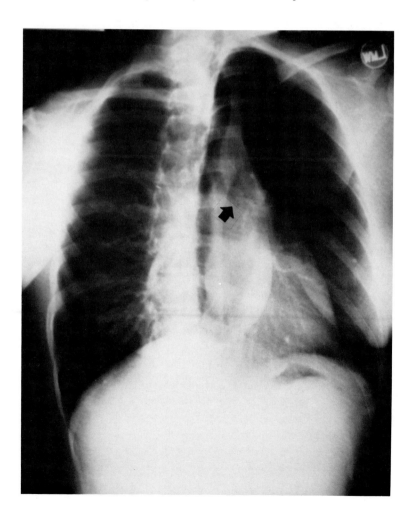

Diagnosis: Bronchial stenosis complicating healed endobronchial tuberculosis.

Discussion: Infectious involvement of the tracheobronchial tree is a common accompaniment of pulmonary tuberculosis. Ten to 37% of patients with active tuberculosis have bronchoscopic evidence of endobronchial infection, with the highest incidence occurring in patients with cavitary disease. It may be difficult to diagnose the endobronchial component in patients with tuberculosis, since the symptoms are nonspecific and wheezes occur in only 15% of patients. Furthermore, in the setting of undiagnosed tuberculosis, endobronchial infection may simulate cancer, since only 50% of patients are febrile, 20% have clear chest radiographs, weight loss and hemoptysis are common, and the bronchoscopic findings may mimic an endobronchial neoplasm. Although many studies indicate that patients with endobronchial tuberculosis have a high frequency of positive sputum smears for Mycobacteria, recent reports note that in 85% of patients with endobronchial tuberculosis, sputum smears are negative.

The major sequelae of endobronchial tuberculosis is bronchostenosis; tuberculois is the commonest cause of infectious airway stricture, and some degree of bronchostenosis occurs in over 90% of patients with endobronchial tuberculosis, even after appropriate antituberculous therapy. Two major forms of airway stricture occur as a result of endobronchial tuberculosis.

During the acute phase of infection, inflammatory swelling from submucosal tubercles, and shallow mucosal ulceration can narrow the airway. At later stages, bronchial scarring develops, causing fixed strictures involving variable lengths of the bronchus. Tuberculous bronchial stenosis can also occur in patients without endobronchial tuberculosis. In these instances, an infected peribronchial lymph node erodes locally into the airway, causing inflammation and short segments of stenosis.

Diagnosis of bronchial stenosis requires awareness of this possibility in patients with active or healed tuberculosis who demonstrate dyspnea or cough out of proportion to the degree of parenchymal disease. Symptoms may be delayed, occurring as long as 20 years after treatment of tuberculosis. The diagnosis can be confirmed by tomography or CT scanning of the airway; noninfectious patients can undergo bronchoscopy when a malignancy is a diagnostic possibility. Spirometry is usually normal except for prolongation of FEV_3. Management of symptomatic tuberculous bronchial stenosis after chemotherapy requires either bronchoplasty with a sleeve resection or lung resection with a lobectomy or pneumonectomy, depending on the location and length of the stricture. Patients should be evaluated preoperatively by bronchography to define the surgical approach.

Clinical Pearls

1. Over 90% of patients with endobronchial tuberculosis will have some degree of bronchostenosis after antituberculous therapy.

2. Bronchostenosis may develop during active endobronchial tuberculosis or be a late manifestation, occurring years after effective antituberculous therapy.

3. Up to 20% of patients with endobronchial tuberculosis have normal chest radiographs, and a negative acid-fast sputum smear does not rule out the diagnosis.

REFERENCES

1. Lynch JP, Ravikrishnan KP. Endobronchial mass caused by tuberculosis. Arch Intern Med 1980; 140:1090–1091.
2. Caligiuri PA, Banner AS, Jensik RJ. Tuberculous main-stem bronchial stenosis treated with sleeve resection. Arch Intern Med 1984; 144:1302–1303.
3. Ip MSM, So SY, Lam WK, Mok CK. Endobronchial tuberculosis revisited. Chest 1986; 89:727–730.
4. Smith JL, Elliott CG, Schmidt CD, Flinner RL. Bronchial stenosis: a complication of healed endobronchial tuberculosis. West J Med 1986; 144:361–362.

PATIENT 40

A 69-year-old man with fever, pleurisy, dyspnea, and fatigue 3 months after coronary artery bypass surgery

A 69-year-old man presented with a 3-week history of pleuritic chest pain, intermittent fevers, dyspnea on exertion, and fatigue. Three months prior, he had coronary artery bypass surgery with uneventful recovery.

Physical Examination: Temperature 99.4°; respirations 20. Thin, chronically ill appearing male; minimal respiratory distress; dullness, decreased breath sounds, rales bilaterally; pleural friction rub on left.

Laboratory Findings: WBC 12,000/μl, 80% PMNs; ESR 62 mm/h. Chest radiograph: small bilateral pleural effusions. Thoracentesis: serosanguinous fluid; total protein 3.8 g/dl; LDH 220 IU/L; glucose 75 mg/dl; leukocytes 25,000/μl, 50% PMNs; 50% mononuclear cells; pH 7.42. Echocardiogram: small posterior pericardial effusion.

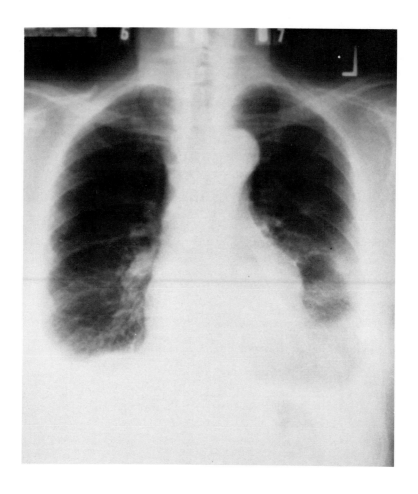

Diagnosis: Postcardiac injury syndrome (PCIS).

Discussion: Postcardiac injury syndrome occurs following a variety of myocardial or pericardial injuries. PCIS has been described following cardiac surgery, myocardial infarction (Dressler's syndrome), blunt chest trauma, percutaneous puncture of left ventricle, and implantation of a pacemaker. It is characterized by fever and signs of pericardial, pleural, and pulmonary parenchymal inflammation days or weeks following the initial injury. Despite recognition of this syndrome for over 30 years, the diagnosis is often elusive and the presentation frequently results in confusion between the syndrome and complications seen in the postinfarction or postsurgical setting; these include congestive heart failure, atelectasis, pneumonia, and pulmonary embolism. PCIS usually develops 3 weeks following injury but has been described 2 to 86 days following the cardiac injury. Recurrent episodes are common. Almost all patients have pleuritic chest pain; the majority have fever, pericardial or pleural rubs, dyspnea, and rales. Hemoptysis is not a part of this syndrome. Laboratory examination usually shows a moderate leukocytosis and an elevated ESR. Patients with PCIS tend to have high titers of anti-myocardial antibodies in serum.

Chest radiograph is virtually always abnormal, with the most common finding being pleural effusion. The effusion is usually unilateral left-sided or bilateral. Pneumonitis is a frequent accompaniment and is usually seen in the left lower lobe. The cardiac silhouette will be enlarged in half of the cases. Echocardiogram frequently shows a posterior pericardial effusion.

The most characteristic aspect of the pleural fluid is that it is bloody or serosanguinous (70%). It is an exudate with a mean leukocyte count of about $10,000/\mu l$, with the differential depending upon the timing of the thoracentesis in relation to the acute injury. pH and glucose are normal. Pleural fluid analysis will aid in the differential diagnosis but cannot differentiate between PCIS and pulmonary infarction.

The syndrome itself is usually self-limited but may require aspirin, nonsteroidal anti-inflammatory drugs, or corticosteroids; anticoagulants are contraindicated. The present patient required moderate doses of corticosteroid therapy for several months for resolution.

Clinical Pearls

1. The absence of pleuritic chest pain virtually excludes the diagnosis of postcardiac injury syndrome.

2. Thoracentesis findings tend to exclude some diagnoses common in the postcardiac or postmyocardial infarction setting, such as congestive heart failure or pneumonia, but cannot differentiate pulmonary infarction from PCIS. Both tend to be bloody, exudative pleural effusions.

3. Postcardiac injury syndrome may occur late (months) following myocardial or pericardial injury and manifest as chronic pleuropulmonary disease with an insidious course.

REFERENCES
1. Dressler W. The post-myocardial-infarction syndrome: a report of 44 cases. Arch Intern Med 1959; 103:28–42.
2. Engle MA, McCabe JC, Ebert PA, Zabriskie J. The postpericardiotomy syndrome and antiheart antibodies. Circulation 1974; 49:401–406.
3. Stelzner TJ, King TE Jr, Antony VB, Sahn SA. The pleuropulmonary manifestations of the postcardiac injury syndrome. Chest 1983; 84:383–387.

PATIENT 41

A 65-year-old woman with a history of breast cancer presenting with a persistent cough

A 65-year-old woman presented complaining of a dry, hacking cough. She denied smoking or any previous pulmonary condition. She actively participated in vigorous sports and had no lapses in consciousness, recent general anesthesia, or foreign body aspiration. Her previous health was unremarkable except for breast cancer treated by a radical mastectomy 22 years earlier. The cancer had not recurred during careful follow-up.

Physical Examination: Vital signs normal. Thorax: well-healed mastectomy scar; decreased breath sounds at the right upper lobe region; cardiac normal.

Laboratory Findings: Routine blood tests normal; sputum cytology negative. Chest radiograph demonstrated partial atelectasis of the right upper lobe.

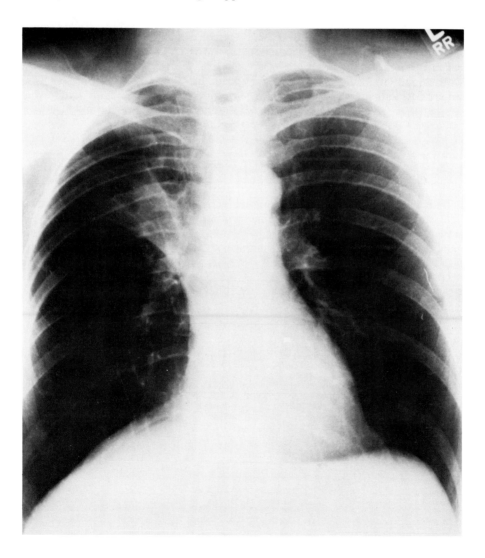

Diagnosis: Endobronchial metastasis from adenocarcinoma of the breast causing right upper lobe atelectasis.

Discussion: Endobronchial metastases complicate the course of 2 to 5% of patients with extrathoracic solid malignancies. Most commonly reported in patients with neoplasms of the colon, kidney, and breast, airway metastases occur in a wide range of tumors, including melanoma, thyroid cancer, uterine leiomyosarcoma, and ovarian adenocarcinoma. Among these diverse cell types, however, breast cancer is the extrathoracic neoplasm that most frequently metastasizes to the endobronchium.

Although endobronchial tumor deposits in patients with breast cancer may often accompany widespread metastases, they also rarely appear as the initial manifestation of cancer or as the sole evidence of tumor recurrence after primary therapy. In the latter situations, the occurrence of nonspecific respiratory symptoms or postobstructive pneumonia may not initially suggest the presence of breast cancer.

Breast cancer has the notable characteristic of recurring after prolonged intervals of clinical quiescence, with patients incurring cutaneous, bone or pleural metastases after 20 years or longer of subclinical disease. Likewise, endobronchial metastases may occur, as noted in the present patient, several decades after the original diagnosis and do not necessarily herald the development of a second primary malignancy.

Clinical manifestations of endobronchial metastases are common to all forms of bronchial obstruction. Cough, hoarseness, wheezing, and rarely hemoptysis are notable symptoms. The chest radiograph may appear normal in the absence of complete airway obstruction, or demonstrate atelectasis, postobstructive pneumonia, or pleural effusions. Since sputum cytologic examination rarely detects the airway tumor, bronchoscopy is required to document airway obstruction and obtain biopsy specimens.

The optimal therapy for endobronchial metastases from breast cancer is uncertain, since no large series of patients has been evaluated. Successful therapy has been reported, however, using systemic chemotherapy or radiation therapy. Although patient survival is variable, a prolonged period from diagnosis of the primary tumor to detection of the endobronchial metastasis is a favorable clinical factor. The present patient underwent systemic chemotherapy with resolution of the endobronchial obstruction and no evidence of further tumor recurrence during 2 years of therapy.

Clinical Pearls

1. Extrathoracic neoplasms metastasize to the endobronchium in 2 to 5% of patients.
2. Breast cancer is the most common extrathoracic solid tumor to spread to the airways.
3. Breast cancer may involve the endobronchium after several decades of clinical remission.

REFERENCES
1. Krutchik AN, Tashima CK, Buzdar AU, Blumenschein GR. Endobronchial metastases in metastatic breast carcinoma. West J Med 1978; 129:177–180.
2. McNamee MJ, Scherzer HH. Endobronchial involvement in metastatic breast carcinoma. Conn Med 1982; 46:244–248.
3. Shepherd MP. Endobronchial metastatic disease. Thorax 1982; 37:362–365.

PATIENT 42

A 15-year-old boy presenting with fever and crushing chest pain

A 15-year-old boy felt entirely well until he noted the sudden onset of severe "crushing" pain in his left chest and upper flank associated with shortness of breath and fever to 102°. The pain lasted several hours, remitting completely only to recur the next day when he sought medical evaluation. Previous health history was entirely normal.

Physical Examination: Pulse 110; respirations 25; temperature 100°. The patient appeared in extreme pain, gripping his left chest and avoiding deep breaths. Splinting respirations without rubs; cardiac normal; abdomen tender in left upper quadrant; extremities normal.

Laboratory Findings: Hct 38%, WBC 7,700/μl; urinalysis normal. ABG (room air): pH 7.54, PCO_2 27 mmHg, PO_2 106 mmHg. Chest radiograph normal; ECG normal; perfusion lung scan normal.

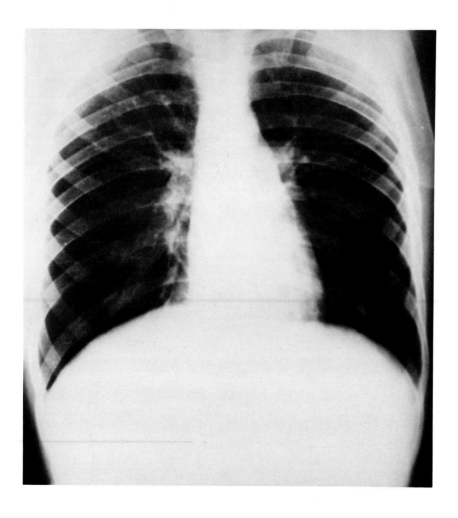

Diagnosis: Coxsackie B virus pleurodynia (Bornholm disease). Other possible diagnoses include pleurisy from various etiologies or splenic infarction.

Discussion: This patient had a sudden and alarmingly severe episode of chest pain with pleuritic qualities that prompted the consideration of pulmonary emboli. The normal perfusion lung scan excluded this possibility, however, and the absence of splenomegaly, abdominal tenderness, or an underlying medical condition decreased the likelihood of a splenic infarction. Pleurisy could not be readily excluded initially, so an ANA titer was drawn and the patient was carefully followed for development of additional pleuropulmonary signs and symptoms. The patient's subsequent course and viral cultures confirmed the diagnosis of pleurodynia.

The Coxsackie virus serotypes B1 to 6 are the most common etiologies of pleurodynia, but echovirus B1, 6, 9, 16, and 19 and Coxsackie A viruses 4, 6, 9, and 10 have been implicated in sporadic outbreaks. The disease occurs most frequently in the summer and fall months following the seasonal distribution of enteroviral disease. Person-to-person spread of the illness is common, with epidemics of pleurodynia occurring 10 to 20 years apart in local regions.

The disease begins as an acute febrile illness with the abrupt onset of fever up to 40° C and either chest or abdominal pain. The pain is described as crushing, sharp, knife-like, or gripping and may be exacerbated by movement or deep breathing, thereby imparting a pleuritic quality. Severe abdominal pain may mimic an acute abdominal process, leading to an exploratory laparotomy. Although clinicopathologic correlates are sparse, the pain appears to arise from the intercostal or abdominal muscles rather than from pleural or peritoneal inflammation. Coxsackie virus, however, has not been clearly isolated from muscle specimens.

A notable feature of the chest pain in pleurodynia is its paroxysmal nature. The pain occurs abruptly, lasting 2 to 10 hours, then remits as the patient becomes afebrile only to recur hours or days later. Subsequent episodes of pain usually decrease in severity. Often the physical examination will detect muscle tenderness or swelling with hyperesthesia over the site of pain.

Most episodes of pleurodynia occur in children, with the peak incidence between the ages of 5 and 15 as opposed to other enteroviral diseases that concentrate in younger age groups. Although most patients do not have a typical viral prodrome before the onset of muscular pain, 25% of patients may experience headaches with fatigue, myalgia, and sore throat.

The diagnosis of pleurodynia is aided by noting the paroxysmal nature of the chest and abdominal pain, the absence of radiographic chest abnormalities, and a clustering of illness in a household or regional epidemic. Routine laboratory studies are usually normal and aid diagnosis only in making other clinical possibilities such as pneumonia, pulmonary infarction, or pericarditis less likely. The diagnosis can be confirmed either by culturing the virus from throat or stool specimens or by demonstrating a rise in viral neutralizing antibody titers in acute and convalescent sera.

Patients typically recover fully from pleurodynia after 7 to 9 days, although 25% of patients may experience a relapse, usually within several days after becoming asymptomatic. Complications are uncommon but may include meningitis or orchitis in 5% of patients and rare occurrences of pericarditis.

The present patient's stool culture was positive for Coxsackie B2, and acute/convalescent viral titers confirmed the diagnosis. He recovered without incident by the fifth day of illness but relapsed 3 days later with transient mild chest pain.

Clinical Pearls

1. The source of pain in pleurodynia is skeletal muscle rather than pleura, and the chest radiograph is subsequently normal.

2. The majority of patients (75%) with pleurodynia do not have associated viral symptoms.

3. Patients often relapse with chest pains several days after becoming asymptomatic.

REFERENCES
1. Moore M, Kaplan MH, McPhee J, et al. Epidemiologic, clinical, and laboratory features of Coxsackie B1–B5 infections in the United States, 1970–79. Public Health Rep 1984; 99:515–522.
2. Grist NR, Bell EJ. Further studies of enterovirus infections in cardiac disease and pleurodynia. Scand J Infect Dis 1970; 2:1–6.

PATIENT 43

A 61-year-old man with non-Hodgkin's lymphoma and bilateral pleural effusions

A 61-year-old man with a 2-year history of non-Hodgkin's lymphoma (poorly differentiated lymphocytic) was referred for bilateral pleural effusions and dyspnea on exertion. At diagnosis, the patient had peripheral lymphocytosis and CT scan evidence of splenomegaly and retroperitoneal lymphadenopathy. Pleural effusions had been present for 18 months, and he had required multiple therapeutic thoracenteses for relief of dyspnea, orthopnea, and cough. Approximately 14 months prior to admission, he received chemotherapy consisting of cyclophosphamide, vincristine, and prednisone without resolution of the pleural effusions.

Physical Examination: Temperature 98.4°; respirations 20. No acute distress; absence of peripheral lymphadenopathy; evidence of a large left and small right pleural effusion; splenomegaly without hepatomegaly.

Laboratory Findings: WBC 30,500/μl, 87% lymphocytes, 13% PMNs; Hct 36%; platelet count 84,000/μl. Chest radiograph: bilateral pleural effusions, large left and small right. Left thoracentesis: serosanguinous, nucleated cells 1281/μl, 71% lymphocytes, 27% macrophages, RBC 42,000/μl, total protein 4 g/dl, LDH 120 IU/L. Cytology positive for lymphoma. Pleural biopsy consistent with lymphomatous infiltrate of the pleura.

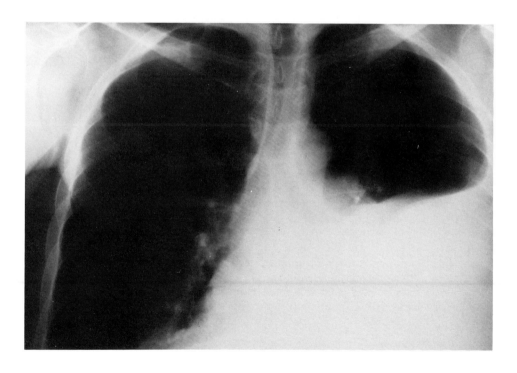

Diagnosis: Non-Hodgkin's lymphoma with pleural effusions.

Discussion: Approximately 10% of malignant pleural effusions are due to lymphomas. At diagnosis, pleural effusions are rare in Hodgkin's disease but not infrequent in non-Hodgkin's lymphoma. A pleural effusion may be the only chest radiographic finding in patients with non-Hodgkin's lymphoma; however, it is unusual for the pleural effusion to be the only clinical manifestation of the disease. While direct lymphomatous invasion of the pleura appears to be an uncommon and late finding in Hodgkin's disease, it has been described with relative frequency in non-Hodgkin's lymphoma. As non-Hodgkin's lymphoma progresses, the incidence of pleural effusions increases and approaches 30%. At autopsy, a 30 to 60% incidence of pleural effusion and a 10 to 30% incidence of pleural nodular or infiltrative lesions have been noted.

The predominant mechanism for the formation of pleural fluid in non-Hodgkin's lymphoma appears to be direct pleural invasion, whereas in Hodgkin's disease impaired lymphatic drainage secondary to mediastinal adenopathy is the primary mechanism. Thus, the yield of pleural fluid cytology and pleural biopsy tends to be high with non-Hodgkin's lymphoma but is generally unrewarding in Hodgkin's disease.

The most common presenting symptom in patients with lymphoma and pleural effusions is dyspnea; cough, chest pain, and orthopnea are present in less than 25% of patients. Similar to patients with carcinomatous pleurisy, about 20% of patients with lymphomatous pleural effusions are relatively asymptomatic at the time that the effusion is discovered.

The pleural effusion in non-Hodgkin's lymphoma usually is a unilateral, serous exudate but can be sanguinous, chylous, transudative, or bilateral. The presence of hemorrhagic fluid usually indicates direct pleural involvement, and a transudate may be seen early in the course of impaired lymphatic drainage of the pleural space. The pleural fluid cell count usually is low, with a predominance of lymphocytes, at times approaching 100%. The glucose and pH are usually normal but may be low; low pH, low glucose lymphomatous effusions usually are chronic and associated with extensive pleural infiltration with tumor.

The presence of a pleural effusion in lymphoma is a poor prognostic sign. Survival will vary from a few months to several years, depending upon response to therapy; a prolonged survival has been observed in patients with pleural effusions who responded to chemotherapy. The most effective modality of therapy depends upon the clinical constellation. If the patient has mediastinal adenopathy without parenchymal or pleural nodules, there is a good likelihood of controlling the effusions by either mediastinal radiation or chemotherapy. Chemotherapy may be effective with parenchymal or pleural disease in association with a pleural effusion. Chylous, lymphomatous effusions appear to respond well to radiation therapy. If these measures are not effective, pleurodesis should be attempted.

The pleural effusions in the present patient were unresponsive to chemotherapy. He underwent left tetracycline pleurodesis and had minimal recurrence of the pleural effusion at 3 months with resolution of dyspnea.

Clinical Pearls

1. It is not uncommon for a pleural effusion to be present at the time of diagnosis in patients with non-Hodgkin's lymphoma and be the only abnormal chest radiographic finding.

2. Direct lymphomatous infiltration of the pleura appears to be the predominant mechanism for pleural effusion in non-Hodgkin's lymphoma; therefore, a high yield on pleural fluid cytology and pleural biopsy can be anticipated.

3. The presence of a pleural effusion in lymphoma is a poor prognostic sign, with survival varying from a few months to several years, depending upon the response to radiation or chemotherapy.

REFERENCES

1. Xaubet A, Diumenjo MC, Marin A, et al. Characteristics and prognostic value of pleural effusions in non-Hodgkin's lymphomas. Eur J Respir Dis 1985; 66:135–140.
2. Jenkins PF, Ward MJ, Davies P, Fletcher J. Non-Hodgkin's lymphoma, chronic lymphatic leukemia and the lung. Br J Dis Chest 1981; 75:22–30.
3. Das DK, Gupta SK, Ayyagari S, et al. Pleural effusion in non-Hodgkin's lymphoma. A cytomorphologic, cytochemical, and immunologic study. Acta Cytol 1987; 31:119–124.

PATIENT 44

A 62-year-old man with diffuse pulmonary nodules, right upper lobe density, and apical pleural thickening

A 62-year-old man was admitted to the hospital for a prostatectomy. The admission chest radiograph was abnormal and pulmonary consultation was obtained. The patient was a long-term smoker, but denied chest symptoms, fever, or weight loss. His occupational history included sandblasting jobs 20 years earlier.

Physical Examination: No lymphadenopathy; clear chest; no murmurs; abdomen soft without organomegaly; no clubbing.

Laboratory Findings: Admission blood tests normal. Chest radiograph showed bilateral nodular interstitial infiltrates with a localized right upper lobe density confirmed by tomography, apical pleural thickening, and hilar calcification. A chest radiograph 1 year earlier was similar except for the absence of the right upper lobe lesion. Sputum cytology, fungal smears, and acid-fast smears were negative.

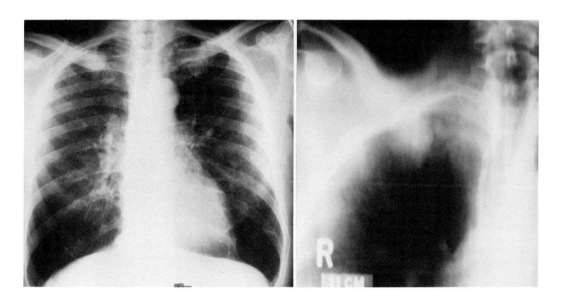

Diagnosis: Silicotuberculosis.

Discussion: Silicosis is a known predisposition for pulmonary tuberculosis. Patients with rapidly progressive silicosis are at the greatest risk, but even patients with minimal disease or a normal chest radiograph with prior silica exposure history have a higher incidence of tuberculous infection compared to the normal population. Pulmonary tuberculosis is often difficult to diagnose in this clinical setting. Marked radiographic abnormalities due to the underlying silicosis may obscure a nidus of tuberculous infection. Conversely, silicotic pulmonary masses or cavitation may be incorrectly ascribed to tuberculosis.

The pathogenesis of the heightened susceptibility to tuberculosis in silicosis is unclear. Laboratory investigation demonstrates that animals exposed to silica develop tuberculous infections with a smaller inoculum, tend to have higher counts of recovered organisms, and have a greater propensity for hematogenous and lymphatic spread. Additional experimental evidence suggests that silica ingestion hampers the bactericidal capacity of macrophages against tuberculosis organisms and accelerates their intracellular replication.

Silicotuberculosis responds poorly to therapy, partially because of the impaired function of silica-laden macrophages but also because of the poor penetrance of antituberculous drugs into silicotic nodules. Treatment failures after 18 to 24 months of older standard regimens containing isoniazid, p-aminosalicylic acid, ethambutol, and/or streptomycin supported recommendations for lifetime isoniazid after initial therapy. Incorporation of rifampin and pyrazinamide into short-course antituberculous regimens, however, may alter these recommendations. These drugs can eliminate organisms sequestered within macrophages, thereby reducing the role of host defenses in the eradication of tuberculosis. At least one recent study indicates that short-course chemotherapy incorporating rifampin or pyrazinamide is as effective in patients with silicotuberculosis as it is in uncomplicated pulmonary tuberculosis.

The bilateral diffuse nodular infiltrate with hilar calcifications in the present patient who had a sandblasting history suggested silicosis. The right upper lobe density could have represented lung cancer but proved to be tuberculosis by fiberoptic bronchoscopy with transbronchial biopsy. A conglomerate silicotic lesion was unlikely because of the density's isolated location and rapid development over a 1-year period. The present patient was treated with isoniazid, rifampin, ethambutol, and pyrazinamide for 9 months, with partial resolution of the right upper lobe density and conversion of sputums to negative.

Clinical Pearls

1. Silica exposure predisposes to pulmonary tuberculosis even when the chest radiograph does not detect silicosis.
2. Silicotuberculosis is relatively resistant to therapy because of impaired function of silica-laden macrophages; however, the potent sterilizing properties of rifampin and pyrazinamide may provide effective short course chemotherapy.

REFERENCES
1. Escreet BC, Langton ME, Cowie RL. Short-course chemotherapy for silicotuberculosis. South Africa Med J 1984; 66:327–330.
2. Morgan EJ. Silicosis and tuberculosis. Chest 1979; 75:202–203.
3. Lin T-P, Suo J, Lee C-N, et al. Short-course chemotherapy of pulmonary tuberculosis in pneumoconiotic patients. Am Rev Respir Dis 1987; 137:808–810.

PATIENT 45

A 57-year-old man with a 5-day history of progressive dyspnea, orthopnea, and pedal edema

A 57-year-old man complained of a 5-day history of progressive dyspnea, orthopnea, and pedal edema. He lost 20 pounds during the previous 4 months while noting low-grade fevers and night sweats. His past history was notable for 80 pack/years of smoking and childhood tuberculosis treated in a sanitarium.

Physical Examination: Pulse 140; blood pressure 100/90 with a 40 mmHg pulsus paradox. Cardiac impulse not palpable, distant heart sounds, no rub, elevated neck veins. Slight dullness at both lung bases. Pedal edema present.

Laboratory Findings: Serum Na 129 mEq/L; Hct 39%; electrocardiogram normal except for low voltage QRS complexes. Chest radiograph showed an enlarged cardiac silhouette with bilateral pleural effusions. Echocardiogram confirmed a large pericardial effusion.

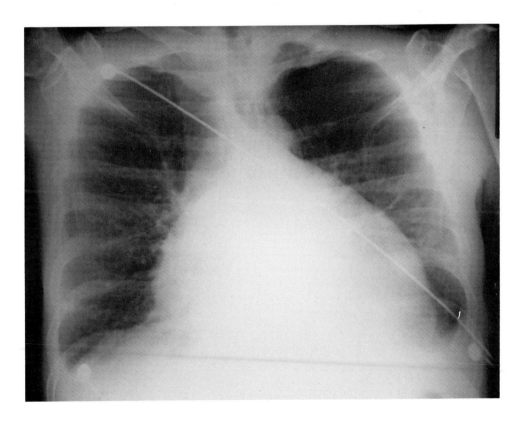

Diagnosis: Malignant pericardial effusion with tamponade.

Discussion: Pericardial effusion from involvement of the pericardium with an underlying malignancy is a common clinicopathologic occurrence. Cancer is the single most frequent cause of cardiac tamponade, accounting for 16 to 41% of instances. Furthermore, in as many as 3% of general autopsies and 12% of autopsies in patients with known cancers, some degree of malignant seeding of the pericardial surface is noted. The mechanisms of malignant pericardial fluid generation relate either to tumor implantation on the pericardial serosal surface or malignant obstruction of the lymphatics that drain the pericardial space. Most investigators consider that the latter mechanism is more important because the pericardial lymphatics are poorly developed, requiring most fluid to be drained by the epicardial lymphatics. These cardiac lymphatic chains are almost always found to be involved with tumor in the setting of malignant pericardial effusions.

Despite the pathologic evidence for their frequent occurrence, malignant pericardial effusions are usually asymptomatic and cardiac tamponade as an initial presentation of an underlying cancer, as occurred in this patient, is distinctly rare. When symptoms are present, they are usually nonspecific, comprising dyspnea, palpitations, fatigue or cough, and are obscured by the symptoms of the primary malignancy or cancer therapy. Indeed, only 30% of patients with malignant pericardial effusions are correctly diagnosed antemortem.

Although initially asymptomatic, a high clinical suspicion for malignant pericardial effusions is warranted, since they eventually contribute to the mortality of cancer patients in 85% of occurrences. Lung cancer is the most common primary neoplasm associated with pericardial metastases, accounting for 35% of patients with malignant pericardial effusions. Breast cancer contributes to an additional 22% of patients followed by leukemia, lymphoma, sarcoma, and melanomas.

The majority of patients with pericardial metastases have enlarged cardiac silhouettes, although effusions may develop rapidly, causing tamponade before the pericardial sac can expand. Once suspected, echocardiography is the most reliable test for confirmation of a malignant pericardial effusion. The therapeutic approach to a symptomatic effusion is partly determined by the existing expertise in an institution. Pericardiocentesis effectively resolves tamponade in 87% of patients, but because of the 5% major complication rate, it should be performed in the cardiac catheterization laboratory by skilled physicians. Cytologic evidence of cancer in aspirated fluid is present in 79% of patients. Subxyphoid pericardiotomy is the favored technique in many institutions because it is 100% effective with minimal complications in relieving tamponade and requires only local anesthesia.

Most symptomatic malignant pericardial effusions require efforts to resolve the long-term problem of fluid reaccumulation after initial pericardiocentesis. Placement of an intrapericardial catheter with sclerotherapy by the instillation of tetracycline is 80% effective. Subxyphoid pericardiotomy is effective in 100% of patients. A pericardial window requires general anesthesia and should not be necessary unless surgical exploration is required for biopsy diagnosis. One should note that pericardial biopsies are positive in malignant pericardial effusions in only 55% of patients. Radiation therapy may resolve recurrent pericardial effusions in patients with lymphoma but proves less effective for carcinomas.

The present patient underwent right heart catheterization, confirming cardiac tamponade, with equalization of right-sided vascular pressures. One liter of bloody fluid was removed by pericardiocentesis, improving the patient's symptoms. The fluid was cytologically positive for adenocarcinoma.

Clinical Pearls

1. Cancer is the most common single cause of pericardial tamponade.
2. Lung and breast cancers are the most common cancers involving the pericardium.

REFERENCES

1. Press OW, Livingston R. Management of malignant pericardial effusion and tamponade. JAMA 1987; 257:1088–1092.
2. Fraser RS, Viloria JB, Wang N-S. Cardiac tamponade as a presentation of extracardiac malignancy. Cancer 1980; 45:1697–1704.
3. Haskell RJ, French WJ. Cardiac tamponade as the initial presentation of malignancy. Chest 1985; 88:70–73.

PATIENT 46

A 54-year-old farmer with dyspnea on exertion, nonproductive cough, fever, and chills of 1 month's duration

A 54-year-old farmer presented with a 1-month history of increasing dyspnea on exertion, nonproductive cough, occasional fevers, and intermittent chills. He occasionally worked in silos and had symptoms of coughing following entrance into the silo. The last time of silo exposure was 2 months prior to admission.

Physical Examination: Temperature 98°; respirations 18; no acute distress; minimal basilar rales.

Laboratory Findings: CBC and chemistries normal. ABG (room air): pH 7.43; PCO_2 39 mmHg, PO_2 75 mmHg. Chest radiograph: diffuse nodular opacities.

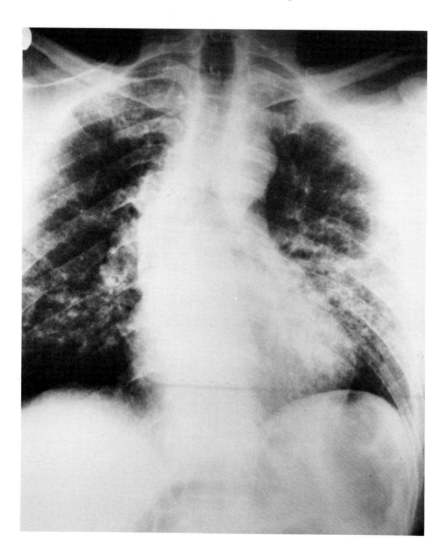

Diagnosis: Silo-filler's disease.

Discussion: It has been known for almost 200 years that nitrogen dioxide (NO_2) can cause acute, fatal lung injury but it was not known until 1949 that high concentrations of NO_2 were present in silo gas and were the cause of silo accidents. The term silo-filler's disease was first used in 1956 by Lowry, who described milder forms of the disease. NO_2 in silo gas is derived from the nitrates within plants. During silo storage, plant nitrates are fermented into nitrites and oxygen; the nitrites combine with organic acids to form nitrous acid (HNO_2). HNO_2 decomposes into nitrous oxide (NO), nitrogen tetroxide (N_2O_4), and nitrogen pentoxide (N_2O_5). NO_2 and its dimer, N_2O_4, are responsible for the pulmonary injury. Large amounts of NO_2 are formed during the first week following filling of the silo, with concentrations ranging from 200 to 4000 ppm. With adequate ventilation, gases usually disappear quickly.

There are three clinical phases of NO_2 inhalation: (1) the superacute phase, (2) acute phase, and (3) subacute and chronic phase. The superacute phase is rare, with severe hypoxemia leading to immediate death. The acute phase occurs within a few hours of exposure and is characterized by cough, dyspnea, bronchospasm, headache and chest pain; pulmonary edema may develop. If the patient survives, he enters a relatively asymptomatic period (possibly with mild dyspnea) of 2 to 5 weeks. Subsequently, he develops fevers, cough, and progressive dyspnea. The chest radiograph characteristically shows multiple nodular densities. Bronchiolitis obliterans has been documented in patients dying in this phase of NO_2 inhalation. Treatment for bronchiolitis obliterans is corticosteroid therapy. The prognosis with early diagnosis and treatment is generally good unless the inflammatory process has progressed to an irreversible stage. Long-term sequelae of NO_2 inhalation probably are related to the extent of exposure and the severity of the bronchiolitis obliterans.

The present patient had an excellent response to corticosteroids, with early resolution of symptoms and later clearing of the chest radiograph.

Clinical Pearls

1. The oxides of nitrogen are moderately insoluble in water (compared to chlorine and ammonia), allowing relatively long exposures to toxic concentrations, which enable distribution to the small airways and alveoli and set the stage for severe inflammation.

2. If the patient survives the initial pulmonary edema, after 1 to 2 weeks he enters a latent period (2–6 weeks) of relative well-being. Fever and chills may herald the relapse, which is associated with increasing dyspnea.

3. The characteristic chest radiograph pattern of the bronchiolitis obliterans stage is ill-defined, large nodular opacities distributed diffusely.

4. If treated early in the bronchiolitis obliterans stage, there usually is a good response to corticosteroids.

REFERENCES

1. Lowry T, Schulman LM. Silo-filler's disease. A syndrome caused by nitrogen dioxide. JAMA 1956; 162:153–160.
2. Ramirez RJ, Dowell AR. Silo-filler's disease: nitrogen dioxide induced lung injury: long term follow-up and review of the literature. Ann Intern Med 1971; 74:569–576.
3. Becklake MR, Goldman HI, Bosman AR, Freed CC. The long term effects of exposure to nitrous fumes. Am Rev Tuberc 1957; 76:398–409.

PATIENT 47

A 44-year-old man with a 6-month history of progressive dyspnea on exertion, weight loss, and clubbing

A 44-year-old man presented with the chief complaint of progressive dyspnea on exertion and weight loss for 6 months. He had a 50 pack/year history of cigarette smoking and admitted to cough and sputum production without hemoptysis. Twenty two years ago, the patient worked for one and a half years in an asbestos factory making blankets.

Physical Examination: Respirations 24; chronically ill appearing male in no acute distress; bilateral clubbing; flat percussion note and decreased fremitus bilaterally with rales at both bases.

Laboratory Findings: PFTs: FVC 2.07 L (38% of predicted), FEV$_1$ 2.00 L (49% of predicted), FEV$_1$/FVC ratio 97%, total lung capacity (66% of predicted); DLCO 44% of predicted. ABG (room air): pH 7.45, PCO$_2$ 35 mmHg, and PO$_2$ 75 mmHg; desaturation with exercise. Chest radiograph: bilateral pleural thickening and pulmonary fibrosis most severe in the lower lobes. CT scan: severe bilateral pleural fibrosis and interstitial lung disease.

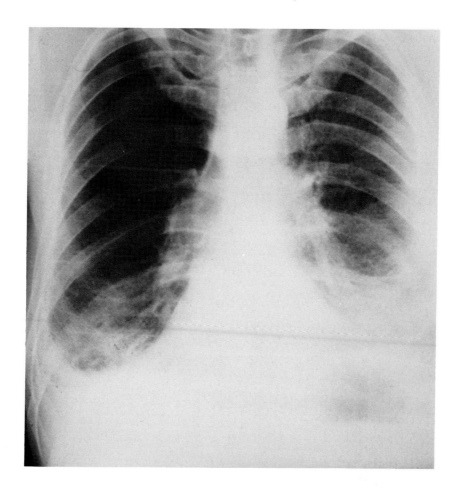

Diagnosis: Progressive pleural fibrosis secondary to asbestos exposure (hyalinosis complicata).

Discussion: Asbestos pleural effusion is the earliest manifestation of asbestos-induced pleuropulmonary disease and generally occurs within the first 10 to 20 years following exposure to asbestos. The majority of patients are asymptomatic but others present with pleuritic chest pain. The effusion will resolve over a 3- to 4-month period but may recur on the same or contralateral side. Blunting of the costophrenic angle is the usual sequelae of the inflammatory insult. However, a small number of patients progress to severe bilateral pleural fibrosis, succumbing to respiratory failure and death due to severe restrictive lung disease.

The patient presenting with unilateral pleural disease poses more of a diagnostic dilemma than the patient with disease involving both pleural spaces. A unilateral effusion, with or without pleural thickening in an asbestos worker who smokes cigarettes, heightens the suspicion of malignancy, particularly carcinoma of the lung. Thoracentesis in the patient with an asbestos pleural effusion usually reveals a serosanguinous exudate that may have eosinophilia and does not contain either malignant cells or asbestos bodies.

The pleural biopsy usually shows nonspecific pleuritis without evidence of asbestos bodies. When there is evidence of ipsilateral volume loss or a parenchymal lesion, bronchoscopy is indicated. With bilateral pleural effusions, a primary malignancy below the diaphragm is a consideration. However, in the setting of asbestos exposure, the clinician should think of progressive pleural fibrosis as the cause of the patient's symptoms. Mesothelioma is always a consideration in these individuals; however, these tumors usually present unilaterally and greater than 30 years following exposure. An open pleural and lung biopsy will document severe fibrosis, usually with evidence of asbestos (ferruginous) bodies in the lung, and generally exclude the diagnosis of mesothelioma. A decision as to whether or not the patient may benefit from decortication needs to be made. Only individuals with a paucity of parenchymal fibrosis have the possibility of benefiting from decortication.

The present patient had moderately severe parenchymal fibrosis, and it was thought that he would not benefit from decortication.

Clinical Pearls

1. Progressive pleural fibrosis due to asbestos exposure can occur relatively acutely and progress rapidly years after exposure to asbestos and lead to respiratory failure.
2. CT scan of the thorax may help in the clinical decision concerning decortication.
3. Decortication will only be successful in relieving symptoms if clinically significant interstitial fibrosis (asbestosis) is not present.

REFERENCES

1. Wright PH, Hanson A, Kreel L, Capel LH. Respiratory function changes after asbestos pleurisy. Thorax 1980; 35:31–36.
2. McGavin CR, Sheers G. Diffuse pleural thickening in asbestos workers: disability and lung function abnormalities. Thorax 1984; 39:604–607.
3. Miller A, Teirstein AS, Selikoff IJ. Ventilatory failure due to asbestos pleurisy. Am J Med 1983; 75:911–919.

PATIENT 48

A 28-year-old woman with fever and a right upper lobe lung cavity

A 28-year-old woman from North Carolina complained of cough, fever, and weight loss. Three years previously, she was treated for pulmonary tuberculosis but ran out of her medications when she moved 4 months after initiating therapy with unknown drugs.

Physical Examination: Temperature 38°; rales and rhonchi in the right upper lobe.

Laboratory Findings: Normal CBC and electrolytes; sputum demonstrated multiple acid-fast organisms. Chest radiograph showed a right upper lobe cavitary infiltrate.

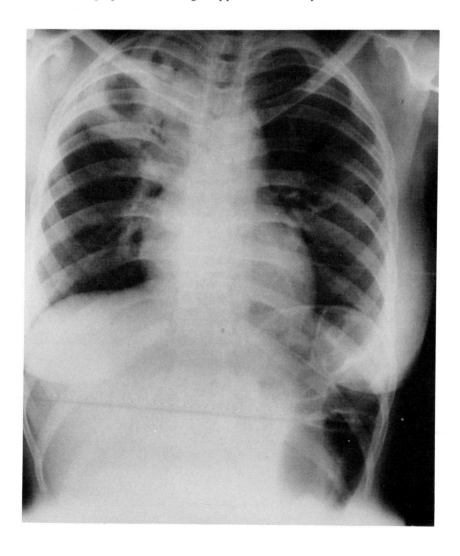

Diagnosis: Isoniazid (INH) resistant pulmonary tuberculosis.

Discussion: Modern chemotherapy has dramatically improved the clinical course of pulmonary tuberculosis, with 98% of patients being cured with short course drug regimens. Drug-resistant organisms, however, continue to challenge the clinician by greatly complicating therapy and worsening prognosis. Drug resistance is either primary or secondary. Primary drug resistance occurs when the host becomes infected with resistant organisms. Secondary resistance develops when patients with initially sensitive organisms undergo unsuccessful antituberculous therapy. The probability of secondary drug resistance increases if patients discontinue medications prematurely, take their drugs episodically, or receive inadequate drug regimens initially.

Consideration of the historical and epidemiologic features of the patient's clinical presentation aids in gauging the probability of drug resistance before sensitivities are available. Patients with prior antituberculosis therapy have a higher incidence of drug resistance compared to previously untreated patients (26% vs. 13%) as do patients from high tuberculosis incidence areas (42% vs. 13%). Awareness of the incidence of resistant organisms in the patient's community and the sensitivity profile of the organisms from a known contact source further assist in evaluating for drug resistance.

Patients with a low risk of drug-resistant tuberculosis are effectively treated with combinations of INH and rifampin (RM) with or without pyrazinamide (PZA). The addition of PZA for the first 2 months of treatment shortens the required duration of chemotherapy from 9 to 6 months. When drug resistance is suspected, patients can either be observed until sensitivities are available or initiated on antituberculous therapy if they are symptomatic or communicable. If therapy is initiated, two-drug regimens with INH or RM are inadequate because secondary drug resistance occurs most commonly with INH. Since at least two effective drugs must always be employed in tuberculosis, the presence of INH resistance would destroy the efficacy of RM in later regimens.

Unfortunately, the efficacy of three-drug regimens consisting of INH, RM, and PZA in suspected drug-resistant tuberculosis is questionable: the RM/PZA combination is unproven in long-term followup studies, and PZA is not as effective as ethambutol (EMB) in preventing secondary resistance to RM. Therefore, many experts suggest initiating therapy with INH, RM and PZA in instances of suspected drug-resistant tuberculosis supplemented by a fourth drug, EMB or streptomycin (SM). Since SM is the second most common drug to develop resistant organisms and is less well tolerated than EMB, EMB is an ideal addition. If the patient's isolates prove to be sensitive, the EMB can be discontinued and the patient treated for 6 months. If INH resistance is present, RM, PZA, and EMB can be continued for 12 months as a proven effective regimen.

The present patient was started on INH, RM, PZA, and EMB. Subsequent culture results indicated resistance to INH. She subsequently responded to a three-drug regimen with RM, PZA, and EMB.

Clinical Pearls

1. INH is the most common drug to which drug resistance develops in tuberculosis.
2. RM and PZA have not been proven effective in long-term studies as an effective antituberculous regimen.
3. When drug resistance is suspected from historical and epidemiologic features, a rational drug regimen is the combination of INH, RM, PZA, and EMB.

REFERENCES
1. Davidson PT. Drug resistance and the selection of therapy for tuberculosis. Am Rev Respir Dis 1987; 136:258–265.
2. Bass JB, Farer LS, Hopewell PC, Jacobs RF. Treatment of tuberculosis and tuberculosis infection in adults and children. Am Rev Respir Dis 1986; 134:355–363.

PATIENT 49

A 64-year-old man with a several week history of back pain, lytic defects of the vertebral bodies, and a pleural-based pulmonary lesion

A 64-year-old man was admitted to the hospital for evaluation of back pain of several weeks' duration and an abnormal chest radiograph. The pain was localized to the lumbar area, and exacerbated by movement but was not radicular.

Physical Examination: Vital signs normal; well nourished; limited movement due to back pain.

Laboratory Findings: WBC 5900/μl, 55% PMNs, 40% lymphocytes; Hct 28% with normal RBC indices; ESR 70 mm/h; serum creatinine 1.7 mg/dl; calcium 10.2 mg/dl. Serum electrophoresis normal; urine electrophoresis: peak of a lambda light chain; bone marrow: focal collection of immature plasma cells. Chest radiograph: homogeneous pleural-based lesion in the right apex; Spine films: punched-out lesions in vertebral bodies; osteoporosis. CT scan: apical pleural based lesion. Needle biopsy of the thoracic lesion was performed.

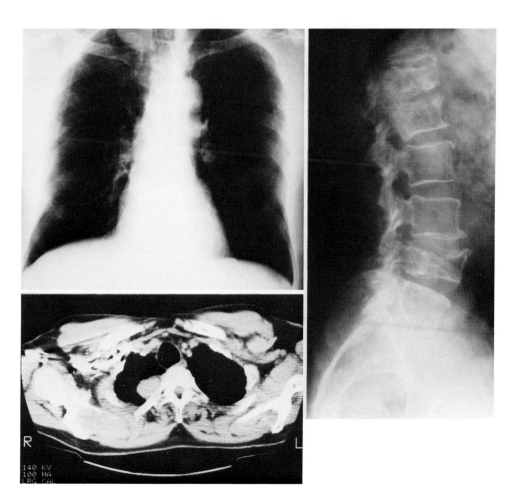

Diagnosis: Multiple myeloma with intrathoracic plasmacytoma.

Discussion: Multiple myeloma is a malignancy of plasma cells that is commonly associated with bone destruction, marrow failure, recurrent infections, hypercalcemia, and renal failure. It is a disease of the middle-aged and elderly, with a median onset at 60 years.

Multiple myeloma may involve the thorax with: skeletal involvement with pathologic fractures, osteolytic lesions, or osteoporosis; pulmonary infiltrates, most commonly infectious but also secondary to plasma cell infiltration; plasmacytomas, intramedullary and extramedullary; and pleural effusions. In a large review of nearly 1000 patients with multiple myeloma, 46% had abnormal chest radiographs during the course of their illness and 25% had a chest radiograph abnormality at initial diagnosis.

Intrathoracic plasmacytomas occur in about 10% of patients with multiple myeloma. The tumor may be found on initial presentation or develop during the course of the disease. Most intrathoracic plasmacytomas are intramedullary and associated with rib destruction. Extramedullary intrathoracic plasmacytomas occur in about 1% of patients with multiple myeloma. Patients presenting with an isolated thoracic plasmacytoma without evidence of multiple myeloma generally progress to disseminated disease; however, there are reports of absence of disease up to 8 years following the diagnosis of plasmacytoma. When multiple myeloma does develop in patients with isolated plasmacytomas, the prognosis, in general, is better. Extramedullary plasmacytomas can involve the lung parenchyma, mediastinum, hilar and mediastinal lymph nodes, tracheobronchial tree, and pleura. Pleural effusions secondary to multiple myeloma are rare (less than 1% incidence) and can be diagnosed by cytologic examination of the fluid or by pleural biopsy.

Histologically, a plasmacytoma demonstrates a monotonous pattern of plasma cells. Radiographically, a homogeneous, well-demarcated mass with extension into the thorax with an associated osteolytic lesion of the rib is most common. Plasmacytomas have a characteristic extrapleural pattern; that is, an extremely sharp convex contour facing the lung with the horizontal diameter of the lesion often almost identical to the vertical length. The superior and inferior edges are tapered and even slightly concave toward the lung, with the widest component of the lesion being opposite the center of attachment. Extramedullary plasmacytomas may be indistinguishable from primary parenchymal lesions.

In the present patient, needle biopsy of the thoracic lesion demonstrated immature plasma cells, confirming the diagnosis of an extramedullary plasmacytoma presumably originating from the parietal pleura.

Clinical Pearls

1. Chest radiograph reveals abnormalities in approximately half of the patients with multiple myeloma during the course of their illness and is abnormal in about 25% of patients at the time of the initial diagnosis.

2. Thoracic abnormalities due to multiple myeloma include skeletal lesions, intra- and extramedullary plasmacytomas, pulmonary infiltrates due to pneumonia or myeloma, and myeloma pleural effusions.

3. Intrathoracic plasmacytomas are characteristic extrapleural lesions seen as a homogeneous mass with a well-defined border with a convexity toward the lung and superior and inferior tapering, widest diameter at the center, and almost equal diameters in horizontal and vertical length.

4. Isolated plasmacytomas are rare, and evidence of disseminated disease is usually present at the time of diagnosis of a plasmacytoma. Most patients with an isolated plasmacytoma develop disseminated disease but some may have the localized process only, which can be treated with either resection or radiation therapy.

REFERENCES

1. Herskovic T, Andersen HA, Bayrd ED. Intrathoracic plasmacytomas. Presentation of 21 cases and review of the literature. Dis Chest 1965; 47:1–6.
2. Kintzer JS, Rosenow EC III, Kyle RA. Thoracic and pulmonary abnormalities in multiple myeloma. A review of 958 cases. Arch Intern Med 1978; 138:727–730.

PATIENT 50

A 61-year-old woman with chronic bilateral leg edema and the insidious onset of dyspnea

A 61-year-old woman with a history of hypertension and bilateral leg edema for several years was admitted to the hospital with the insidious onset of dyspnea. She had no risk factors for coronary artery disease and the history was negative for angina or previous myocardial infarction. There was a history of chronic sinusitis and recent nonproductive cough.

Physical Examination: Temperature 98.6°; pulse 88 and regular; respirations 20; blood pressure 150/110. Healthy-appearing and in no acute distress but somewhat unkempt with the exception of brightly polished red nails. Mild AV nicking. Chest examination: bilateral pleural effusions. Cardiac examination normal. No hepatomegaly or ascites; 2+ edema of both legs.

Laboratory Findings: WBC 9000/μl, normal differential; Hct 45%. ABG (room air): pH 7.47, PCO$_2$ 30 mmHg, PO$_2$ 84 mmHg. Chest radiograph: bilateral pleural effusions without parenchymal lesions. Thoracentesis: straw-colored fluid, nucleated cells 4950/μl, 80% lymphocytes, 15% mesothelial cells, 5% PMNs; total protein 5.9 g/dl, glucose 110 mg/dl, LDH 68 IU/L. Gram and AFB stain negative; bacterial, fungal and tuberculous cultures negative; cytology negative. Pleural biopsy: chronic pleuritis with lymphocytic and plasma cell infiltration.

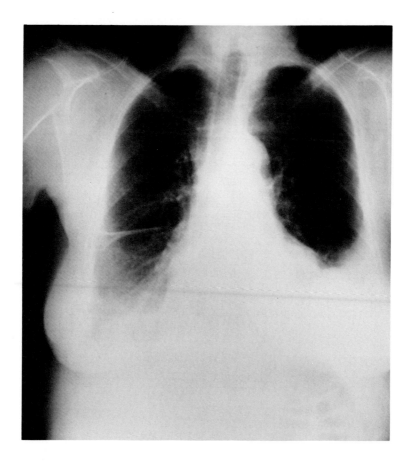

Diagnosis: Yellow nail syndrome (YNS).

Discussion: The association of slow-growing discolored nails and peripheral edema was coined the YNS by Samman and White in 1964. Two years later the complete triad of yellow nails, lymphedema and pleural effusion was described. Since that time, approximately 100 patients with the YNS have been reported. The associated bronchiectasis and sinusitis are now known to be part of the syndrome, which is best described as the triad of yellow nails, lymphedema and respiratory tract involvement, with all three features not necessarily being present. In a review of 62 patients with YNS, 53 had yellow nails, 45 lymphedema, 24 pleural effusions, 20 chronic pulmonary infections and 11 sinus infections. Of the 62 patients; 24 had the combination of yellow nails and lymphedema; 17 had yellow nails, lymphedema and pleural effusions; 14 had yellow nails alone; 8 had lymphedema and pleural effusion; and no patients had yellow nails and pleural effusions only.

The etiology of YNS is impaired lymphatic drainage due to a decreased number of hypoplastic and dilated lymphatics. The median age of onset of symptoms is 40 years, with some patients being born with lymphedema and others developing symptoms as late as age 65. In about one-third of patients, yellow nails and lymphedema are the initial symptoms. The nails are slow-growing with yellow to yellow-green discoloration, thickening, onycholysis, and over-curvature both in the transverse and longitudinal plane. About one-third of patients provide a history of 10 to 20 years of recurrent chronic bronchitis, often associated with bronchiectasis, chronic sinusitis, or pneumonia; pleural effusions may be the presenting respiratory manifestation in about one-third of patients.

The chest radiograph may show bilateral or unilateral pleural effusions that vary from small to massive. The effusions are not transient, persist in relatively constant volume, and recur within days to months following thoracentesis. The pleural fluid usually is a straw-colored exudate, often with a protein value greater than 4.0 g/dl and an LDH concentration greater than 200 IU/L. Pleural fluid glucose is similar to blood glucose and the pleural fluid pH is approximately 7.40. The RBC is usually less than $10,000/\mu l$ with a low number of leukocytes (usually less than $1000/\mu l$); there is a predominance of lymphocytes, usually greater than 80%.

Diagnosis is not difficult when the complete triad is present. However, symptoms seldom appear simultaneously and the full triad may never occur. In the presence of lymphedema and pleural effusions, but without yellow nails, the diagnosis should be regarded as one of exclusion. At times due to the color and disfiguration of the nails, some women use opaque nail polish and obscure this finding from the unsuspecting observer.

Treatment has been symptomatic, with anecdotal reports of successful therapy. In patients with symptomatic pleural effusions, pleurectomy and chemical pleurodesis have been successful in controlling the effusions. Partial or complete recovery of the nail symptoms occurs in about 30% of patients, with occasional relapses. The lymphedema and pleural effusions are chronic and persistent, and spontaneous recovery has not been reported.

The present patient had tetracycline pleurodesis on the right, which was successful and improved her exercise tolerance.

Clinical Pearls

1. Respiratory tract involvement including pleural effusions, bronchiectasis, sinusitis, and pneumonia are an integral component of the yellow nail syndrome.

2. Yellow nail syndrome should be considered in the differential diagnosis of the "asymptomatic" patient with chronic bilateral pleural effusions.

3. Women frequently cover discolored and disfigured nails with opaque nail polish and obscure this important clinical finding from the unsuspecting observer.

4. The most common constellation of findings at the time of diagnosis appears to be yellow nails and lymphedema; the isolated combination of yellow nails and pleural effusions appears to be extremely uncommon.

REFERENCES
1. Samman PD, White WF. The yellow nail syndrome. Br J Dermatol 1964; 76:153–157.
2. Pavlidakey GP, Hashimoto K, Blum D. Yellow nail syndrome. J Am Acad Dermatol 1984; 11:509–512.
3. Nordkild P, Kromann-Andersen H, Struve-Christensen E. Yellow nail syndrome—the triad of yellow nails, lymphedema, and pleural effusions. Acta Med Scand 1986; 219:221–227.

PATIENT 51

A 43-year-old woman with a 2-month history of nonproductive cough, dyspnea, and pulmonary nodules

A 43-year-old black woman was well until 2 months prior to admission when she began to experience a nonproductive, nocturnal cough associated with dyspnea. She also reported occasional wheezing that responded to inhaled beta-agonists, but denied fever, constitutional symptoms, or travel out of South Carolina.

Physical Examination: Temperature 98.6°; pulse 84; respirations 16. Healthy-appearing and in no acute distress. Skin: no lesions. Chest: vesicular breath sounds. Abdomen: no tenderness, masses, or organomegaly.

Laboratory Findings: WBC 8000/μl with normal differential, Hct 39%. Liver function tests normal. Total protein 7.0 g/dl, albumin 3.8 g/dl, calcium 9.5 mg/dl. Chest radiograph: multiple patchy nodular densities throughout both lung fields; no hilar or mediastinal adenopathy or pleural disease. Pulmonary function tests: FVC 2.57 L (92% of predicted), FEV_1 1.84 L (82% of predicted), FEV_1/FVC ratio 71%, DL/VA ratio 5.30. Fiberoptic bronchoscopy with transbronchial lung biopsy: no endobronchial lesions; increased vascular pattern of the mucosa. Transbronchial lung biopsies (6 biopsies): chronic inflammation and focal fibrosis without granulomas; no evidence of malignancy. An additional procedure was performed.

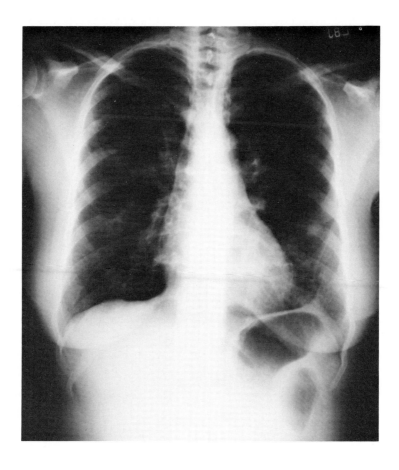

Diagnosis: Nodular sarcoidosis.

Discussion: During the course of the disease, over 90% of patients with sarcoidosis have chest radiographic abnormalities. Lymphadenopathy occurs in 75 to 85% of patients at some time during their illness, with bilateral hilar adenopathy being the most common finding. Parenchymal abnormalities occur in more than 60% of patients, with 20% showing only parenchymal abnormalities on the initial radiograph. There appears to be an inverse relationship between adenopathy and parenchymal lesions, as it is typical for the adenopathy to diminish while the parenchymal lesions increase. This is in contrast to lymphoma, in which adenopathy and parenchymal involvement often progress together. The reticulonodular pattern is characterized by fine linear densities and small nodules. Up to 25% of patients with a reticulonodular pattern progress to fibrosis, characterized by persistent linear densities and loss of volume with retraction and distortion. Less common parenchymal patterns of sarcoidosis are the acinar pattern and multinodular patterns. Patients with an acinar pattern may demonstrate air bronchograms; the majority of these patients have persistent infiltrates and many progress to fibrosis. Nodular densities initially described in the 1950s represent a rare radiographic manifestation of sarcoidosis. The lesions may occur in the absence of adenopathy and are frequently multiple, from 5 to 40 mm in diameter, and distributed diffusely throughout both lung fields. The borders may be sharp or irregular and fluffy. The differential diagnosis of the multinodular pattern includes metastatic carcinoma, fungal disease, tuberculosis, hamartomas, septic emboli, lymphoma, Wegener's, rheumatoid nodules, and amyloidosis. The presentation of the patient in conjunction with the chest radiograph will limit the differential diagnosis. Patients with nodular sarcoidosis are frequently asymptomatic or have only mild, nonspecific symptoms. The indistinct fluffy margins are less characteristic of metastatic malignancy, and the presence of cavitation would be more likely with septic emboli, Wegener's, and rheumatoid nodules than with sarcoidosis.

Transbronchial lung biopsy, because of its low morbidity, high diagnostic yield, and specificity, is one of the initial diagnostic procedures for obtaining histologic confirmation in patients with suspected sarcoidosis. The diagnostic yield appears to increase from stage I to stage III sarcoidosis and to diminish in the fibrocystic form of the disease. If four or more transbronchial biopsies are obtained, the yield of noncaseating granuloma in all stages is about 75%, with a range of 50 to 100%.

The present patient had a nondiagnostic transbronchial lung biopsy with an adequate number of good samples of lung tissue. She chose to undergo open lung biopsy rather than repeat bronchoscopy. The open lung biopsy showed noncaseating granulomas that were negative on stain and culture. The patient has been followed for the past year without treatment; her chest radiograph, pulmonary function and clinical status have remained stable.

Clinical Pearls

1. Less than 5% of patients with sarcoidosis present with a multinodular chest radiograph pattern with or without hilar adenopathy.

2. Patients with nodular sarcoidosis are frequently asymptomatic, an important clinical point in the differential diagnosis when considering metastatic malignancy, septic emboli, or Wegener's granulomatosis.

3. Transbronchial lung biopsy should be used as one of the initial diagnostic tests for obtaining histologic confirmation in the patient with suspected sarcoidosis, as it has a low morbidity and a high diagnostic yield ($> 75\%$, range 50–100%) and specificity.

REFERENCES

1. Felson B. Uncommon roentgen patterns of pulmonary sarcoidosis. Dis Chest 1958; 44:357–367.
2. Kirks DR, Greenspan RH. Sarcoid. Radiol Clin North Am 1973; 11:279–294.
3. Puar HS, Young RC Jr, Armstrong EN. Bronchial and transbronchial lung biopsy without fluoroscopy in sarcoidosis. Chest 1985; 87:303–306.

PATIENT 52

A 23-year-old man with a metallic taste in his mouth, headache, and fever several hours following intravenous self-injection of a substance

A 23-year-old man with a history of intravenous drug use came to the emergency room 8 hours after injecting a "small amount" of a substance he had purchased by mail order. He complained of a metallic taste in his mouth, headache, and fever. Specifically, he denied respiratory or other neurologic symptoms.

Physical Examination: Temperature 100.4°; pulse 110; respirations 20; blood pressure 130/80; no acute distress. Chest examination: equal bilateral expansion, no adventitious sounds. Cardiac examination: negative except for a regular tachycardia. Neurologic examination normal. Skin: needle tracks in the left arm.

Laboratory Findings: WBC 9400/μl with normal differential, Hct 38%. Electrolytes, liver function tests, BUN, and creatinine: normal. Electrocardiogram: sinus tachycardia. ABG (room air): pH 7.43, PCO_2 36 mmHg, PO_2 90 mmHg. Chest radiograph is shown below.

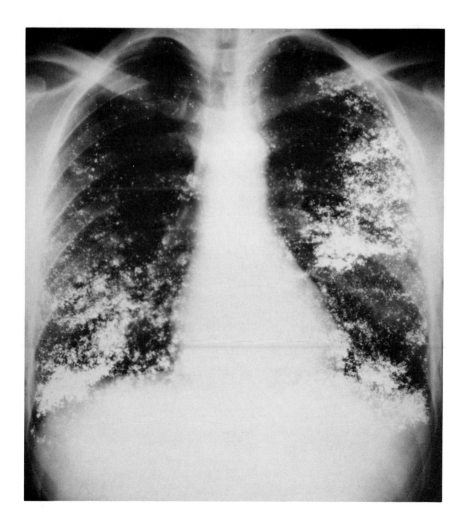

Diagnosis: Intravenous elemental mercury injection with pulmonary embolization.

Discussion: If deposited in tissues, metallic mercury is considered to be relatively inert. However, inhalation, ingestion, or injection of metallic mercury can produce toxicity. Acute inhalation of vaporized mercury can be fatal from pulmonary edema and also is associated with renal tubular degeneration and necrosis of the GI tract mucosa. Chronic inhalation is primarily an industrial and laboratory hazard that can produce anemia, renal tubular damage, colitis, and peripheral neuritis. Ingestion of metallic mercury has been associated with appendicitis and fistulas.

The toxicity of the intravenous injection of mercury probably is modified by several factors, one being blood solubility and conversion to the ionic form. The possible consequences of intravascular mercury injection include obstruction to the vascular tree, local tissue inflammation, and systemic toxicity. Intraarterial injection has resulted in ischemia of the digits and retinal and cerebral artery occlusion. Following intravenous injection, there may be dyspnea, chest pain, hypoxemia, and pulmonary function abnormalities; however, the patient may have no acute respiratory symptoms and present only with a metallic taste in the mouth, headache and fever.

Mercury globules may lead to foreign body granulomas without signs of systemic toxicity. There appears to be a poor correlation between systemic toxicity and mercury blood levels.

Right heart catheterization following intravenous mercury injection has demonstrated normal pressures, and angiography has shown normal pulmonary vasculature. However, lesions demonstrated in systemic arteries suggest that the mercury is able to pass through the pulmonary circulation. Some reports have documented clearing of the chest radiograph over an unspecified period of time, with the globules most likely being distributed in other organs where their presence is not as evident. Others have demonstrated no change in the chest radiograph over 1 year. A single report showed no change in serial physiologic studies over a period of a year and a half.

In most reports, metallic mercury has been demonstrated by radiograph either at the site of introduction or as pulmonary emboli. On chest radiograph, there are multiple, tiny, dense spherules, usually diffusely distributed, or, at times, restricted to several dependent areas. These lesions may appear as scattered densities of various sizes or as beaded chains that conform to the pulmonary arterioles. Mercury also may be noted at the apex of the right ventricle, either within the endocardium or as a free intraluminal pool. Diagnosis of mercury embolization is suggested by the density, size, and characteristic spherical shape of the mercury droplets. Birdshot and shrapnel have angular margins; emboli following lymphangiography exhibit a diffuse haze and are less radiodense; and aspirated barium or bronchographic contrast media result in a more linear appearance.

The present patient's symptoms, fever and tachycardia, resolved over the next three days.

Clinical Pearls

1. Symptoms following intravenous injection of elemental mercury may be dyspnea, chest pain, hypoxemia, fever, headache, tachycardia, and a metallic taste in the mouth. However, the patient may be relatively asymptomatic. The degree of the symptoms depends on the dose injected and underlying pulmonary status.

2. The chest radiograph characteristically shows multiple, dense spherules throughout both lungs conforming to the pulmonary arterioles. Identification of associated intracardiac mercury and mercury in the abdominal vessels and subcutaneous tissue of the extremities is confirmatory.

3. The chest radiograph may remain unchanged for an extended period but may resolve, presumably from the passage of the mercury globules through precapillary shunts or pulmonary capillaries resulting in deposition in systemic sites. There appears to be no significant effect on pulmonary function.

REFERENCES

1. Conrad ME Jr, Sanford JP, Preston JA. Metallic mercury embolization. Clinical and experimental. Arch Intern Med 1957; 100:59–65.
2. Ambre JJ, Welsh MJ, Svare CW. Intravenous elemental mercury injection: blood levels and excretion of mercury. Ann Intern Med 1977; 87:451–453.
3. Chitkara R, Seriff NS, Kinas HY. Intravenous self-administration of metallic mercury in attempted suicide. Report of a case with serial roentenographic and physiologic studies over an 18 month period. Chest 1978; 73:234–236.

PATIENT 53

**A 34-year-old man with a 3-week history of decreased visual acuity,
hemoptysis, fever, bloody nasal discharge, and a pulmonary cavity**

A 34-year-old man was referred because of an abnormal chest radiograph. He was in good health until approximately 3 weeks prior when he noticed "scratchy, irritated" eyes and a decrease in visual acuity. He medicated himself with over-the-counter eyedrops and sought medical attention when he developed minimal hemoptysis. Further questioning disclosed nasal discharge with occasional blood-streaking and intermittent low-grade fever. He also complained of "ear congestion" and right anterior substernal chest discomfort.

Physical Examination: Temperature 100.8°; respirations 20; marked scleral inflammation; bilateral serous otitis media; bloody crusted lesions in the nasal septum; amphoric breathing right anterior chest; cardiac examination normal; abdomen: non-tender without hepatosplenomegaly; neurologic examination normal.

Laboratory Findings: WBC 9300/μl, 78% PMNs, 12% lymphocytes, 5% monocytes, 5% eosinophils, Hct 33% with normal indices, platelet count 450,000/μl, BUN 21 mg/dl, creatinine 0.7 mg/dl, ESR 78 mm/h, rheumatoid factor 1:128. ANA negative; PPD positive; urinalysis: 3 WBCs/hpf. Chest radiograph: large, thick-walled cavity in the right upper lobe. Nasal septal biopsy: acute and chronic inflammation. Fiberoptic bronchoscopy: larynx and airways showed no lesions but there was mild nonspecific airway inflammation. Transbronchial biopsy of the right upper lobe lesion showed acute and chronic inflammation. A diagnostic procedure was performed.

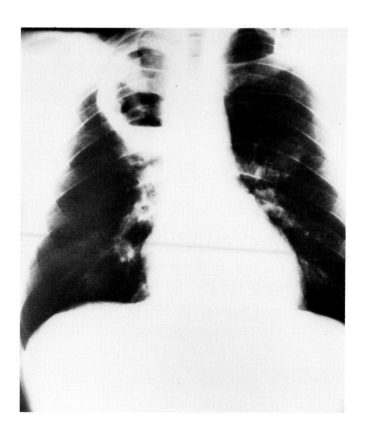

Diagnosis: Wegener's granulomatosis with episcleritis, nasal septal ulceration, serous otitis media, sinusitis, and a solitary cavitary lung lesion.

Discussion: Classic Wegener's is a disease characterized by necrotizing granulomatous vasculitis of both the upper and lower respiratory tracts in association with glomerulonephritis; the vasculitis involves both small arteries and veins. A localized form of Wegener's, limited primarily to the upper and lower respiratory tracts, does occur. Because Wegener's frequently is a multisystem disease, the differential diagnosis includes a wide spectrum of diseases: vasculitides such as systemic lupus and polyarteritis nodosa, granulomatous diseases such as sarcoidosis, granulomatous and vasculitic diseases such as allergic granulomatosis, infectious diseases such as blastomycosis, malignancy, and the pulmonary-renal syndromes such as Goodpasture's.

The characteristic patient is a male in the fifth decade of life who presents with symptoms referable to the upper respiratory tract, such as nasal or postnasal drainage, sinus pain, or nasal mucosal ulceration. Cough, chest pain (both pleuritic and nonpleuritic), hemoptysis, fever (either due to the underlying disease or secondary infection), and anorexia and weight loss also may be presenting symptoms.

Multiple nodules appear to be the most common radiographic finding but solitary nodules can occur. The nodules usually are well-defined, round, and from 1 to 5 cm in diameter, without lobar predilection. Cavitation is frequent, ranging from minimal to almost complete evacuation of the lesion. The cavity walls have been described as both thick and thin. Regression of lesions in one area of the lung and progression in other areas should suggest the possibility of Wegener's.

The diagnosis can be made by biopsy of any involved organ. The limited form of Wegener's that lacks renal involvement may be an early form of the disease and tends to have a more favorable prognosis. The use of cyclophosphamide has resulted in remarkable improvement in prognosis and it is recommended that the drug be continued for at least 1 year following complete remission.

The present patient had an open lung biopsy which demonstrated the characteristic pathologic features of Wegener's. He had an excellent clinical response to cyclophosphamide and is currently on a low dose of the drug 18 months following its initiation.

Clinical Pearls

1. Signs and symptoms referable to the nose and sinuses are the most common presenting complaints of patients with Wegener's.

2. The most common chest radiographic pattern is multiple cavitary nodules; however, up to 25% of patients may present with a solitary cavitary nodule.

3. Spontaneous regression of lesions in one area of the lung with progression in other areas should heighten the suspicion for Wegener's.

REFERENCES

1. Fauci AS, Wolff SM. Wegener's granulomatosis: studies in 18 patients and a review of the literature. Medicine 1973; 52:535–561.
2. Carrington CB, Liebow AA. Limited forms of angiitis and granulomatosis of Wegener's type. Am J Med 1966; 41:497–527.
3. Gohel VK, Dalinka MK, Israel HL, Libshitz HI. The radiological manifestations of Wegener's granulomatosis. Br J Radiol 1973; 46:427–432.

PATIENT 54

A 25-year-old man with a several-week history of cough, dyspnea, weight loss, lymphadenopathy, and persistent hemorrhage from a lymph node biopsy site

A 25-year-old black man was admitted to a local hospital with a several-week history of cough, dyspnea on exertion, fever, and weight loss. On examination, he was noted to have diffuse lymphadenopathy. A supraclavicular lymph node biopsy was obtained which showed noncaseating granuloma with negative AFB and fungal stains. Following the biopsy, the patient had continuous "oozing" from the biopsy site. Subsequently, a platelet count was found to be 7000/μl. He was transferred to our institution.

Physical Examination: Temperature 102°; "oozing" from lymph node biopsy site. Chest examination unremarkable. Abdomen: no hepatosplenomegaly or masses. Skin: numerous petechiae and ecchymoses.

Laboratory Findings: WBC 4700/μl with normal differential; Hct 34%; platelet count 7000/μl; total protein 5.8 g/dl; albumin 3.3 g/dl. Liver function tests normal; angiotensin converting enzyme 40 U; anti-platelet antibodies positive; bone marrow biopsy: megakaryocytic hyperplasia; PPD skin test negative; controls negative. Chest radiograph: bilateral hilar and right paratracheal adenopathy.

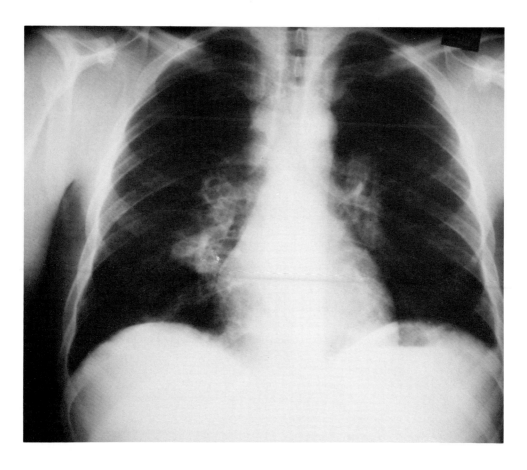

Diagnosis: Sarcoidosis with autoimmune thrombocytopenia.

Discussion: First described in 1938, approximately 50 patients have been reported with sarcoidosis and thrombocytopenia. It is estimated that 2% of patients with sarcoidosis develop thrombocytopenia. The mechanisms for this phenomenon include hypersplenism, bone marrow involvement with granulomas, and antibody-mediated immune destruction of platelets. Patients with hypersplenism frequently have signs of portal hypertension, a moderate reduction in platelet count, and varying degrees of leukopenia and anemia. Following splenectomy, peripheral blood counts return toward normal. Other patients with sarcoidosis and thrombocytopenia do not have splenomegaly but have moderate to severe thrombocytopenia. There are two categories of these patients. One group presents with an insidious course of minimal to moderate bleeding involving the mucous membranes, skin, and genitourinary tract without pancytopenia. The second group may present with the acute onset of bleeding, which may involve not only the skin and mucous membranes but the central nervous system as well; leukocyte counts usually are normal with moderate anemia and severe reductions in platelet counts to less than $10,000/\mu l$. These patients usually are in the second to fourth decades, with no sex predominance. Splenomegaly may or may not be present, mortality is high with supportive treatment alone, and there appears to be a good response to splenectomy. Bone marrow biopsy shows a normal or increased number of megakaryocytes, suggesting that the problem is not one of thrombopoiesis. It appears that these patients have increased peripheral destruction of platelets. Indirect evidence for autoimmune thrombocytopenia includes a decreased survival time of transfused platelets and response to corticosteroids. In addition, platelet-associated IgG has been demonstrated in patients with severe thrombocytopenia and sarcoidosis.

In sarcoidosis there is an accumulation of helper T cells at active disease sites with a predominance of suppressor T cells in the circulation. Helper T lymphocytes in the lungs are stimulatory for the proliferation of B lymphocytes and synthesis with hypergammaglobulinemia, a common finding in sarcoidosis. A consequence of B cell activation may be the production of antibodies that have an affinity for platelet antigens.

When severe thrombocytopenia develops in sarcoidosis, treatment needs to be instituted promptly, as these patients are at risk for having a fatal central nervous system bleed. Corticosteroids should be instituted immediately. If hypersplenism is present, splenectomy should be performed if there is refractoriness to corticosteroids. Intravenous human gammaglobulin has been found to be effective in increasing the platelet count, as this immunoglobulin probably competes with the IgG-coated platelets for clearance by the reticuloendothelial system. High doses of intravenous gammaglobulin may be tried before splenectomy if there is a corticosteroid failure.

The present patient was treated with platelet transfusions and corticosteroids, with an increase in the platelet count to $85,000/\mu l$.

Clinical Pearls

1. Thrombocytopenia is an unusual complication of sarcoidosis and can occur through three mechanisms: (1) hypersplenism; (2) bone marrow involvement with granulomas; and (3) antibody-mediated immune platelet destruction.

2. Antibody-mediated immune platelet destruction may be associated with severe thrombocytopenia (platelet counts $< 10,000/\mu l$) and platelet-associated IgG.

3. Patients with sarcoidosis and severe thrombocytopenia should be treated promptly with corticosteroids; if thrombocytopenia is refractory to corticosteroids, high doses of intravenous gammaglobulins may be tried prior to splenectomy.

REFERENCES

1. Jersild M. The syndrome of Heerfordt (uveo-parotid fever). a manifestation of Boeck's sarcoid. Acta Med Scand 1938; 97:322–328.
2. Dickerman JD, Holbrook PR, Zinkham WH. Etiology and therapy of thrombocytopenia associated with sarcoidosis. J Pediatr 1972; 81:758–764.
3. Lawrence HJ, Greenberg BR. Autoimmune thrombocytopenia in sarcoidosis. Am J Med 1985; 79:761–764.
4. Henke M, Engler H, Engelhardt R, Lohr GW. Successful therapy of sarcoidosis-associated thrombocytopenia refractory to corticosteroids by a single course of human gamma globulins. Klin Wochenschr 1986; 64:1209–1211.

PATIENT 55

A 35-year-old man with confusion, ataxia, and an abnormal chest radiograph

A 35-year-old man was admitted for evaluation of altered mental status. One week before admission, his family noted forgetfulness followed by confusion and a stumbling gait. The patient denied headaches, a smoking history, or drug usage.

Physical Examination: Vital signs normal; skin unremarkable; no lymphadenopathy; lung examination normal; neurologic examination: abnormal with confusion, anesthesia of the right lower face, and ataxia.

Laboratory Findings: CBC and electrolytes normal. Chest radiograph: bilateral hilar adenopathy. CT scan of head: hydrocephalus with a lesion in the pontine-cerebellar angle. PPD and anergy panel skin tests: nonreactive.

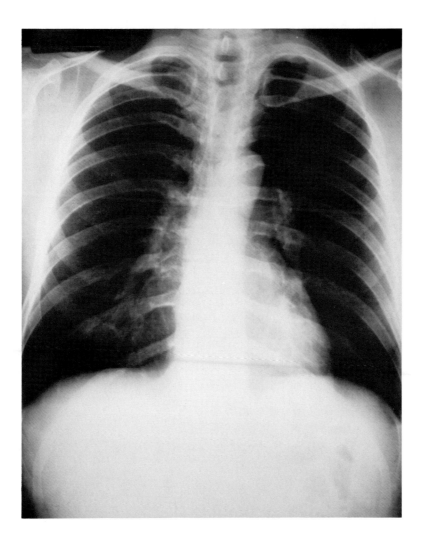

Diagnosis: Sarcoidosis with central nervous system involvement.

Discussion: Sarcoidosis is a multisystem granulomatous disorder that presents with pulmonary manifestations in the majority of patients. Occasionally, extrapulmonary symptoms may overshadow the more typical and recognizable pulmonary features of the disease.

The nervous system is one of the most important extrapulmonary sites of involvement in sarcoidosis because of the potential for serious and disabling symptoms with long-term morbidity. Occurring in up to 5% of sarcoid patients, neurologic disease can occur anywhere in the nervous system. Peripheral involvement most commonly develops in the cranial nerves, promoting symptoms that include facial palsy and anesthesia, anosmia, visual disturbances, and hearing deficits. Peripheral nerve involvement occurs less frequently but may be longer lasting than the usually transient cranial nerve dysfunction.

Central nervous system sarcoid creates major potential for serious disability and can present anywhere in the CNS. Several reports suggest that diabetes insipidus is the most common lesion, occurring in 35% of patients with CNS sarcoid. These studies often did not confirm depleted reserves of antidiuretic hormone, and subsequent investigations indicate that most instances of polyuria in CNS sarcoid relate to altered thirst from hypothalamic lesions. Granulomatous inflammation of the hypothalamus is also the major mechanism of hypopituitarism in sarcoid, since direct pituitary destruction occurs in the minority of instances. Although these endocrine disturbances usually occur in patients with widespread disease involving the lung, skin, and liver, 6% of patients with CNS sarcoid may have normal chest radiographs.

CNS sarcoid may also present as meningeal or intracerebral space-occupying lesions, as occurred in the present patient. In these instances the presence of focal neurologic symptoms, cerebrospinal fluid pleocytosis with elevated protein, and a mass defect on radiographic studies may mimic an intracranial neoplasm. A CNS tuberculoma is also in the differential diagnosis.

Neurologic involvement in sarcoidosis is an indication for corticosteroid therapy. Lesions present for less than 1 year tend to regress on therapy. Older lesions may stabilize but often do not improve, thereby creating an urgency for early diagnosis and rapid initiation of therapy. Endocrine disturbances, except for alterations in thirst, typically do not resolve with corticosteroids.

The present patient's chest radiograph was interpreted as bilateral hilar adenopathy, suggesting the possibility of sarcoidosis. Fiberoptic bronchoscopy with transbronchial biopsies demonstrated multiple noncaseating granulomas that were negative on special stains for fungi or mycobacteria. The patient was treated with prednisone, 80 mg a day, with gradual improvement of the neurologic symptoms and normalization of the chest radiograph over the subsequent 2 months.

Clinical Pearls

1. Up to 5% of patients with sarcoidosis have neurologic involvement.
2. As many as 6% of patients with CNS sarcoid have normal chest radiographs.
3. Polyuria is a common manifestation of CNS sarcoid that more commonly relates to hypothalamic thirst disturbances rather than to diabetes insipidus.

REFERENCES
1. Stuart CA, Neelon FA, Lebovitz HE. Hypothalamic insufficiency: The cause of hypopituitarism in sarcoidosis. Ann Intern Med 1978; 88:589–594.
2. Cariski AT. Isolated CNS sarcoidosis. JAMA 1981; 245:62–63.

PATIENT 56

A 24-year-old man with a history of acute myelogenous leukemia presenting with fever, cough, and bilateral infiltrates during induction chemotherapy

A 24-year-old man was hospitalized while undergoing induction therapy for acute myelogenous leukemia. During the interval of bone marrow suppression, he became febrile and developed a cough.

Physical Examination: No skin abnormalities; fundi normal. Chest: scattered rhonchi. Cardiac: no murmurs.

Laboratory Findings: WBC 800/μl with 40% polymorphonuclear cells; Hct 28%; platelet count 95,000/μl. ABG (room air): pH 7.42; PCO$_2$ 38 mmHg; PO$_2$ 75 mmHg. Chest radiograph showed multiple bilateral nodular infiltrates. Sputum was rusty in appearance and revealed no predominant organisms on routine or special stains. After progression of the infiltrates to multiple cavities, pulmonary consultation was obtained.

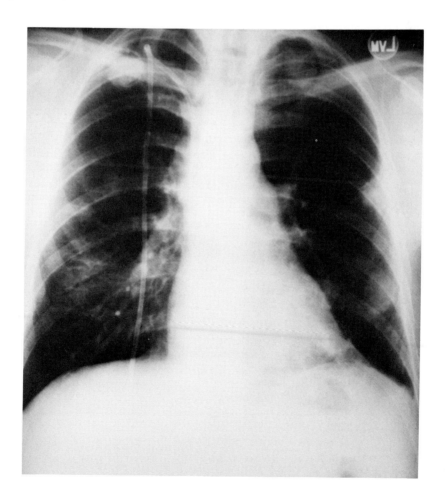

Diagnosis: Invasive pulmonary aspergillosis.

Discussion: Aspergillus species are common pathogens in immunocompromised patients, being second only to Candida as a cause of invasive mycosis. A ubiquitous saprophyte in soil and the hospital environment, Aspergillus is acquired via inhalation of airborne spores. Hematologic malignancies, granulocytopenia, and prolonged antibiotic therapy, as occurred in the present patient, are the most common risk factors; however, patients with lymphoma, organ transplants, and corticosteroid or cytotoxic chemotherapy also have lowered host defenses against Aspergillus infection.

The early pathologic lesions of pulmonary Aspergillosis are 1 to 3 cm nodules (target lesions) and comprise a central zone of tissue necrosis with a rim of hemorrhage adjacent to a thrombosed artery. These lesions may cavitate or progress to diffuse pulmonary consolidation. In 10 to 25% of patients dissemination occurs, with the brain being the most common site of metastatic infection.

Diagnosis of invasive aspergillosis is suspected in any immunocompromised patient with fever without defined source. Typical signs and symptoms include cough with or without sputum production, pleuritic chest pain, evidence of sinusitis or mastoiditis, and pulmonary rales or rhonchi. Rarely patients may be asymptomatic, presenting with a stable pulmonary nodule. Of note is the preservation of gas exchange in most patients with marked radiographic abnormalities, which is possibly attributable to the thrombosis of vasculature supplying infected lung zones, thereby preserving matching of ventilation with perfusion.

The radiographic manifestations of aspergillosis mirror the pathologic findings. Multiple bilateral nodular infiltrates represent the target lesions of early disease. These lesions progress to cavitation, diffuse alveolar infiltrates, or pleural based wedge-shaped infiltrates. The latter finding underlies the recommendation to consider aspergillosis in any immunocompromised patient with radiographic evidence of pulmonary infarction without accompanying clinical symptoms of thromboembolic disease. Chest CT scans show a characteristic pattern of a nodule with a surrounding "halo" of hyperlucency.

When suspected, the diagnosis of invasive aspergillosis must be aggressively pursued because of the 70% mortality. Sputum cultures are positive in less than 10% of patients and may represent saprophytic colonization. However, positive sputum cultures in immunocompromised patients with pulmonary infiltrates warrant initiation of antifungal therapy. Positive surveillance nasal cultures for Aspergillus in patients with leukemia may identify aspergillosis as the probable etiology of subsequent pulmonary infiltrates. Aspergillus precipitins are of no value in this setting, although tests for serodiagnosis of Aspergillus antigen are sensitive and specific but not widely available. In most centers, bronchoscopy or open lung biopsy is required to confirm the diagnosis. Broncho-alveolar lavage is particularly valuable in patients with bleeding diatheses and can provide specimens for culture, staining, and antigen detection.

After diagnosis and initiation of amphotericin B, a major complication is massive hemoptysis from pulmonary necrosis. Patients with cavitary infiltrates are at greatest risk for hemoptysis, which typically develops after peripheral neutrophil counts recover, allowing greater tissue inflammation and destruction.

The present patient underwent bronchoscopy, with transbronchial biopsy and bronchoalveolar lavage demonstrating *Aspergillus fumigatus* on pathologic and lavage specimens. He responded to amphotericin B.

Clinical Pearls

1. Radiographic manifestations of pulmonary infarction without associated symptoms of pulmonary embolism in a patient with leukemia suggest invasive aspergillosis.

2. Hemoptysis is a major complication of pulmonary aspergillosis that tends to occur after recovery of peripheral neutrophil counts.

REFERENCES

1. Gerson SL, Talbot GH, Hurwitz S, et al. Discriminant scorecard for diagnosis of invasive pulmonary aspergillosis in patients with acute leukemia. Am J Med 1985; 79:57–64.
2. Yu VL, Muder RR, Poorsattar A. Significance of isolation of Aspergillus from the respiratory tract in diagnosis of invasive pulmonary aspergillosis. Am J Med 1986; 81:249–254.
3. Albelda SM, Talbot GH, Gerson SL, et al. Pulmonary cavitation and massive hemoptysis in invasive pulmonary aspergillosis. Influence of bone marrow recovery in patients with acute leukemia. Am Rev Respir Dis 1985; 131:115–120.

PATIENT 57

A 63-year-old man with pain in the right shoulder, axilla, arm, and hand of 4 months' duration

A 63-year-old man with a 35 pack-year history of cigarette smoking was referred with a 4-month history of pain in the right shoulder which, at times, radiated anteriorly to the axilla and pain in the medial aspect of the right arm and hand. He had chronic cough and sputum production which was unchanged over several years. He denied hemoptysis, exposure to tuberculosis, or a previous PPD skin test.

Physical Examination: Vital signs normal; no acute distress; ptosis of the right eyelid; right pupil 2 mm, left pupil 4 mm; diminished breath sounds without adventitious sounds; minimal loss of sensation in the right 5th finger and the ulnar aspect of the 4th finger and ulnar border of the palm.

Laboratory Findings: WBC 8500/μl with normal differential, Hct 45%; routine chemistries normal. Chest radiograph: mass in the right apex, no hilar or mediastinal adenopathy. CT scan: right apical mass, no mediastinal or hilar adenopathy. Fiberoptic bronchoscopy was performed.

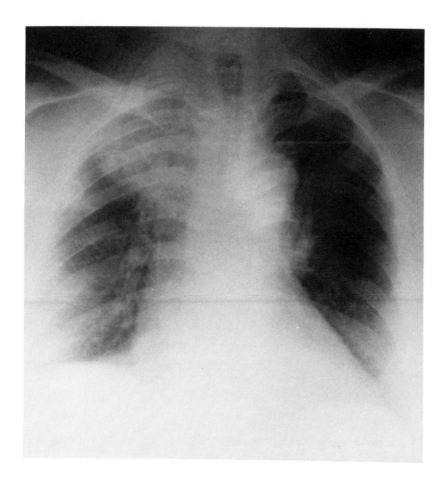

Diagnosis: Superior sulcus tumor (Pancoast tumor).

Discussion: Tumors in the apex of the lung with pain in the shoulder, ulnar neuropathy, Horner's syndrome, and vertebral invasion were first reported in the 1830s by a London surgeon. Almost 100 years later H.K. Pancoast characterized the radiographic features of this tumor. He defined such tumors as occurring at the thoracic inlet, producing constant pain in the ulnar distribution, and having associated Horner's syndrome.

A Pancoast tumor must be differentiated from the usual lung cancers of the upper lobe, as this tumor has a propensity to invade locally but not to metastasize, as is the tendency for carcinomas in other locations. Several centers have reported 5-year survival rates approaching 50% with preoperative radiation therapy and radical resection. This is in contrast to the low 5-year survival rate with most lung carcinomas in other locations.

Superior sulcus tumors originate in the apex of the lung and may be mistaken as pleural thickening. As the tumor spreads contiguously, local invasion of nerve and bone produces pain early in the course of the disease, sometimes before the mass is prominent radiographically. Symptoms associated with lung cancer of the upper lobe, such as hemoptysis or change in cough and sputum production, are notably absent, as are signs of mediastinal tumor invasion.

The typical patient presents with intense pain in the shoulder or scapula area which, at times, radiates to the anterior chest, proximal arm, or axilla. The pain, which at first is not impressive, tends to become more constant and severe and results in a visit to the physician several months following its onset. Ulnar neuropathy and Horner's syndrome may be present, depending on the stage of disease at presentation.

The chest radiograph shows an ill-defined apical lesion. CT scan will confirm the presence of the tumor and identify destructive bone lesions and the status of the mediastinum. The vertebral bodies are involved in approximately half of patients. The histologic diagnosis can be established by fiberoptic bronchoscopy or percutaneous needle biopsy with a cervical approach. Superior sulcus tumors may be squamous cell, adenocarcinoma, or large cell undifferentiated carcinoma.

The most successful therapy is low-dose preoperative radiation (3000 rads) followed by radical resection, which has led to 5-year survivals of 30 to 50%. Prognosis appears to depend on involvement of mediastinal lymph nodes. If these nodes are involved, survival is usually less than a year, with no patient surviving for more than 3 years. Without nodal involvement, the 5-year survival increases markedly.

The present patient was found to have squamous cell carcinoma of the lung by transbronchial biopsy. He received radiation therapy (3000 rads) followed 4 weeks later by surgical resection. The patient is alive 15 months postoperatively without symptoms and evidence of recurrence.

Clinical Pearls

1. Patients with superior sulcus tumor usually present with shoulder or scapula pain and, at times, have a barely perceptible apical lesion on chest radiograph.

2. The clinical manifestations of this tumor are due to the location in the superior pulmonary sulcus, which is adjacent to the first and second thoracic and eighth cervical roots, the stellate ganglion of the sympathetic chain, and the roots of the brachial plexus. Involvement of these structures causes pain in the shoulder and scapula area and the ulnar distribution of the arm, forearm and fingers, Horner's syndrome, and anhidrosis.

3. The presence or absence of mediastinal and hilar lymphadenopathy appears to be the most important factor in prognosis.

4. Preoperative radiotherapy followed 2 to 4 weeks later by resection has resulted in 5-year survivals of up to 50% in patients with negative mediastinal and hilar nodes.

REFERENCES

1. Pancoast HK. Superior pulmonary sulcus tumor: tumor characterized by pain, Horner's syndrome, destruction of bone and atrophy of hand muscles. JAMA 1932; 99:1391–1396.
2. Shaw RR, Paulsen BL, Kee JL Jr. Treatment of the superior sulcus tumor by irradiation followed by resection. Ann Surg 1961; 154:29–40.
3. Paulson BL. Carcinomas in the superior pulmonary sulcus. J Thorac Cardiovasc Surg 1975; 70:1095–1104.
4. Shahian DM, Neptune WB, Ellis FH Jr. Pancoast tumors: improved survival with preoperative and postoperative radiotherapy. Ann Thorac Surg 1987; 43:32–38.

PATIENT 58

A 46-year-old woman with bone pain and multiple pulmonary nodules with left hilar adenopathy

A 46-year-old woman was evaluated for bone pain and an abnormal chest radiograph. Four years earlier, she developed cutaneous malignant melanoma on her shoulder (Clark level IV) with negative lymph nodes. She underwent wide resection and adjuvant therapy with BCG vaccine. She did well until developing pain over her forearms and lower legs after being lost to follow-up for 1 year.

Physical Examination: Vital signs normal; skin normal except for a well-healed skin graft; lymph nodes negative; chest normal; abdomen no organomegaly; tenderness over tibial ridges and distal ulna.

Laboratory Findings: Routine blood and liver function tests normal; sputum cytology negative. Chest radiograph demonstrated multiple bilateral pulmonary nodules with left hilar adenopathy.

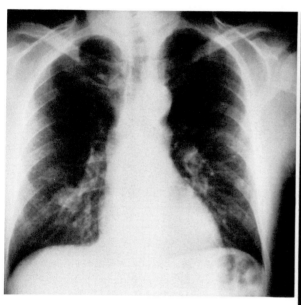 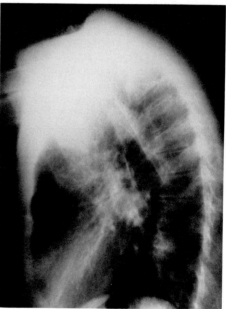

Diagnosis: Metastatic malignant melanoma with hypertrophic osteoarthropathy.

Discussion: During the last decade, the clinical significance of malignant melanoma has expanded because of a doubling of its frequency to 2% of all malignancies and the resistance of disseminated disease to chemotherapy protocols. The challenge is to improve prognosis—the majority of patients with malignant melanoma die within 10 years. The increasing incidence specifically challenges the pulmonologist, since 16% of patients have some form of intrathoracic metastases.

Metastatic melanoma to the lung presents several pulmonary manifestations. Pulmonary nodules may appear as solitary or multiple with occasional diffuse miliary nodules; 50% of patients with pulmonary nodules due to malignant melanoma also have enlarged hilar and mediastinal lymph nodes that are involved secondarily from lymphatics draining the nodules. Malignant pleural effusions also occur, but endobronchial metastases are rare. Symptoms include weight loss, cough, and shortness of breath with occasional paraneoplastic syndromes such as hypertrophic osteoarthropathy, as demonstrated by the present patient.

Therapy for disseminated malignant melanoma is discouraging. Cytotoxic protocols using DTIC result in response rates of only 13 to 18%, and combination drug protocols showing 40% response rates have not withstood the challenge of large prospective trials. The resistance of melanoma to standard cytotoxic agents has generated a proliferation of research that has recently employed newer agents such as interferon and viral oncolysate, a potential immunostimulant.

Because disseminated melanoma responds poorly to chemotherapy, and many patients with pulmonary metastases die of lung involvement, investigators have pursued pulmonary metastasectomy as a therapeutic modality. First reported in 1939, resection of pulmonary metastases has been shown to improve long-term, tumor-free survival in certain nonmelanoma malignant cell types. Tumors, such as soft tissue sarcoma, osteosarcoma, hypernephroma, and nonseminomatous testicular tumors, demonstrate hematogenous spread with the pulmonary capillary bed filtering the malignant cells. Such malignancies appear to disseminate in a step-wise fashion, first involving one organ, such as the lung, before spreading widely. If metastases limited to the lung are removed, tumor-free survival can be improved, as clearly demonstrated for osteogenic sarcoma.

The utility of resection of pulmonary nodules due to malignant melanoma is less well supported. Melanoma usually spreads to the lung synchronous with other viscera rather than as an initial single stage of dissemination. Since partial resection of metastatic disease is of no value, patients with melanoma involving other organs need to be excluded from pulmonary resection. Similarly, pulmonary resection should be complete, avoiding omission of radiographically occult nodules. Since plain chest films miss 20 to 50% of metastatic melanoma pulmonary nodules, preoperative CT scanning should be employed. Tumors involving the pleura, chest wall, or diaphragm have a markedly decreased survival and should not be considered for resection.

After careful staging and control of the primary tumor, resection is considered if metastatic melanoma appears localized to the lung nodules. Several groups have demonstrated that rapidly growing melanomas do not respond well to resection, and recommend repeating a CT scan 40 to 60 days after biopsy confirmation of the tumor. If the metastases appear radiographically stable, resection is performed; if the doubling time is faster than 40 to 60 days, chemotherapy is instituted. The present patient underwent percutaneous needle aspiration, confirming metastatic melanoma, but refused further evaluation.

Clinical Pearls

1. Plain chest films do not detect 20 to 50% of pulmonary metastases from malignant melanoma.

2. Up to 16% of patients with malignant melanoma have some form of pulmonary involvement.

3. Malignant melanoma metastatic to the lung usually involves other viscera, decreasing the utility of pulmonary metastasectomy.

REFERENCES

1. Chiles C, Ravin CE. Intrathoracic metastasis from an extrathoracic malignancy: a radiologic approach to patient evaluation. Radiol Clin North Am 1985; 23:427–437.
2. Wellner LJ, Putman CE. Imaging of occult pulmonary metastases: State of the art. CA 1986; 36:48–58.
3. Seegar J, Richman SP, Allegra JC. Systemic therapy of malignant melanoma. Med Clin North Am 1986; 70:89–94.

PATIENT 59

A 34-year-old man with blunt chest trauma and mediastinal emphysema

A 34-year-old man was admitted in coma to the intensive care unit after being involved in an automobile accident. He was found slumped over the steering wheel and was intubated at the scene because of depressed respirations.

Physical Examination: Vital signs stable. Large bruise over the sternum with subcutaneous emphysema over the anterior chest extending into the neck. Diffuse rhonchi with equal breath sounds; a "crunching" sound present with each heart beat. The endotracheal tube contained a small amount of fresh blood. The patient was unconscious, responding with withdrawal from painful stimuli.

Laboratory Findings: Chest radiograph revealed mediastinal and subcutaneous emphysema without evidence of pneumothorax or broken bones. The endotracheal tube was appropriately positioned.

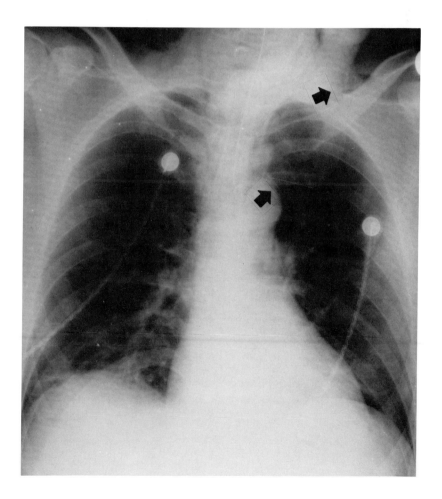

Diagnosis: Traumatic disruption of the intrathoracic trachea.

Discussion: Although major injury to the tracheobronchial tree is relatively rare, it has become more common during the last several decades largely due to an increase in high-speed traffic accidents. Because of its 30% mortality rate and uncommon occurrence, high clinical suspicion and awareness of the typical clinical presentation are required to diagnose tracheobronchial disruption.

Disruption of the intrathoracic trachea and bronchi usually results from blunt thoracic trauma with rapid deceleration as occurs with steering wheel injuries. The exact pathogenesis of injury is uncertain, but three mechanisms appear likely. First, the lungs are relatively mobile in the chest, whereas the trachea and mainstem bronchi are stiff and fixed in the mediastinum. During a rapid deceleration injury, the lungs continue forward and shear the trachea and bronchi usually at a point within 2 cm of the carina. Second, the usual closed position of the glottis at the time of anticipated impact causes chest compression that raises airway pressure beyond the elastic strength of the tracheobronchial walls. Lastly, anteroposterior chest compression causes lateral expansion of the thorax, which separates the two lungs from the midline, resulting in lateral traction of the bronchi at the carina.

The clinical manifestations of tracheobronchial disruption are diverse. With a complete disruption of the airway, pneumothorax is present, with the lung occasionally sagging in the thorax rather than the more typical collapse toward the hilum. Chest tube resuscitation may show a massive air leak and failure of lung reexpansion. Pneumothorax may be lacking if an airleak does not rupture into the pleural space. Dissection of air through the mediastinum into the adjacent cervical planes may result in a pneumomediastinum with subcutaneous emphysema, as in the present patient. Additional signs and symptoms include dyspnea, hemoptysis, and a mediastinal "crunch" noted during thoracic auscultation. In 10% of instances, patients may lack airway symptoms or an air leak, and the diagnosis is suspected entirely on the basis of the severity of thoracic trauma. In these instances, fractures of the first and third ribs indicate a tremendous crushing injury, suggesting associated tracheobronchial disruption.

When suspected, the diagnosis should be urgently evaluated to assess the degree of airway disruption. If the injury remains undiagnosed and not primarily repaired, subsequent airway healing and granulation may result in tracheal or bronchial strictures that cause obstructive atelectasis. Fiberoptic bronchoscopy is the most reliable diagnostic technique, allowing examination of the tracheobronchial tree for complete airway laceration or small tears.

If tracheobronchial disruption is detected by bronchoscopy, thoracic surgical consultation is required to determine the therapeutic approach. Occasionally, small tears of the membranous portion of the trachea or bronchi may be managed with a tracheotomy, allowing reduction of airway pressures and air leaks. If rupture is present, thoracotomy is urgently required to permit primary repair. Results are usually excellent, except when an accompanying respiratory failure requires mechanical ventilation with high airway pressures that may disrupt the surgical anastomosis.

The present patient underwent fiberoptic bronchoscopy demonstrating a laceration of the distal trachea one cm above the carina. He underwent early median sternotomy with end-to-end anastomosis of the trachea, subsequently fully recovering from his cerebral contusion.

Clinical Pearls

1. Blunt chest trauma with deceleration injuries is the most common cause of tracheobronchial disruption.

2. Pneumothorax, mediastinal emphysema, subcutaneous emphysema, and hemoptysis are clinical signs of tracheobronchial injury.

3. In the absence of airway symptoms or an air leak, chest trauma sufficiently severe to fracture the first three ribs is cause to exclude tracheobronchial disruption.

REFERENCES

1. Shackford SR. Blunt chest trauma: The intensivist's perspective. J Intens Care Med 1986; 1:125–136.
2. Bertelsen S, Howitz P. Injuries of the trachea and bronchi. Thorax 1972; 27:188–194.
3. Scully RE, Galdabini JJ, McNeely BU. Case records of the Massachusetts General Hospital. N Engl J Med 1981; 19:1155–1160.
4. Eastridge CE, Hughes FA Jr, Pate JW, et al. Tracheobronchial injury caused by blunt trauma. Am Rev Respir Dis 1970; 101:230–237.

PATIENT 60

A 40-year-old man with weight loss, productive cough, hemoptysis, and a hereditary disorder

A 40-year-old man was referred because of weight loss, productive cough, and hemoptysis. A hereditary disorder was diagnosed at age five. He had a 25 pack-year history of cigarette smoking and a positive PPD skin test.

Physical Examination: Temperature 98°; short male in no acute distress; multiple cutaneous lesions, particularly over the anterior chest; dark lesion in the iris. Chest examination: minimal scattered rhonchi without other adventitious sounds.

Laboratory Findings: WBC 7000/μl with normal differential; Hct 35%; ESR 40 mm/h. Liver function tests, electrolytes, calcium and phosphorus normal. Chest radiograph (3 months prior): multiple nodular lesions projected over lung fields (below left). The patient had the majority of these skin lesions removed shortly after the chest radiograph was obtained. A repeat chest radiograph (below right) was obtained and a diagnostic procedure performed.

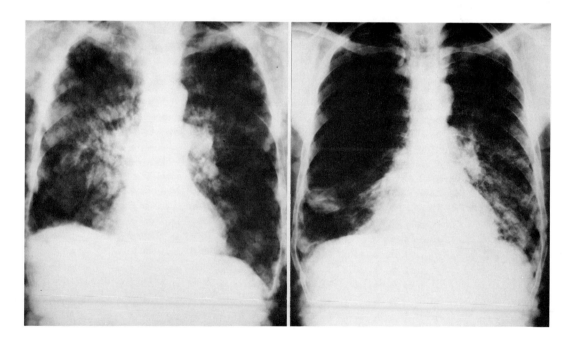

Diagnosis: Adenocarcinoma of the lung in a patient with neurofibromatosis (von Recklinghausen's disease).

Discussion: Neurofibromatosis is a hereditary autosomal dominant (1 in 3000 births), progressive, hamartomatous disorder that primarily involves the ectoderm and mesoderm. It is one of the neurocutaneous disorders along with tuberous sclerosis and ataxia-telangiectasia that has pulmonary manifestations. Von Recklinghausen's disease usually is first recognized by the presence of multiple cafe-au-lait spots or cutaneous neurofibromas. A lisch nodule (melanocytic hamartoma of the iris) is seen in almost all patients over 5 years of age. Other findings include an increased incidence in schwannomas, interstitial lung disease, lateral meningoceles, dural ectasia, and kyphoscoliosis, and risk of malignancy.

Neurofibromas are composed of all elements of the nerve, including Schwann cells, nerve fibers, and fibroblasts. The involved nerve is expanded and diffusely infiltrated by tumor. Schwannomas, in contrast, are encapsulated and lie on the surface of the nerve rather than infiltrate it.

The chest radiograph usually reveals multiple rounded densities that represent skin nodules projected over the lung fields. With only a few lesions, the radiograph may be misinterpreted as that of pulmonary parenchymal nodules; skin lesion markers or tomograms can resolve the issue. With multiple cutaneous lesions projected over the lung fields, a pulmonary nodule may be overlooked. Due to the increased rate of malignancy in neurofibromatosis, pulmonary nodules should be diligently sought. Chest CT is helpful in excluding pulmonary metastatic disease in patients with known primary malignant lesions.

Other lesions that may be seen on chest radiograph include: (1) solitary neurofibromas or schwannomas involving the sympathetic chain, vagus, phrenic, or intercostal nerves that may present as an extrapleural mass, paraspinal mass, or mediastinal mass; (2) lateral meningocele seen as a discrete mass in the intrathoracic paravertebral area; (3) interstitial lung disease of the reticulonodular variety usually more extensive in the bases, postulated to be due to a mesenchymal defect resulting in a primary deposition of collagen rather than to a post-inflammatory reparative process (incidence variable); (4) thoracic skeletal abnormalities, including scoliosis with or without kyphosis (incidence 10%); (5) posterior scalloping of the vertebral bodies; and (6) twisted rib deformity.

Patients are at increased risk for malignancy usually due to benign nerve tumors that have undergone malignant transformation into neurofibrosarcomas (incidence 5%). CT is helpful in identifying and defining the extent of nonpalpable neurofibrosarcomas and may be particularly helpful in identifying a parenchymal nodule among multiple projected skin lesions over the thorax. The diagnosis of malignancy is often difficult and delayed, contributing to poor survival rate.

In the present patient, repeat chest radiograph showed a large lesion in the right lower lung field. Fiberoptic bronchoscopy with transbronchial biopsy revealed adenocarcinoma. CT scan of the chest showed no abnormal mediastinal or hilar nodes. The patient had a right lower lobectomy and is disease-free 18 months following surgery.

Clinical Pearls

1. In patients with neurofibromatosis, multiple skin nodules projected over the thorax may obscure a pulmonary nodule; CT of the thorax will help in this differentiation.

2. There is an increased incidence of malignancy most commonly due to the malignant transformation of benign nerve tumors into neurofibrosarcomas, which then may metastasize to the lungs. In patients with a known neurofibrosarcoma, chest CT will be helpful in excluding pulmonary metastases.

3. Interstitial lung disease of the reticulonodular variety is associated with neurofibromatosis (approximately 5%, reported range 1 to 29%) and may be due to a primary deposition of collagen rather than an inflammatory process.

REFERENCES
1. Davies PDB. The diffuse pulmonary involvement in von Recklinghausen's disease: a new syndrome. Thorax 1963; 8:198.
2. Schabel SI, Schmidt GE, Vujic I. Overlooked pulmonary malignancy in neurofibromatosis. J Can Assoc Radiol 1983; 31:135–136.
3. Sack GH Jr. Malignant complications of neurofibromatosis. Clin Oncol 1983; 9:17–23.
4. Aughenbaugh GL. Thoracic manifestations of neurocutaneous diseases. Radiol Clin North Am 1984; 22:741–756.

PATIENT 61

A 49-year-old woman with a 6-month history of dyspnea, weight loss, fatigue, easy bruising, and recent hemoptysis

A 49-year-old woman was transferred for evaluation of hemoptysis. She was well until 6 months prior to admission when she noticed increasing dyspnea on exertion, which progressed to dyspnea at rest. Approximately 1 week prior to admission, she had hemoptysis. She had lost 40 pounds, and had fatigue and easy bruising. She was not a cigarette smoker.

Physical Examination: Temperature 97.6°, pulse 112; respirations 36. Obese female in moderate respiratory distress; numerous ecchymoses; no lymphadenopathy. Chest examination: decreased breath sounds in both bases; no breast masses. Cardiac examination: normal except for tachycardia. Pelvic and abdominal examinations: normal.

Laboratory Findings: WBC 10,700/μl, 56% PMNs, 10% bands, 15% lymphocytes, 6% eosinophils, 3% metamyelocytes, 2% myelocytes, 4% nucleated red blood cells; Hct 36%; platelet count 43,000/μl; PT and PTT normal; fibrinogen 415 mg/dl. Chest radiograph: decreased lung volumes, silhouette sign of the left hemidiaphragm with increased opacity in the left retrocardiac region; left hilar prominence; increased interstitial markings bilaterally. Lateral decubitus: small free-flowing pleural effusions bilaterally. ABG (room air): pH 7.52, PCO_2 17 mmHg, PO_2 65 mmHg. A bone marrow aspirate and biopsy were performed.

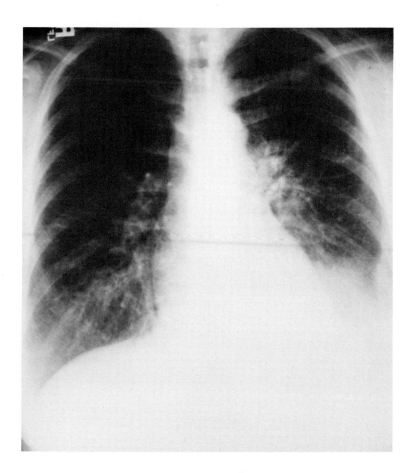

Diagnosis: Adenocarcinoma of the lung with lymphangitic metastasis and involvement of the bone marrow.

Discussion: Lymphangitic metastasis to the lungs is most common in carcinoma of the breast, lung, and stomach, and is seen with increased frequency in thyroid, pancreatic, and laryngeal carcinoma. Lymphangitic carcinomatosis has been observed in up to 40% of patients with breast cancer at autopsy. Two possible pathogenetic mechanisms for lymphangitic carcinomatosis are: (1) pulmonary vascular embolization with subsequent tumor invasion through the blood vessel walls and into adjacent lymphatics; and (2) less commonly, retrograde lymphatic invasion from mediastinal and hilar lymph nodes. Radiographic differentiation of these two mechanisms is virtually impossible, although the absence of hilar and mediastinal node involvement may suggest hematogenous spread. Once the mediastinal lymph nodes become infiltrated with metastatic cells, the lymphatics may become functionally obstructed and the valves rendered incompetent.

The diagnosis of lymphangitic carcinomatosis can be suspected from the chest radiograph. An increase of bronchovascular markings, which tend to be coarse and irregular and most prominent in the lower lobes, is characteristic. There may be a nodular component, making the pattern reticulonodular. At autopsy, hilar and mediastinal lymph nodes are virtually always involved but may not be detected radiographically. Invasion of the septa or edema of the septa from lymphatic obstruction may produce septal lines (Kerley B). Rarely, the chest radiograph may be normal when the patient presents with marked dyspnea. A lung scan that shows multiple, irregular, peripheral perfusion defects caused by tumor emboli in small arteries and arterioles is compatible with the diagnosis; ventilation scans are normal.

Patients usually present with progressive dyspnea that is incapacitating by the time there is definitive radiographic disease. Hypoxemia with hypocapnia and respiratory alkalosis is universally present. Pulmonary function studies show a restrictive ventilatory defect; however, the diffusing capacity may be the only abnormal finding. Lymphangitic carcinomatosis is a cause of subacute cor pulmonale. The survival of patients with lymphangitic carcinomatosis is short, in the range of a few weeks to few months. Anecdotes of lung radiation and combination chemotherapy inducing remission and prolonged survival in patients with breast carcinoma have been reported.

Bone marrow biopsy in the present patient demonstrated poorly differentiated adenocarcinoma with the majority of the marrow space containing either nests of malignant cells or benign fibrous tissue. Mammography was negative. Bronchoscopy was not performed because of the patient's decision that intubation not be performed. She died on the eighth hospital day, 4 days following intracerebral hemorrhage due to thrombocytopenia. Postmortem examination showed adenocarcinoma of the left lower lobe metastatic to the hilar and mediastinal lymph nodes and involving the lymphatics of both lungs.

Carcinoma of the lung is one of the solid tumors most often associated with myelophthisic anemia; invasion of the bone marrow by tumor impairs both erythropoiesis and thrombopoiesis, with neutrophil production being normal or decreased. Myelophthisis causes distortion of the microcirculation of the marrow with premature release of normoblasts and immature myeloid cells.

Clinical Pearls

1. Carcinoma of the breast, stomach, lung, pancreas, thyroid, and larynx are the most common sites of origin of a predominantly lymphangitic metastatic pattern in the lungs.

2. Patients may present with severe dyspnea due to lymphangitic carcinomatosis and have a normal chest radiograph. A perfusion lung scan showing multiple irregular peripheral defects and a normal ventilation scan may be present with a normal chest radiograph.

3. A characteristic radiographic pattern is irregular reticular opacities most prominent in the lower lobes, hilar and mediastinal adenopathy, pleural effusions, and septal lines; at times, nodular densities may predominate.

REFERENCES

1. Hauser TE, Steer A. Lymphangitic carcinomatosis of the lungs: 6 case reports and a review of the literature. Ann Intern Med 1951; 34:881–898.
2. Harold JT. Lymphangitis carcinomatosa of the lungs. Q J Med 1952; 21:353–360.
3. Green M, Swanson L, Kern W, et al. Lymphangitic carcinomatosis: lung scan abnormalities. J Nucl Med 1976; 17:258–260.
4. Emirgil C, Zsoldos S, Heinemann H. Effect of metastatic carcinoma to the lung on pulmonary function in man. Am J Med 1964; 36:382–394.

PATIENT 62

A 39-year-old man presenting with ascites, edema, dyspnea, and bilateral pleural effusions 15 years after orchiectomy and mediastinal radiation therapy for a seminoma

A 39-year-old man was admitted with a several-week history of ascites, bilateral leg edema, dyspnea on exertion, orthopnea, and cough. Past history revealed an orchiectomy for seminoma of the left testicle followed by radiation therapy to the mediastinum and periaortic area 15 years prior. Radiation therapy consisted of 30 treatments over 45 days that included 4200 rads to the anterior mediastinum and 2600 rads to the posterior mediastinum.

Physical Examination: Temperature 98.6°; pulse 96 and regular; respirations 20; blood pressure 120/80 with a pulsus paradoxus of 15; no acute distress; neck vein distention at 45° with collapse on inspiration; diastolic knock present; evidence of a large right pleural effusion; hepatomegaly; ascites; bilateral peripheral edema.

Laboratory Findings: WBC 4,400/μl; Hct 41%; LDH 152 IU/L, SGOT 33 IU/L. Chest radiograph: large right pleural effusion and a small left effusion. Cardiac silhouette normal. Right heart catheterization: right atrial pressure 22 mmHg, right ventricular pressure 35/20 mmHg, pulmonary artery 35/20 mmHg (mean 25 mmHg), pulmonary capillary wedge pressure 22 mmHg, cardiac output 4.2 L/min. Thoracentesis: clear yellow fluid, nucleated cells 200/μl, 70% lymphocytes, 20% macrophages, protein 4.0 g/dl, PF/S ratio .52, LDH 55 IU/L, pH 7.45, glucose 108 mg/dl, cytology negative.

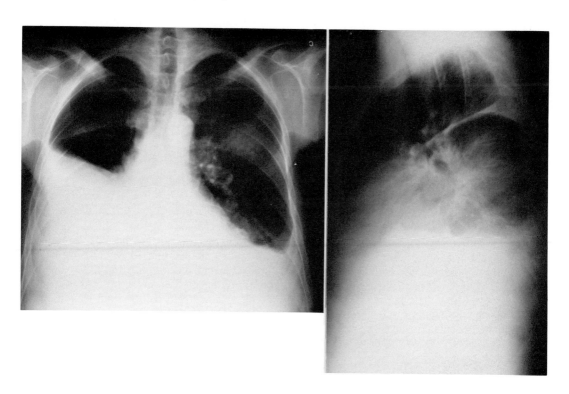

Diagnosis: Constrictive pericarditis secondary to radiation therapy with bilateral pleural effusions.

Discussion: The diagnosis of constrictive pericarditis requires a high index of suspicion following a detailed history and meticulous physical examination. The history may include malignancy (mesothelioma, lung and breast cancer or lymphoma and leukemia), uremia, radiation therapy to the mediastinum, or infectious pericarditis (viral, bacterial, or tuberculous). Less common causes are SLE, rheumatoid disease, and trauma.

Presenting manifestations include unexplained weight gain, fatigue, dyspnea on exertion, peripheral edema, and ascites. The abdomen always appears enlarged due to hepatomegaly and ascites. Also, there is always jugular vein distention with evidence of diastolic collapse. The carotid pulse frequently is small in amplitude. Auscultation may reveal an extra heart sound (diastolic knock) early in diastole before the classic S3 is appreciated. EKG typically shows nonspecific ST and T wave changes. The chest radiograph usually reveals a normal cardiac silhouette, may show pericardial calcification (best seen on the lateral view), and generally shows pleural effusions, usually bilateral.

It was thought that radiation therapy rarely produced myocardial or pericardial disease. However, it appears that when doses of > 4000 rads are administered to the anterior mediastinum, the incidence of radiation-induced heart disease is approximately 3 to 7%. The most striking feature pathologically is fibrosis with thickening of the parietal pericardium. Pericardial effusion is usually found. Myocardial injury is characterized by diffuse interstitial fibrosis. It may be difficult to distinguish pericardial disease alone from combined pericardial and myocardial involvement.

The radiation fields, dose, and fractionation are of help in implicating the likelihood of radiation-induced heart disease. Pericardial tolerance may be as low as 1500 rads if over 50% of the heart is included in the radiation field; however, a greater number of rads appears to be tolerated with less direct heart radiation. The timing of radiation pericardial damage is not the same as for radiation pneumonitis. Approximately 60% of pericardial changes are detected from 4 to 12 months following completion of therapy, 20% detected from 1 to 2 years following therapy, and 20% more than 2 years after the completion of radiation therapy.

In a known malignancy, development of a pericardial effusion is of concern, and the pericardial fluid needs to be evaluated as any newly diagnosed effusion. Bloody pericardial fluid suggests a malignant process; however, the absence of tumor cells does not exclude the diagnosis. Radiation-induced pericardial effusion usually is a serous exudate without other distinguishing characteristics. Pleural effusions from constrictive pericarditis result from increased hydrostatic pressures, as the patient has diastolic equalization of pressures with both pulmonary and systemic venous hypertension. It has been documented that combined venous hypertension is associated with a high incidence of pleural effusions. The effusions, therefore, should be transudative in nature; however, chronic transudative effusions in a patient on diuretic therapy may lead to increased total protein concentrations in the exudative range.

The present patient underwent pericardiectomy because of worsening symptoms and experienced partial relief. Underlying myocardial fibrosis probably accounted for the suboptimal response to pericardiectomy.

Clinical Pearls

1. Patients who receive > 4000 rads to the anterior mediastinum are at risk for the development of constrictive pericarditis.

2. In contrast to patients with radiation pneumonitis, who always present within the first 6 months following completion of therapy, almost half of patients with radiation-induced pericardial disease present at least 1 year following therapy.

3. Patients with constrictive pericarditis commonly have bilateral pleural effusions that are usually transudative in nature but may have an elevated pleural fluid protein, especially if the effusion is chronic and the patient is receiving diuretics.

REFERENCES

1. Lidshitz HI, Southard ME. Complications of radiation therapy: the thorax. Semin Roentgenol 1974; 9:41–49.
2. Stewart JR, Fajardo LF. Radiation-induced heart disease. Clinical and experimental aspects. Radiol Clin North Am 1971; 9:511–531.
3. Morton DL, Kagan AR, Roberts WC, et al. Pericardiectomy for radiation-induced pericarditis with effusion. Ann Thorac Surg 1969; 8:195–208.

PATIENT 63

A 49-year-old man with fever, chills, night sweats, purulent sputum, and hemoptysis of 2 months' duration

A 49-year-old man was admitted with a 2-month history of cough with purulent sputum production, hemoptysis, anorexia, malaise, fever, chills, and night sweats. He was treated by his local physician with multiple antibiotics for pneumonia, initially a right-sided unilobar process. Antibiotic treatment resulted in minimal clinical improvement and subsequent exacerbation. Fiberoptic bronchoscopy with biopsies were nondiagnostic and cultures for AFB and fungi were negative. There was chest radiographic progression with multilobar involvement on the right and cavitation. Open lung biopsy showed nonspecific inflammation. Antibiotics and corticosteroids were instituted. He was admitted to our hospital 3 weeks later with worsening symptoms.

Physical Examination: Temperature 101°; pulse 110; respirations 36; appeared chronically ill, cachectic, and in moderate respiratory distress; white plaques in oropharynx on an erythematous base; bilateral basilar rales with diffuse wheezing; neurologic exam normal.

Laboratory Findings: WBC 30,600/μl, 75% PMNs, 5% bands, 15% lymphocytes, Hct 35%. ABG (room air): pH 7.49, PCO$_2$ 34 mmHg, PO$_2$ 53 mmHg. Chest radiograph: bilateral alveolar infiltrates diffusely throughout the right lung and involving the left lower lobe with cavitation and air-fluid levels on the right. A transbronchial biopsy and BAL were performed.

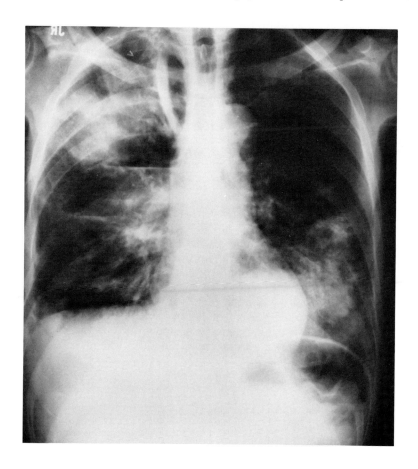

Diagnosis: Nocardia pneumonia.

Discussion: Nocardia, a soil inhabitant, is not normally found in the oropharynx or intestinal tract; therefore, isolation of the organism from sputum or exudate generally indicates infection. Man usually becomes infected by inhalation of the organism; however, there is no proof of man-to-man or animal-to-man transmission. Nocardia occurs in both normal and immunocompromised hosts. Groups particularly susceptible to nocardiosis are those with hematologic malignancies, other malignant diseases, sarcoidosis, and alveolar proteinosis. Transplant recipients, patients receiving corticosteroids, and those having prolonged neutropenia also are at increased risk.

Following the initial infection in the lungs, the pneumonitis advances to a necrotic stage, resulting in multiple abscess formation. The chest wall may be involved by direct extension, and lymphohematogenous spread may result in lesions in the brain, skin, bone, and liver.

The clinical spectrum of nocardia ranges from an acute, fulminant disease to one of insidious onset and chronicity. The most typical presentation is of a subacute pneumonitis that is progressive. Patients usually report cough productive of purulent and often blood-tinged sputum, persistent fevers, and night sweats. Chest pain usually reflects extension to the pleura. Leukocytosis and anemia are common. The underlying disease often masks nocardia, which tends to run a more fulminant course in the immunocompromised host. The chest radiograph varies, depending on the stage of disease. Patterns include (1) single or multiple large nodules, (2) thick-walled cavities, (3) subsegmental or lobar consolidation with a tendency toward cavitation, and (4) a miliary pattern.

The diagnosis depends upon culturing the organism from sputum, pleural fluid, or other exudate. Serologic tests are of no clinical value. Multiple specimens should be cultured and the laboratory notified that nocardia is suspected. Problems that may make recovery difficult are (1) contamination with other bacteria, (2) slow growth, and (3) loss of the organism during the concentration procedure for identification of mycobacteria. The diagnosis of nocardiosis can be inferred by identifying gram-positive branching filaments that are weakly acid-fast in the specimen.

Nocardia pneumonia should be in the differential diagnosis of any chronic pneumonia, which also includes tuberculosis, atypical mycobacteria, actinomycosis, anaerobic lung abscess, and fungal diseases. Fiberoptic bronchoscopy with transbronchial biopsy and bronchoalveolar lavage should be done in patients with undiagnosed chronic pneumonia.

Any of the sulfonamides, sulfadiazine, sulfisoxazole, or trimethoprim-sulfamethoxazole, is appropriate therapy. It is important that peak serum levels be maintained between 10 and 20 mg/dl. To prevent relapse, especially in the immunocompromised individual, a prolonged course of therapy (from 6 to 12 months) is necessary. Abscesses or empyema should be drained. Even with appropriate treatment, there is a 25% mortality. Factors that portend a poor prognosis include (1) a short duration of symptoms; (2) corticosteroid or cytotoxic drug therapy; and (3) presence of central nervous system involvement.

The present patient was treated with sulfadiazine, 8 g daily (peak serum levels 14–16 mg/dl), with good clinical response.

Clinical Pearls

1. Nocardia should be considered in the differential diagnosis of any patient with chronic pneumonia, especially those unresponsive to conventional antibiotic therapy.

2. Risk factors for nocardia pneumonia include organ transplantation, corticosteroid therapy, alveolar proteinosis, sarcoidosis, neutropenia, and malignancy.

3. The laboratory should be notified that nocardia is suspected so that they will take special precautions to optimize identification of the organism.

4. Isolation of nocardia from the sputum in a patient with new pulmonary infiltrates highly suggests the diagnosis, as nocardia is not a normal inhabitant of the oropharynx.

REFERENCES

1. Palmer DL, Harvey RL, Wheeler JK. Diagnostic and therapeutic considerations in *Nocardia asteroides* infection. Medicine 1974; 53:391–401.
2. Young LS, Armstrong D, Blevens AN, Lieberman P. *Nocardia asteroides* infection complicating neoplastic disease. Am J Med 1971; 53:356–367.
3. Neu HC, Silva M, Hazen E, Rosenheim SH. Necrotizing nocardial pneumonitis. Ann Intern Med 1967; 66:274–284.

PATIENT 64

A 26-year-old man with wheezing, fever, chills, and pulmonary infiltrates

A 26-year-old white male was referred for evaluation of poorly controlled asthma. He had a history of rhinitis, eczema and occasional wheezing as a child; symptoms resolved during adolescence. During the previous 2 years, he had several emergency room visits and was hospitalized on three occasions for severe asthma. These episodes were characterized by fever, chills, wheezing, expectoration of brownish sputum, and infiltrates on chest radiograph. He was treated for an exacerbation of asthma due to pneumonia and had gradual improvement.

Physical Examination: Temperature 100°; respirations 20; no acute distress. Chest examination: minimal scattered expiratory wheezes. Remainder of examination unremarkable.

Laboratory Findings: WBC 11,000/μl, 18% eosinophils. Sputum smear: multiple eosinophils with rare PMNs. Sputum culture: positive for *Aspergillus fumigatus*; positive precipitating antibodies to *Aspergillus fumigatus*; positive prick-test to Aspergillus; serum IgE 3300 ng/ml. Chest radiograph: numerous round and elliptical opacities in a perihilar distribution with a predominance in the upper lobes; several of the densities with a "Y" or "V" configuration pointing toward the hilum; homogeneous densities in the right lower lobe; several ring shadows.

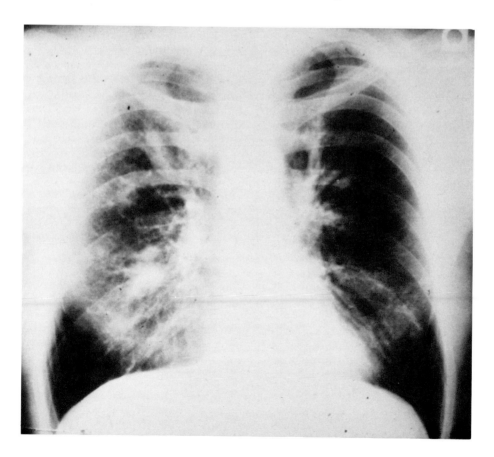

Diagnosis: Allergic bronchopulmonary aspergillosis (ABPA).

Discussion: First described in England in 1952 by Hinson and colleagues, ABPA has been diagnosed frequently in this country but diagnosis often is delayed, as the presentation mimics simple asthma, bacterial pneumonia, or, on occasion, the granulomatous diseases. In contrast to the usual asthmatic, these individuals frequently require high-dose, prolonged corticosteroid therapy to establish a remission.

ABPA should be considered in any asthmatic exacerbation associated with fever and chills, fleeting or fixed pulmonary infiltrates, or expectoration of brownish plugs; some have mild symptoms despite extensive chest radiographic abnormalities. Radiographically, the dilated mucus-plugged proximal bronchi appear as elliptical or oval opacities more common in the upper lobes. Depending on the extent of bronchial involvement, the mucous plugs may form a "Y" or "V" shadow on the radiograph, with the leg of the "Y" and point of the "V" directed toward the hilum. Tomography, and possibly CT scan, can define proximal saccular bronchiectasis with a normal peripheral bronchial tree, in contrast to the usual form of bronchiectasis in which the peripheral bronchi are predominantly affected with central sparing. Other radiographic features include homogeneous consolidation or evidence of previous bronchial disease in the form of parallel lines or ring shadows that represent proximal bronchiectasis. When mucoid impaction is present, the lung distal to the obstruction is usually air-containing, probably due to collateral ventilation, and may show segmental atelectasis and cavitation. The radiographic differential diagnosis includes tuberculosis, bacterial pneumonia, Loffler's syndrome, and bronchocentric granulomatosis.

The criteria for the diagnosis of ABPA include: asthma, a history of pulmonary infiltrates, a positive prick-test to *Aspergillus fumigatus* antigen, positive precipitating antibodies to *Aspergillus fumigatus* during an acute attack, and an increased serum IgE ($>$ 2000 ng/ml) unless the patient is on corticosteroids. Criteria strongly suggestive of the diagnosis include saccular proximal bronchiectasis and elevated specific IgE and IgG against *Aspergillus fumigatus*. Blood and sputum eosinophilia, expectoration of brown plugs, and growth of Aspergillus from the sputum are usually found.

ABPA is not an invasive disease but is caused by an altered host response to colonization of the Aspergillus antigens in the proximal bronchi. A variety of immunologic mechanisms appear to be responsible and include IgE-mediated hypersensitivity, antigen-antibody immune complex reactions and, possibly, cell-mediated delayed hypersensitivity, alternate pathway complement activation and antibody-dependent cellular cytotoxicity.

Corticosteroids, the treatment of choice, should be given at moderate dosages of 0.5 to 1.0 mg/kg for 2 to 4 weeks, depending on clinical response. Alternate-day steroids should then be maintained for an additional 3 months and tapered gradually over the ensuing 3 months. Serum IgE levels require close monitoring, as a rise signals an exacerbation, which may be associated with minimal symptoms. The initial resolution of the chest radiograph may take several weeks; follow-up radiographs should be obtained on a regular basis, as the disease may continue without symptoms.

Clinical Pearls

1. A high index of suspicion for ABPA should be maintained in any asthmatic with febrile exacerbations and transient or fixed pulmonary infiltrates on chest radiograph.

2. In the proper clinical setting, the diagnosis is confirmed by positive prick-test for *Aspergillus fumigatus,* positive precipitating antibodies to *Aspergillus fumigatus,* and a total serum IgE level $>$ 2000 ng/ml. Proximal bronchiectasis and elevated specific IgE and IgG against Aspergillus are strongly suggestive.

3. Corticosteroids are the cornerstone of therapy and need to be continued for at least 6 months to prevent exacerbation; the IgE level should be monitored closely, as it is a signal of exacerbation and may precede the clinical symptoms.

REFERENCES

1. Hinson KFW, Moon AA, Plummer NS. Bronchopulmonary aspergillosis. A review and a report of 8 new cases. Thorax 1952; 7:317–333.
2. McCarthy DS, Pepys J. Allergic bronchopulmonary aspergillosis. Clinical immunology: clinical features. Clin Allergy 1971; 1:261–286.
3. Rosenberg M, Patterson R. Clinical and immunologic criteria for the diagnosis of allergic bronchopulmonary aspergillosis. Ann Intern Med 1977; 86:405–414.

PATIENT 65

A 32-year-old woman with recurrent cough, fever, purulent sputum, and a right middle lobe infiltrate

A 32-year-old woman was admitted with increasing cough, fever, and purulent sputum for 3 days. She had a severe episode of measles with pneumonia during childhood, but did well until 3 years previously when she began having recurrent episodes of cough, purulent sputum, and "walking pneumonias."

Physical Examination: Temperature 102°; blood pressure 121/77. Diffuse rhonchi with rales in the right lateral and anterior thorax; cardiac normal.

Laboratory Findings: Hct 36%; WBC 12,900/μl with 90% PMNs. Sputum Gram stain: multiple leukocytes with large numbers of diverse organisms. Admission chest radiograph demonstrates a right middle lobe infiltrate (below right). A previous chest radiograph 6 months earlier was normal except for increased bronchial markings in the right middle lobe (below left).

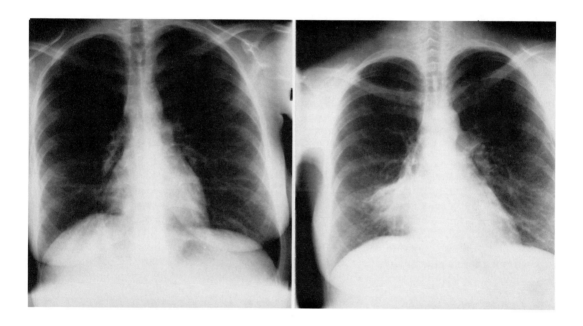

Diagnosis: Right middle lobe bacterial pneumonia due to underlying bronchiectasis.

Discussion: Although less common in the antibiotic era, bronchiectasis is still a major source of morbidity and mortality. Defined as an abnormal dilatation of the bronchi, bronchiectasis is categorized as cylindrical or saccular. Cylindrical bronchiectasis describes bronchi that fail to taper normally as they bifurcate to the lung periphery. Saccular bronchiectasis refers to bronchi that not only fail to taper but may be larger toward the periphery, demonstrating saccular outpouchings. Saccular bronchiectasis denotes permanent injury to the airway subsequent to severe infection; cylindrical disease may be reversible, occurring temporarily for 1 to 4 months in 40% of patients treated for bacterial pneumonia, which underlies the recommendation not to perform bronchography for 4 months in a patient with resolving pneumonia.

Bronchiectasis results from bronchial injury subsequent to severe infection. Most infections are viral or secondary bacterial pneumonias and occur during childhood when airways are relatively small and fragile. Adults may acquire bronchiectasis from necrotizing bacterial pneumonias, such as those due to *Klebsiella pneumoniae,* and from tuberculous or fungal infections. Bronchiectasis may result from congenital disorders such as cystic fibrosis, Kartagener's syndrome, yellow nail syndrome, or Williams-Campbell syndrome (deficiency of bronchial cartilage). Obstructive airway lesions or corrosive gas inhalations may also predispose to bronchiectasis. Bronchiectasis most commonly involves the left lung, with lobar frequency descending in the order of left lower lobe, lingula, right lower lobe, and right middle lobe.

Many patients have anatomic evidence of bronchiectasis without associated symptoms; therefore, the incidental demonstration of bronchiectasis is not a reason to initiate therapy. When symptoms do occur, they may become disabling, with cough, purulent sputum, hemoptysis, and recurrent episodes of pneumonia. Initial therapy is medical with antibiotics and inhaled bronchodilators. Chest physical therapy with percussion, postural drainage, vibration, and directed coughing accelerates sputum clearance but does not provide any immediate or delayed improvement of measurable pulmonary function in any clinical condition with bronchiectasis except cystic fibrosis.

Patients with disabling symptoms or progressive bronchiectasis should be considered for surgery. Localized disease that can be completely removed by segmentectomy, lobectomy, bilobectomy, or pneumonectomy presents the greatest probability of responding to surgery; partial resection of only the "worst" regions of diffuse bronchiectasis invariably results in continued symptoms with diminished functional pulmonary reserve. Preoperative staging of the extent of bronchiectasis, therefore, is crucial and requires carefully performed bilateral bronchograms with visualization of all segmental bronchi. Computerized tomography is useful for diagnosing and monitoring the progression of bronchiectasis in symptomatic patients when bronchography is refused or contraindicated. Since the sensitivity and specificity of CT scanning at a segmental level are only 66% and 92% respectively, it is less valuable in preoperative staging.

The present patient rapidly improved with parenteral then oral antibiotics. Subsequent episodes of productive cough were managed with inhaled bronchodilators, antibiotics, and chest physiotherapy. She did well for 3 years until exacerbations of bronchiectasis became more frequent and two more episodes of right middle lobe pneumonia occurred. She underwent bilateral bronchography, demonstrating localized right middle lobe bronchiectasis, followed by a lobectomy that eliminated her symptoms.

Clinical Pearls

1. Cylindrical bronchiectasis may be a temporary finding in 40% of patients with treated pneumonia and may persist for up to 4 months.

2. Surgery for bronchiectasis should be reserved for patients with sharply localized bronchiectasis in one or two adjacent lobes.

3. The sensitivity of CT scanning in the diagnosis of bronchiectasis is 66%.

REFERENCES

1. Cooke JC, Currie DC, Morgan AD, et al. Role of computed tomography in diagnosis of bronchiectasis. Thorax 1987; 42:272–277.
2. Annest LS, Kratz JM, Crawford FA. Current results of treatment of bronchiectasis. J Thorac Cardiovasc Surg 1982; 83:546–550.
3. Mazzocco MC, Owens GR, Kiriloff LH, Rogers RM. Chest percussion and postural drainage in patients with bronchiectasis. Chest 1985; 88:360–363.

PATIENT 66

A 69-year-old man with confusion, respiratory failure, and diffuse pulmonary infiltrates

A 69-year-old man was admitted with confusion and profound dyspnea. He had a history of chronic low back pain that was particularly severe during the previous 2 weeks, confining him to bed and necessitating over-the-counter pain medications. On the day of admission, he complained of dizziness and became markedly short of breath.

Physical Examination: Respirations 30; pulse 120; blood pressure 120/70 (falling with sitting); temperature 101°. Dry mucous membranes; bibasilar rales with scattered wheezes; cardiac normal without gallop; confused male without focal abnormalities.

Laboratory Findings: Serum sodium 139 mEq/L, potassium 3.4 mEq/L, chloride 113 mEq/L, bicarbonate 8 mEq/L, BUN 42 mg/dl, creatinine 1.5 mg/dl. ABG (room air): pH 7.42, $PaCO_2$ 13 mmHg, PaO_2 33 mmHg, protime 13/11.5 sec; Hct 48%; WBC 12,800/μl. Chest radiograph revealed diffuse, bilateral alveolar infiltrates. Urinalysis 2+ proteinuria. The patient was intubated and placement of a Swan-Ganz catheter demonstrated the pulmonary capillary wedge pressure to be 7 mmHg.

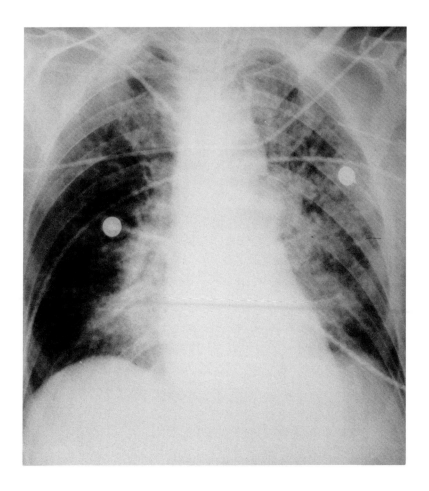

Diagnosis: Salicylate-induced noncardiogenic pulmonary edema.

Discussion: Noncardiogenic pulmonary edema is a serious complication of several drug intoxications that include heroin, barbiturates, propoxyphene, ethchlorvynol, methadone, and salicylates. The relationship of salicylates with respiratory failure was first noted in the 1950s with observations that children receiving high-dose aspirin for rheumatic carditis occasionally developed pulmonary edema. The entity was subsequently reported in patients without underlying cardiac dysfunction and confirmed to be noncardiogenic in origin on the basis of normal pulmonary capillary wedge (Pcw) pressures. The incidence of salicylate-induced pulmonary edema is uncertain; however, one series observed respiratory failure in 28% of patients admitted with serum salicylate levels greater than 30 mg/dl.

The clinical features of salicylate-induced pulmonary edema suggest the diagnosis. The patient is typically a middle-aged or elderly smoker with concurrent medical problems who presents with dyspnea, bilateral diffuse alveolar infiltrates, and altered mental status ranging from confusion to coma. Respiratory failure usually develops during the course of chronic aspirin ingestion when the patient inadvertently becomes toxic, rather than after a purposeful drug overdose, and is characterized by rales without signs of congestive heart failure. Characteristic clinical and laboratory features of salicylism may suggest the diagnosis, although the presence of respiratory failure may obscure the significance of these findings. These features include volume depletion, Kussmaul respiration, a mixed acid-base disturbance (an anion gap metabolic acidosis and respiratory alkalosis), a mild coagulopathy, and proteinuria.

The pathogenesis of salicylate-induced pulmonary edema is not easily defined. Although altered mentation is a common associated finding, respiratory failure in salicylate toxic patients without neurologic abnormalities diminishes the potential role of neurogenic pulmonary edema. Since aspirin is a potent inhibitor of cyclooxygenase, an enzyme important in prostaglandin and leukotriene balance, salicylate toxicity may either deplete the lung of compounds that maintain vascular integrity (prostacyclin) or promote generation of agents that enhance membrane permeability (leukotrienes).

The outcome is generally favorable if the diagnosis is rapidly determined and appropriate therapy aggressively initiated. When a patient presents with noncardiogenic pulmonary edema of uncertain etiology with clinical features of salicylism, the diagnosis should be promptly evaluated with serum salicylate measurements. Salicylate levels greater than 40 mg/dl are required for the development of respiratory failure. Management centers on respiratory support that may range from face mask oxygen to intubation with mechanical ventilation, depending on the severity of respiratory insufficiency. Gastric lavage and instillation of charcoal impede further absorption of retained aspirin, and alkaline diuresis with careful attention to fluid balance accelerates elimination of the drug. Patients with exceptionally high serum salicylate levels or renal insufficiency may benefit from hemodialysis or charcoal hemoperfusion.

The combination of respiratory failure, confusion, and a mixed acid-base disturbance with metabolic acidosis and respiratory alkalosis suggested salicylism in the present patient. A serum salicylate level assayed on blood drawn in the emergency room was 65 mg/dl. Subsequent results of sputum and blood cultures were negative for pathogens. He required high inspired oxygen concentrations with positive end-expiratory pressure for 5 days, but gradually improved after undergoing alkaline diuresis.

Clinical Pearls

1. The constellation of noncardiogenic pulmonary edema with a mixed acid-base disturbance, proteinuria, and altered mental status suggests the diagnosis of salicylism.
2. Salicylate-induced pulmonary edema usually occurs in middle-aged patients with a history of chronic aspirin use who become inadvertently toxic.
3. Pulmonary edema does not occur when serum salicylate levels are below 40 mg/dl.

REFERENCES
1. Heffner JE, Sahn SA. Salicylate-induced pulmonary edema. Clinical features and prognosis. Ann Intern Med 1981; 95:405–409.
2. Heffner JE, Starkey T, Anthony P. Salicylate-induced noncardiogenic pulmonary edema. West J Med 1979; 130:263–266.
3. Bowers RE, Brigham KL, Owen PJ. Salicylate pulmonary edema: the mechanism in sheep and review of the clinical literature. Am Rev Respir Dis 1977; 115:261–268.

PATIENT 67

A 46-year-old man with recurrent pneumothoraces for 27 years and cystic pulmonary lesions

A 46-year-old white male was transferred 2 days following the development of a tension pneumothorax. At age 19, he had had a left recurrent, spontaneous pneumothorax, for which a pleurectomy was performed. Ten years later he developed dyspnea upon exertion and was noted to have an abnormal chest radiograph. The diagnosis of sarcoidosis was established by transbronchial lung biopsy.

Physical Examination: Afebrile; normal vital signs. Chest examination: right chest tube in place with minimal air leak, hyperresonant to percussion, distant breath sounds without adventitious sounds. Cardiac examination: no evidence of congestive heart failure or cor pulmonale; no cyanosis, clubbing, or edema.

Laboratory Findings: WBC 8800/μl, 90% PMNs, 6% monocytes, 3% lymphocytes; Hct 47%. ABG (room air): pH 7.43, PCO_2 41 mmHg, PO_2 75 mmHg. Pulmonary function studies 2 months prior to admission: FVC 3.84 L (70% of predicted), FEV_1 1.50 L (37%), FEV_1/FVC ratio 39%. Chest radiograph: multiple, large, bullous lesions, fibrotic changes, and pleural thickening in the left apex; chest tube in the right pleural space without evidence of pneumothorax. Electrocardiogram: without right ventricular hypertrophy.

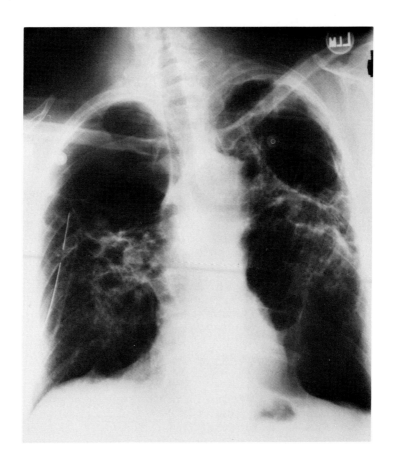

Diagnosis: Fibrocystic sarcoidosis with recurrent pneumothorax treated with pleurectomy.

Discussion: Fibrosis develops in 20 to 25% of patients with sarcoidosis and parenchymal abnormalities. The initial reticulonodular pattern develops progressively over several years, leading to posterior and superior retraction and distortion of lung parenchyma. The chest radiograph characteristically shows perihilar contracted fibrosis with a predominance of upper lung zone bullous and bronchiectatic changes. The chest radiograph may be similar to that seen in upper lobe tuberculosis, silicosis, and fungal diseases. When the patient with sarcoidosis reaches this stage of fibrosis, he usually has developed dyspnea on exertion. Once the cystic lesions appear radiographically, they tend to increase in size and number; they do not spontaneously regress. At this stage of the disease, absence of noncaseating granuloma on biopsy is not uncommon. Earlier chest radiographs show progressive cystic changes in the presence of hilar and mediastinal lymphadenopathy and are helpful in the radiologic differential diagnosis.

Patients with end-stage fibrotic lung disease from any etiology are at increased risk for pneumothorax due to the large number of bullae that form on or near the pleural surface. As fibrosis worsens and bronchiolar scarring occurs, further airway obstruction ensues, leading to progressively enlarging bullous lesions. An acute increase in intraairway pressure may rupture the strategically placed bullous lesions, resulting in pneumothorax. Once a pneumothorax develops, the individual has a 30 to 50% chance of having a recurrent ipsilateral pneumothorax, usually within 2 years, and a 10 to 15% chance of a contralateral occurrence. Following a second pneumothorax, the chance of recurrence is 50 to 80%. In up to 10% of patients, simultaneous, bilateral pneumothoraces can occur.

Tube thoracostomy is the primary method of management in patients with a large or symptomatic primary spontaneous pneumothorax and is always indicated for secondary spontaneous pneumothorax (secondary to underlying lung disease), unless it is extremely small and there is evidence that the air leak has ceased. The insertion of a chest tube generally leads to rapid reexpansion of the lung, even if there is a continued air leak. It rarely is necessary to insert more than one chest tube. The most common cause of failure of the initial thoracostomy tube is occlusion of the tube by fibrin or blood. Patients who have a persistent air leak for many days despite a well-placed and functioning chest tube

or those with recurrent pneumothoraces should undergo thoracotomy if they are surgical candidates. At thoracotomy, the bleb can either be excised or oversewn and pleural symphysis produced by pleural abrasion or parietal pleurectomy. First described in 1956 by Gaensler, parietal pleurectomy is highly effective for the treatment of recurrent pneumothorax, with a failure rate of less than 1%. Complications have been reported in up to 10% of patients, the most common being intrapleural hemorrhage, contralateral pneumothorax, and bronchopleural fistula. The mortality rate in pleurectomy is less than 3%, slightly greater than the 1% mortality rate from elective thoracotomy. No study is available that compares parietal pleurectomy with pleural abrasion in the treatment of spontaneous pneumothorax. Mortality is similar (up to 3%) but morbidity probably is less. No loss of pulmonary function results from parietal pleurectomy, and the post-pleurectomy chest radiograph shows no sequelae from the surgical procedure. Some surgeons recommend a median sternotomy and bilateral pleural abrasion or pleurectomy in patients with a recurrent pneumothorax because of the high likelihood of contralateral occurrence.

Tension pneumothorax requires immediate action. The symptomatology and rapidity with which cardiovascular collapse occurs depends upon the degree of tension and the underlying cardiopulmonary status of the patient. Patients with interstitial fibrosis and COPD are most devastated by a tension pneumothorax. The treatment is immediate decompression of the pleural space by insertion of a large-bore needle into the second anterior interspace. If the clinical decision is correct, a rush of air will be heard through the needle and there will be an immediate decrease in heart rate, increase in blood pressure, decrease in respiratory rate, and improvement in oxygenation. Following stabilization, insertion of a thoracostomy tube is effective in gaining control of the pneumothorax. The approach to a tension pneumothorax, once the patient is stabilized, is no different from that in a pneumothorax not under tension.

The present patient underwent a right thoracotomy, partial pleurectomy and pleural abrasion. The air leak ceased by the third postoperative day and the chest tubes were removed at day 6. He was discharged on postoperative day 11. The patient continues to be dyspneic on exertion but has had no recurrence of the pneumothorax at 7 months.

Clinical Pearls

1. Twenty to 25% of patients with sarcoidosis develop pulmonary fibrosis that, in some patients, progresses to multicystic disease as a result of bullae and cystic bronchiectasis.

2. Once a spontaneous pneumothorax occurs there is a 30 to 50% chance of ipsilateral recurrence, usually within 2 years, and a 10 to 15% chance of contralateral occurrence.

3. The treatment of recurrent pneumothorax should be either thoracotomy or median sternotomy and unilateral or bilateral parietal pleurectomy or pleural abrasion, if the patient can tolerate a major surgical procedure. In the nonoperable candidate, chemical pleurodesis with tetracycline or talc should be attempted.

REFERENCES

1. Felson B. Uncommon roentgen patterns of pulmonary sarcoidosis. Dis Chest 1958; 34:357–367.
2. Gaensler EA. Parietal pleurectomy for recurrent spontaneous pneumothorax. Surg Gynecol Obstet 1956; 102:293–308.
3. Gobbel WG, Rhea WG, Nelson IA, Daniel RA. Spontaneous pneumothorax. J Thorac Cardiovasc Surg 1963; 46:331–345.
4. Neal JF, Vargas G, Smith DE, et al. Bilateral bleb excision through median sternotomy. Am J Surg 1979; 138:794–797.

PATIENT 68

A 37-year-old man with fever, nonproductive cough, pleurisy, and dyspnea of 3 days' duration

A 37-year-old man presented with a 3-day history of nonproductive cough, pleuritic chest pain, dyspnea with exertion and fever. He was a construction worker without a significant past medical history. Due to chest pain and dyspnea, he was unable to work on the third day following the initiation of symptoms.

Physical Examination: Temperature 100.6°; pulse 110; respirations 28; minimal respiratory distress. Chest examination: flat percussion note, decreased fremitus, and absent breath sounds on the left. Cardiac examination unremarkable. Neurologic examination normal.

Laboratory Findings: WBC 9300/μl; 80% PMNs, 1% bands; 15% lymphocytes; Hct 35%. Liver function tests normal. Chest radiograph: large left pleural effusion with contralateral mediastinal shift, no parenchymal infiltrates in the right lung. Thoracentesis: serous, total protein 5.2 g/dl, LDH 220 IU/L; nucleated cells 3800/μl, 90% PMNs, 8% mononuclear cells, 2% mesothelial cells; glucose 50 mg/dl, pH 7.20; Gram stain negative; AFB stain negative; aerobic and anaerobic cultures negative; tuberculosis and fungal cultures pending; PPD negative; controls positive. A pleural biopsy was performed.

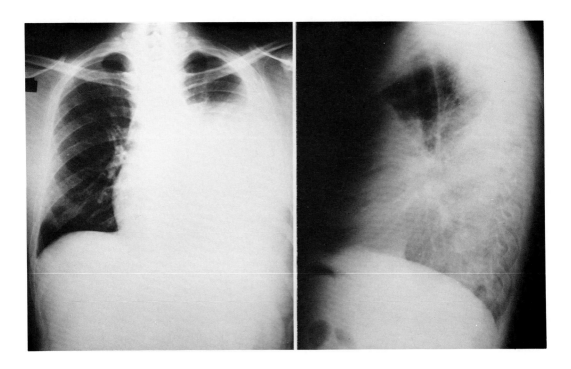

Diagnosis: Tuberculous pleurisy.

Discussion: Although the incidence of pulmonary tuberculosis has declined, TB pleurisy has remained stable in the United States, representing about 4% of newly diagnosed cases per year. Tuberculous pleurisy should be considered in any patient with a unilateral exudative pleural effusion. Even though acute tuberculous pleurisy is a self-limited disease, active pulmonary or extrapulmonary tuberculosis will develop in up to 70% of patients within 5 years if untreated.

Tuberculous pleural effusions occur on an immunologic basis when a subpleural focus of tuberculosis ruptures into the pleural space. Tuberculin protein and tubercle bacilli enter the pleural space from a reactivated focus contiguous to the pleura, by direct extension of post-primary disease, or as a result of hematogenous dissemination; all represent an "active" state of tuberculosis. Tuberculous antigens interact with sensitized T lymphocytes with liberation of lymphokines, which may alter pleural capillary permeability. Post-primary tuberculous pleurisy historically was seen most commonly in children but is occurring with increased incidence in the elderly due to an increasing number of immunologically naive individuals and the reactivation of disease in the immunologically impaired elderly population. Tuberculous pleurisy most commonly occurs 3 to 7 months following the primary exposure.

Tuberculous pleurisy may present as an acute illness simulating bacterial pneumonia or as a more insidious disease first suspected on chest radiograph in a patient with minor constitutional symptoms. Younger patients have a tendency to present with a more acute illness. A nonproductive cough and chest pain, usually pleuritic, are the two most common presenting symptoms. When both cough and pleuritic chest pain are present, pleurisy usually precedes the cough; a pleural friction rub is unusual. Patients are usually febrile and can have temperatures over 104°. Peripheral leukocytosis is unusual. Chest radiograph shows a unilateral small to moderate pleural effusion, although massive effusions are noted in approximately 5% of patients. Coexisting parenchymal disease can be detected radiographically in about one-third of patients. The effusion is almost always on the side of the infiltrate and is a marker of active parenchymal disease.

Intermediate-strength PPD will be negative in up to 30% of patients on admission; most will convert their skin tests to positive if repeated within 6 to 8 weeks. The most probable explanation for a negative PPD with tuberculous pleurisy is that in the acute phase of the disease circulating mononuclear cells suppress the sensitized T lymphocytes in the peripheral blood and skin but not in pleural fluid.

The pleural fluid is a serous exudate with a total protein greater than 4.0 g/dl. The total leukocyte count generally is less than $5000/\mu l$ with a predominance of lymphocytes (90 to 95% lymphocytes). A PMN predominance does occur in the first few days following entry of the tubercle bacillus into the pleural space; this PMN predominance is rapidly replaced by mononuclear phagocytes and lymphocytes. A paucity of mesothelial cells is characteristic, and pleural fluid eosinophilia is rarely observed. A low pleural fluid glucose and pH is found in approximately 20% of patients. The glucose is rarely below 20 mg/dl and the pH ranges between 7.00 and 7.29; a pleural fluid pH greater than 7.40 makes the diagnosis of TB pleurisy unlikely.

AFB smear is positive in less than 10% of patients, whereas culture is positive in about 50% (25 to 70%). Pleural biopsy is the best single test for establishing the diagnosis. Granuloma can be demonstrated in the parietal pleura in 50 to 80% of patients and provides a presumptive diagnosis. Culture of the pleural tissue will grow *M. tuberculosis* 55 to 80% of the time. Combining pleural fluid and pleural tissue studies, the diagnosis can be established in 90 to 95% of patients. Sputum and gastric cultures rarely are positive for *M. tuberculosis* unless parenchymal lesions are present.

Patients with tuberculous pleurisy can be treated with the same regimen used for pulmonary tuberculosis—nine months of daily isoniazid and rifampin. With treatment, the patient usually becomes afebrile within 2 weeks; however, the fever may persist for as long as 6 to 8 weeks. Most resolve the pleural effusion by 6 weeks, but it can persist for 3 to 4 months.

The present patient's pleural biopsy demonstrated granulomas and *M. tuberculosis* grew from both the pleural tissue and pleural fluid. He was treated with INH and rifampin and a single therapeutic thoracentesis. He became afebrile on day 6 and the effusion resolved completely in 8 weeks.

Clinical Pearls

1. Patients with tuberculous pleurisy may present with an illness similar to acute bacterial pneumonia; these usually are younger patients.

2. Up to 30% of patients will have a negative PPD on admission; repeat PPD 6 to 8 weeks later usually will be positive. A negative PPD is due to mononuclear suppressor cells in the peripheral circulation.

3. Approximately 20% of patients with TB pleurisy have a low glucose, low pH effusion; a PMN predominance in pleural fluid may be found if thoracentesis is done within a few days of the acute pleural injury.

4. Tuberculous pleurisy will resolve with or without treatment, but untreated patients have up to a 70% chance of developing active pulmonary or extrapulmonary tuberculosis within 5 years.

REFERENCES

1. Roper WH, Waring JJ. Primary serofibrinous pleural effusion in military personnel. Am Rev Tuberc 1955; 71:616–634.
2. Levine H, Szanto PB, Cugell DW. Tuberculous pleurisy. An acute illness. Arch Intern Med 1968; 122:329–332.
3. Berger HW, Mejia E. Tuberculous pleurisy. Chest 1973; 63:88–90.

PATIENT 69

A 29-year-old woman with the insidious onset of fever, weight loss, cough, dyspnea, and the subacute development of bilateral lung masses during corticosteroid therapy

A 29-year-old woman was referred for evaluation of insidious onset of fever, weight loss, cough, dyspnea, and pulmonary infiltrates of 2 months' duration. She was in excellent health prior to the illness. She was a non-smoker and did not take medications on a regular basis.

Physical Examination: Temperature 101°; respirations 28; no lymphadenopathy or skin lesions. Chest examination: rhonchi most prominent in the upper lung zones. Cardiac examination: no evidence of left or right heart failure. Clubbing absent; neurologic examination normal.

Laboratory Findings: WBC 3500/μl, 65% PMNs, 25% lymphocytes, 5% monocytes, 5% eosinophils; alkaline phosphatase 225 IU/L, angiotensin-converting enzyme 35 U. Chest radiograph: diffuse fibronodular cystic disease with central accentuation and upper lobe volume loss, bilateral apical pleural thickening (below left). Fiberoptic bronchoscopy with endobronchial and transbronchial lung biopsies: lacy, reticular mucosal pattern compatible with sarcoidosis; endobronchial and transbronchial biopsies: noncaseating granuloma. Stains and cultures negative. Pulmonary function studies: FVC 1.31 L (37% of predicted), FEV$_1$ 1.23 L (44% of predicted), FEV$_1$/FVC ratio 94%, DL/VA ratio 3.50; ABG (room air): pH 7.46, PCO$_2$ 37 mmHg, PO$_2$ 79 mmHg.

The diagnosis of sarcoidosis was established. Because of severe systemic symptoms, corticosteroids were instituted (prednisone 40 mg/d). At follow-up examination 1 month later, the patient was clinically improved with lysis of fever, weight gain, and improvement in dyspnea and cough but she had occasional blood-streaked sputum. A chest radiograph was obtained (below right).

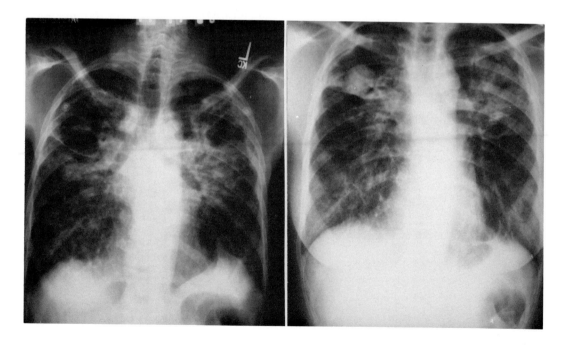

Diagnosis: Bilateral aspergilloma in a patient with sarcoidosis following one month of corticosteroid therapy.

Discussion: There are three clinical settings in which primary aspergillomas occur (where aspergillus infection initiates the cavity process and is followed by aspergilloma): (1) allergic bronchopulmonary aspergillosis (ABPA), (2) chronic necrotizing pulmonary aspergillosis (CNPA), and (3) invasive pulmonary aspergillosis. When ABPA causes bronchiectasis, aspergillomas may develop. In CNPA, an indolent clinical variant of invasive aspergillosis in immunocompetent hosts, aspergillomas are common; with invasive disease, cavity formation may occur and be a subsequent source of a fungus ball. However, most aspergillomas appear to originate from colonization and proliferation of the fungus in a preexisting non-aspergillus lung cavity. Tuberculosis probably is the most common cause of the cavitary lung disease, but in certain parts of the United States, particularly the Southeast, sarcoidosis is a common background for aspergilloma. Cavitating neoplasms, lung abscess, fungal disease, pulmonary infarction, and necrotizing pneumonia also have been reported as predisposing factors for the development of aspergillomas. The pathogenesis of aspergillomas in preexisting cavities has not been well defined. However, the greater the prevalence of aspergillus in the environment and the greater the incidence of cavitary lung disease, the more likely an individual will be colonized by the fungus. Therefore, aspergillomas tend to occur with increased frequency where the incidence of tuberculosis and sarcoidosis is high and the humid environment is conducive to growth of the aspergillus (the southeastern U.S.).

It has been shown experimentally that corticosteroids, in addition to antibiotics, diabetes, radiation, cytotoxic drugs, and malignancies, facilitate the growth of aspergillus in lung tissue. While control animals that inhale aspergillus spores develop transient, purulent bronchitis and bronchopneumonia, which resolve in several days without demonstrable hyphae, corticosteroid-treated animals develop progressive bronchitis and bronchopneumonia that result in death. Corticosteroid-treated animals develop hyphae quickly with an absent macrophage response, which may be responsible for the host's natural resistance to fungal infection. In ABPA, corticosteroids are the treatment of choice, the proposed mechanisms being inhibition of the toxic antigen-antibody inflammatory reaction, reduction of bronchial secretions, and creation of a less favorable environment for the endobronchial growth of aspergillus. Some have suggested that beclomethasone is effective therapy, whereas others suggest that the drug only increases the likelihood of saprophytic growth.

The present patient developed large bilateral aspergillomas after 1 month of moderate-dose corticosteroid therapy. Aspergillus was cultured from the sputum and the patient had precipitating antibodies for aspergillus. It is conceivable that the minimal pleural thickening on the initial radiograph may have been the harbinger of aspergillus colonization, as this radiographic sign has been reported to antedate the appearance of a fungus ball by 2 to 3 years. Thus, corticosteroids could have led to the rapid development of aspergillomas. The other possibility is that there was "limited invasive" disease prior to corticosteroid therapy. Even though sputum or transbronchial biopsy did not show evidence of aspergillus prior to corticosteroid therapy, this could have been a sampling error. In ABPA complicated by bronchocentric granulomatosis, the development of aspergillomas has been described following corticosteroid therapy, and tissue from these patients has shown aspergillus hyphae within granulomatous tissue.

Despite the development of bilateral aspergillomas, the patient had a marked improvement clinically. Corticosteroids were tapered rapidly to 15 mg of prednisone every other day, with maintenance of clinical improvement. The patient has been followed for 6 months on low-dose, alternate-day corticosteroid therapy and has remained clinically well without evidence of either spontaneous lysis or progression of the aspergillomas; there has been no further hemoptysis.

Clinical Pearls

1. Corticosteroids have been associated rarely with invasive pulmonary aspergillosis and disseminated aspergillosis in immunocompetent hosts such as those with bronchial asthma or allergic bronchopulmonary aspergillosis.

2. The rapid development of aspergillomas following corticosteroid therapy suggests either previous colonization or local invasion or the rapid proliferation of hyphae following spore inhalation.

3. Corticosteroids appear to inhibit host defense mechanisms against the aspergillus spores, particularly the pulmonary macrophage, which prevents hyphae formation with colonization or locally invasive disease.

4. Particularly in areas where aspergillus is ubiquitous, patients with aspergillus colonization or preexisting conditions associated with colonization, sputum cultures, serology, and tomograms or CT scan should be done prior to instituting corticosteroids. Furthermore, the indication for corticosteroids needs to be clearly defined.

REFERENCES

1. Sidransky H, Friedman L. The effect of cortisone and antibiotic agents on experimental pulmonary aspergillosis. Am J Pathol 1959; 35:169–179.
2. Israel HL, Ostrow A. Sarcoidosis and aspergilloma. Am J Med 1969; 47:243–250.
3. Anderson CJ, Craig S, Bardana EJ Jr. Allergic bronchopulmonary aspergillosis and bilateral fungal balls terminating in disseminated aspergillosis. J Allergy Clin Immunol 1980; 65:140–144.
4. Lake KB, Browne PM, van Dyke JJ, Ayers L. Fatal disseminated aspergillosis in an asthmatic patient treated with corticosteroids. Chest 1983; 83:138–139.

PATIENT 70

A 63-year-old man with severe substernal chest pain, dyspnea, and dysphagia

A 63-year-old man was admitted with severe substernal pain, dyspnea, and dysphagia of several hours' duration. He was an alcoholic and admitted to a heavy drinking binge the previous night. He awoke with vomiting, retching, and hematemesis.

Physical Examination: Temperature 100.5°; pulse 110; respirations 28; blood pressure 100/60. Thin white male in distress due to substernal chest pain and dyspnea; subcutaneous air felt in the neck and pectoral areas; pain on palpation in the epigastrium; flat percussion note and decreased breath sounds in the left chest.

Laboratory Findings: WBC 18,500/μl, 80% PMNs, 7% bands; amylase 170 IU/L. Supine chest radiograph: normal cardiac silhouette; moderate left pleural effusion. Thoracentesis: turbid fluid, nucleated cells 22,000/μl, 85% PMNs, pH 6.45, glucose 70 mg/dl, total protein 3.7 g/dl. Culture: Bacteroides and Fusobacterium species. Esophagram: extravasation of contrast into the mediastinum.

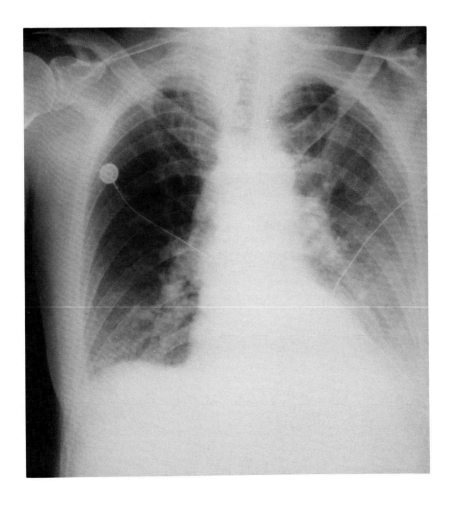

Diagnosis: Spontaneous esophageal rupture (Boerhaave's syndrome).

Discussion: Esophageal rupture is a potentially life-threatening event that requires immediate diagnosis and therapy; however, the correct management remains controversial, probably because of the varied etiologies. The most common cause of esophageal rupture today is iatrogenic. Endoscopy or dilation was the cause of esophageal perforation in 39% of 127 patients seen in a major medical center over the past 50 years.

Patients with spontaneous esophageal rupture have the poorest survival due to a delay in recognition and treatment. Spontaneous rupture occurs when there is an acute rise in intraesophageal pressure generated by an increase in intraabdominal pressure with the glottis in a closed position, as occurs in retching or vomiting. Experimentally, it has been shown that it is the acuteness of the pressure rise rather than the absolute pressure that is critical to causing perforation. The esophageal tear almost always occurs in the distal half of the esophagus just above the esophagogastric junction on the left. Perforation occurs distally because this portion of the esophagus is devoid of striated muscle and deficient in extramural support.

Patients with spontaneous esophageal rupture frequently give a history of severe retching or vomiting or a conscious effort to resist vomiting. However, in some patients the perforation may be silent. Early recognition depends largely on the interpretation of the chest radiograph. Several factors influence chest radiographic findings: (1) time between perforation and chest radiograph examination; (2) site of perforation; and (3) mediastinal pleural integrity. The radiograph taken within minutes of the acute injury is usually unremarkable and may remain normal in up to 10% of patients. Probably one to two hours need to elapse before mediastinal emphysema may be demonstrated radiographically; it is present in less than half of patients. Mediastinal widening may not become obvious for several hours. The presence of a pneumothorax, seen in about 75% of patients, indicates rupture of the mediastinal pleura. Pneumothorax occurs with a 70% incidence on the left, a 20% incidence on the right, and is bilateral in 10%. Mediastinal air is seen early if pleural integrity is maintained, and pleural effusions secondary to mediastinitis tend to occur later. Pleural fluid, with or without associated pneumothorax, occurs in 75% of perforations.

Radiographic confirmation of a presumptive diagnosis of esophageal rupture needs to be accomplished immediately. The choice of contrast medium is either barium sulfate or water-soluble contrast compounds. The advantages of barium include its greater radiographic density, better mucosal adherence, and minimal irritation to the tracheobronchial tree; the disadvantage is its ability to incite a foreign body reaction, granulomas, and fibrosis. Water-soluble agents are rapidly absorbed by the mediastinal pleura and do not incite an inflammatory reaction; drawbacks are greater hypertonicity, marked irritation to the tracheobronchial tree, and a high percentage of false-negative studies. As a rule, the water-soluble agent should be used initially and, if no perforation is seen, a barium study should follow. Esophagrams are positive in about 90% of patients. When the radiographic study is done with the patient upright, rapid passage of the contrast material may not demonstrate the small rent. The study probably should be done with the patient in the appropriate lateral decubitus position.

The pleural fluid findings will depend upon the degree of perforation and the timing of thoracentesis from the injury. Early thoracentesis without mediastinal perforation will result in a serous, sterile exudate with a predominance of PMNs; the pleural fluid amylase and pH will be normal. Once the mediastinal pleura tears, amylase of salivary origin will appear in the fluid in very high concentrations. As the pleural space is seeded with anaerobic organisms from the mouth, the pH will rapidly and progressively fall to about 6.00. Experimentally, it has been shown that pleural fluid leukocyte metabolism, not gastric acid reflux, is the major contributor to the low pH of esophageal rupture effusions. Other findings in the pleural fluid suggestive of esophageal rupture include the presence of squamous epithelial cells and food particles.

The diagnosis of spontaneous esophageal rupture dictates immediate operative intervention. If diagnosed within the first 24 hours, primary closure should be attempted. If primary repair is accomplished within 24 hours of rupture, survival is generally greater than 90%. In addition to the primary closure, antibiotics covering mouth anaerobes, parenteral nutrition, and appropriate drainage of the mediastinum and pleural space constitute the complete therapeutic regimen.

The present patient was taken immediately to the operating room following diagnosis where primary closure was accomplished. Following antibiotics, drainage and parenteral nutrition, the patient recovered.

Clinical Pearls

1. Early suspicion of spontaneous esophageal rupture in the appropriate clinical setting depends upon interpretation of the chest radiograph. Radiographic findings suggesting esophageal rupture include mediastinal or subcutaneous emphysema, left pneumothorax, or left pleural effusion.

2. Immediate confirmation of the diagnosis should be pursued with an esophagram done in the appropriate lateral decubitus position, with a water-soluble agent being used initially. Esophagrams are positive in 90% of patients.

3. Once the mediastinal pleura tears, the pleural fluid has a high amylase (of salivary origin) and a pH that approaches 6.00 (due to anaerobic empyema).

4. Spontaneous esophageal rupture is an emergency and primary closure should be accomplished within 24 hours to ensure a high survival rate.

REFERENCES

1. Parkin GJ. The radiology of perforated oesophagus. Clin Radiol 1973; 24:324–331.
2. Good JT Jr, Antony VB, Reller RB, et al. The pathogenesis of the low pleural fluid pH in esophageal rupture. Am Rev Respir Dis 1983; 127:702–704.
3. Bladergroen MR, Lowe JE, Postlethwait RW. Diagnosis and recommended management of esophageal perforation and rupture. Ann Thorac Surg 1986; 42:235–239.

PATIENT 71

A 42-year-old man with fever, fatigue, arthralgias, and pulmonary nodules

A 42-year-old man was transferred to our hospital for evaluation of pulmonary infiltrates. He was in good health until 2 months prior to admission when he noted arthralgias and effusions of both knees. He subsequently developed progressive fatigue, weakness, a cough productive of mucoid sputum, and low-grade fever and bilateral pulmonary infiltrates without mediastinal adenopathy or pleural disease. There was no history of asthma, drug ingestion, or travel outside of South Carolina.

Physical Examination: Temperature 100.0°; pulse 100; respirations 24. Lethargic, healthy appearing, in no acute distress, no rash or edema; absence of adenopathy. Chest examination: basilar rales without wheezes. Cardiac examination normal; no hepatosplenomegaly; neurologic examination normal.

Laboratory Findings: WBC 20,600/μl, 65% PMNs, 25% eosinophils, 6% lymphocytes. Hct 35%; platelets 825,000/μl; urinalysis: 1+ protein, 1-2 RBCs/hpf. Chest radiograph (left): multiple pulmonary nodular lesions in the right lung field, the largest measuring 5 cm in diameter, alveolar infiltrate in the left middle lung zone, no hilar or mediastinal adenopathy. Pulmonary function studies: FVC 1.44 L (27% of predicted), FEV$_1$ 1.01 L (25%), FEV$_1$/FVC ratio 70%. Stool for ova and parasites negative; hepatitis B surface antigen negative; liver function studies normal; ANA 1:320 with a homogeneous pattern; total serum IgE 363 ng/ml; ESR 122 mm/h. Bronchoscopy and transbronchial biopsy: no endobronchial lesions, erythematous and edematous bronchial mucosa, no alveoli in specimens, bronchial walls had numerous eosinophils without granulomas; bronchial washings showed numerous eosinophils and macrophages. ENT evaluation: without upper airway lesions.

A procedure was performed. Corticosteroids were given but infiltrates progressed (right) and respiratory failure occurred.

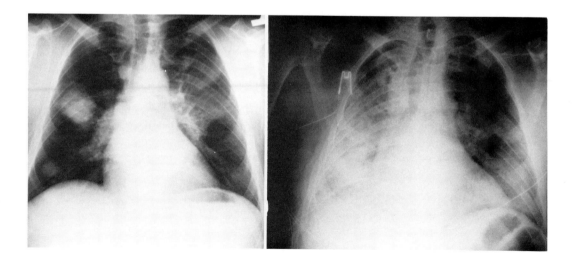

Diagnosis: Eosinophilic pneumonia with respiratory failure.

Discussion: Pulmonary infiltrates with peripheral eosinophilia encompasses a spectrum of diseases ranging from Loffler's syndrome (fleeting pulmonary infiltrates in moderately ill or asymptomatic patients) to the vasculitides (Churg-Strauss syndrome). Between these extremes are diseases such as allergic bronchopulmonary aspergillosis (ABPA), chronic eosinophilic pneumonia, drug reactions, hypereosinophilic syndrome, and parasitic infestation. While some of the illnesses can be diagnosed on clinical grounds (ABPA, drug reactions, and, at times, Churg-Strauss and hypereosinophilic syndrome), others such as chronic eosinophilic pneumonia and, on occasion, hypereosinophilic and Churg-Strauss syndromes, require organ biopsy. Elevated antifilarial titers will diagnose tropical eosinophilia, and ova, larvae, or adult worms may be found in the stool with other parasitic infections. Corticosteroids and, at times, cytotoxic therapy for the vasculitides usually produce a dramatic response in the pulmonary eosinophilia syndromes.

As corticosteroids produce eosinopenia, it follows that corticosteroids are the cornerstone of therapy in these conditions, particularly when the antigen cannot be identified or is unavoidable. Eosinophils have certain beneficial functions in the body such as modulating mast cell-dependent reactions, phagocytosis of intact mast cell granules and IgE antigen complexes, and the ability to produce antibody-dependent or complement-dependent damage to the larval stages of several parasites. However, tissue destruction may be associated with prolonged persistent hypereosinophilia. Major basic protein (MBP) constitutes the core of the eosinophil granule and has been shown to cause damage to a wide variety of mammalian target cells and organs. MBP is ciliastatic and can damage tracheal mucosal cells. It is probable that interstitial eosinophilia can cause parenchymal damage by release of MBP. Other eosinophilic constituents that could be pathogenetic include superoxide ions, lysosomal hydrolase, eosinophil-derived neurotoxin, and possibly arachidonic acid metabolites.

It is possible that in the present patient the eosinophil constituents caused severe pulmonary capillary membrane permeability resulting in ARDS. A paradoxical response to corticosteroid treatment could have occurred from eosinophil lysis, as the acute respiratory failure was temporally related to corticosteroid therapy. It is also possible that steroid therapy was administered too late in the course of the disease, and major lung injury had occurred prior to institution and could not be reversed. Certainly, corticosteroids remain the cornerstone of therapy in pulmonary infiltrates with eosinophilia and, as in any disease state, therapy should be instituted early to prevent irreversible organ damage.

The present patient developed acute hypoxemic respiratory failure (ARDS) despite corticosteroid therapy for eosinophilic pneumonia. Infection or multisystem organ involvement was not demonstrated and the open lung biopsy (the procedure) did not show vasculitis. An acute interstitial pneumonitis was demonstrated, the major inflammatory cell being the eosinophil, with a smaller number of plasma cells, neutrophils, and monocytic cells. Neither necrotizing vasculitis nor larval worms or ova were seen. There was minimal accumulation of eosinophils and macrophages within air spaces. The small bronchi were unremarkable, and the reaction was not bronchocentric. The biopsy was compatible with an acute eosinophilic pneumonia. A specific antigenic stimulus for eosinophilic response in the lung was not demonstrated. Although the responsible antigen can be identified only in ABPA, drug reactions, and parasitic infestations, immunologic abnormalities have been reported in all the illnesses with pulmonary infiltrates and eosinophilia. Elevated serum IgE levels are found characteristically in patients with ABPA, parasitic infestation, and Churg-Strauss syndrome, and have been reported in some patients with chronic eosinophilic pneumonia and hypereosinophilic syndrome.

The patient was started on prednisone and, because of worsening dyspnea, was given 1 gram of methylprednisolone daily for 3 days. Despite corticosteroids, bilateral alveolar infiltrates worsened and refractory hypoxemia ensued, requiring intubation and mechanical ventilation. The patient could not be oxygenated or ventilated adequately, developed barotrauma, and was given a trial of jet ventilation. He died an hypoxic death 9 days following open lung biopsy and 2 months from the onset of his illness. A single report exists of acute respiratory failure developing in a patient with chronic eosinophilic pneumonia; the patient responded to corticosteroids and was weaned from the ventilator by four days.

Clinical Pearls

1. Pulmonary infiltrates with eosinophilia encompass the spectrum of disease from Loffler's syndrome to vasculitis. The diagnosis can be made clinically in Loffler's syndrome, in drug reactions, and in ABPA but requires biopsy confirmation in chronic eosinophilic pneumonia and, at times, in the hypereosinophilic syndrome. Churg-Strauss syndrome may be diagnosed with confidence on clinical grounds; the diagnosis can be confirmed by lung biopsy.

2. Rarely, pulmonary infiltrates with eosinophilia can progress to hypoxemic respiratory failure.

3. Constituents of the eosinophil such as major basic protein, superoxide ions, and lysosomes not only perform beneficial functions but also may be responsible for tissue damage.

4. A paradoxical response to corticosteroids by release of massive amounts of eosinophilic constituents could transiently result in worsening organ function.

REFERENCES

1. Gaensler EA, Carrington CB. Peripheral opacities in chronic eosinophilic pneumonia: the photographic negative of pulmonary edema. AJR 1977; 128:1–13.
2. Libby DL, Murphy TF, Edwards A, et al. Chronic eosinophilic pneumonia: an unusual cause of acute respiratory failure. Am Rev Respir Dis 1980; 122:497–500.
3. Schatz M, Wasserman S, Patterson R. The eosinophil and the lung. Arch Intern Med 1982; 142:515–519.
4. Granthan JG, Meadows JA III, Gleich GJ. Chronic eosinophilic pneumonia. Evidence for eosinophilic degranulation and release of major basic protein. Am J Med 1986; 80:89–94.

PATIENT 72

A 33-year-old man with chronic alcoholism presenting with fever, chills, purulent sputum, pleurisy, pericardial effusion, and respiratory failure

A 33-year-old black male smoker with a history of alcohol abuse was transferred to our hospital because of worsening dyspnea and hypoxemia. He was well until 10 days prior to admission when he had developed symptoms of an upper respiratory tract infection. A few days later there was an abrupt onset of fever and shaking chills; cough and pleurisy ensued. Dyspnea became a prominent symptom over the next 72 hours.

Physical Examination: Temperature 103.4°; pulse 124; respirations 40; blood pressure 100/60. Lethargic and in moderate respiratory distress. Chest examination: flat percussion note, decreased fremitus and bronchial breathing throughout the entire left lung, no evidence of volume loss.

Laboratory Findings: WBC 3200/μl, 80% PMNs, 7% bands; Hct 30%; platelet count 98,000/μl. Sputum: tenacious, dark brown. Gram stain: numerous PMNs with many thick, short, gram-negative rods both in pairs, short chains, and single. Blood cultures pending. Chest radiograph: homogeneous opacification of the left hemithorax with sparing of the costophrenic angle and minimal ipsilateral mediastinal shift. Ultrasound: minimal amount of loculated pleural fluid and small anterior and posterior pericardial effusion. Pericardiocentesis: turbid, nucleated cells 5700/μl, 80% PMNs, total protein 4.3 gm/dl, LDH 300 IU/L, glucose 95 mg/dl, pH 7.34. Gram stain negative; culture negative. ABG (room air): pH 7.50, PCO_2 30 mmHg, PO_2 57 mmHg. Bone marrow biopsy: normal cell lines. Hospital course: because of progressive hypercapnia and respiratory rates exceeding 40/min, elective intubation was performed late on the first hospital day.

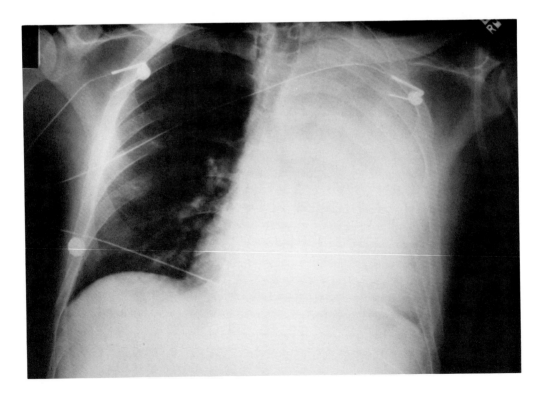

Diagnosis: *Klebsiella pneumoniae* pneumonia with pancytopenia and sympathetic pericardial effusion.

Discussion: Klebsiella pneumonia accounts for less than 1% of all bacterial pneumonias, but is the most common cause of community-acquired, gram-negative, aerobic bacillary pneumonias. In contrast, Klebsiella pneumonia accounts for a substantial number of nosocomial pneumonias, as the nasopharynx of severely ill patients is commonly colonized by this organism. *K. pneumoniae* can be cultured from the oropharynx in up to 5% of healthy adults; however, the rate of colonization increases dramatically in alcoholics, diabetics, and hospitalized patients. The characteristic patient who develops community-acquired Klebsiella pneumonia is a middle-aged or elderly male with a history of alcohol abuse. Other predisposing factors include COPD and, less commonly, diabetes. Klebsiella pneumonia should be suspected in the appropriate clinical setting in nursing home residents, granulocytopenic patients, and patients with carcinoma.

Aspiration of oropharyngeal secretions is the usual route of primary infection. The clinical features may be indistinguishable from those of pneumococcal pneumonia, with the abrupt onset of fever and chills followed shortly by pleurisy and a cough productive of tenacious, dark brown or currant jelly sputum (< 50%). Prostration and marked dyspnea are common. Very often there is a history of a recent upper respiratory tract infection, and epigastric distress and vomiting may be an initial symptom.

Lobar consolidation is the rule and there may be evidence of either volume loss due to mucous plugging from tenacious secretions or contralateral mediastinal shift due to complete alveolar filling with patent bronchi. The "classic" chest radiograph showing lobar consolidation in the right upper lobe with a bulging minor fissure occurs only occasionally. In a majority of patients there is multilobar involvement; necrotization and empyema are common. There may be peripheral leukocytosis but counts are often decreased, a reflection of severe infection in an alcoholic patient with poor bone marrow reserve and folate deficiency.

Most strains of *K. pneumoniae* are sensitive to amikacin and third-generation cephalosporins. In suspected Klebsiella pneumonia, treatment should be initiated with a third-generation cephalosporin in combination with an aminoglycoside, and the regimen modified when sensitivities become available. Strains resistant to first- and second-generation cephalosporins, gentamicin and tobramycin have been reported with increased frequency. Treatment should be continued for 2 to 3 weeks, depending upon the clinical response. Risk factors associated with a high mortality are severe underlying disease, bacteremia, leukopenia, and old age.

The present patient had blood and bone marrow cultures positive for *Klebsiella pneumoniae* but pericardial fluid was sterile. Defervescence occurred after 7 days of treatment with amikacin and a third-generation cephalosporin, with mechanical ventilation discontinued at day 9. CT scan of the chest showed multiple areas of necrotization of the left lung with a small loculated hydropneumothorax. The patient was treated with antibiotics for three weeks. Follow-up examination at 3 months showed partial resolution of the left lung process. The pericardial fluid represented a "sympathetic" effusion, similar to an uncomplicated parapneumonic effusion, as the area of pneumonic infiltrate was juxtaposed to the pericardium.

Clinical Pearls

1. *Klebsiella pneumoniae* is the most frequent cause of a community-acquired, gram-negative, aerobic, bacillary pneumonia and should be suspected in the middle-aged to elderly alcoholic male who presents with prostration and an acute pneumonic history.

2. The characteristic dark brown or currant jelly sputum occurs in less than half of patients, and the characteristic bulging fissure sign or loss of lung volume occurs only occasionally.

3. For suspected Klebsiella pneumonia, amikacin and a third-generation cephalosporin should be instituted, and the regimen modified when sensitivities are available. Treatment should be continued for 2 to 3 weeks, depending on the clinical response.

REFERENCES

1. Ritbo M, Martin F. The clinical and roentgen manifestations of pneumonia due to bacillus mucosus capsulatus (primary Friedlander pneumonia). AJR 1949; 62:211–222.
2. Manfredi F, Daly WJ, Behnke RH. Clinical observations of acute Friedlander pneumonia. Ann Intern Med 1963; 58:642–653.
3. Kessner DM, Lepper MH. Epidemiologic studies of gram negative bacilli in the hospital and community. Am J Epidemiol 1967; 85:45–60.
4. Edmondson EB, Sanford JP. The Klebsiella-enterobacter (aerobacter)-serratia group. A clinical and bacteriological evaluation. Medicine 1967; 46:323–340.

PATIENT 73

A 55-year-old man with recent fever, cough, and dyspnea developing 6 months after right pneumonectomy, radiation therapy, and chemotherapy for squamous cell carcinoma of the lung

A 55-year-old man, status post right pneumonectomy for squamous cell carcinoma 6 months previously, was admitted to the hospital for fever, cough, and dyspnea of several days' duration. Following pneumonectomy, he received 2 cycles of mitomycin (total dose 40 mg), vinblastine, and prednisone, the last course having been completed 3 months prior to admission. He subsequently underwent radiation therapy, completing 4500 rads 2 weeks prior to admission.

Physical Examination: Temperature 102°; pulse 84; respirations 20; no acute distress. Chest examination: rales heard over the left posterior chest. Cardiac examination: no evidence of congestive heart failure or pulmonary hypertension.

Laboratory Findings: WBC 10,600/μl, 77% PMNs, 12% monocytes, 9% lymphocytes; Hct 31%; alkaline phosphatase 15 IU/L. Chest radiograph: changes consistent with previous right pneumonectomy, increase in the interstitial markings in the left lung field, particularly in the base. ABG (room air): pH 7.46, PCO_2 37 mmHg, PO_2 55 mmHg. Pulmonary function tests: FVC 1.88 L (37% of predicted), FEV_1 1.64 L (45% of predicted), with FEV_1/FVC ratio 87%, DL/VA ratio 2.76. CT of chest and abdomen: no evidence of metastatic disease or infiltrates in the left lung. Fiberoptic bronchoscopy with transbronchial lung biopsy was performed.

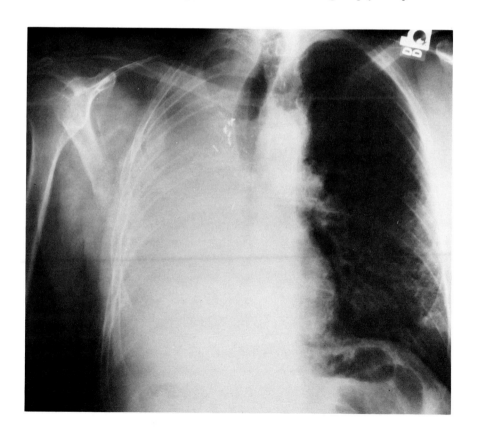

Diagnosis: Mitomycin-induced lung disease precipitated by radiation therapy.

Discussion: In patients with known malignancy who develop a diffuse pulmonary infiltrate, the differential diagnosis includes (1) opportunistic infection, (2) progression of the malignancy, and (3) an adverse effect of therapy, either radiation or chemotherapy. Radiation pneumonitis usually occurs 2 to 6 months following the completion of radiation therapy, with the insidious onset of a nonproductive cough with subsequent blood-streaking and the cardinal symptom of dyspnea, which initially may be present only upon exertion. Fever, which may be high and intermittent, and other constitutional symptoms occur in severe radiation pneumonitis. Chest pain is unusual. Physical signs include tachypnea with a paucity of chest findings. The earliest radiographic change consists of a ground-glass density or obscuration of the pulmonary markings. The infiltrate may be alveolar, nodular, or show frank consolidation. Radiologic changes usually are limited to the margins of the port and create a sharp demarcation between the pneumonitis and normal lung. Changes outside the port are presumably due to oblique radiation and are less impressive than the changes within the port. It is unusual for changes of radiation pneumonitis to occur radiographically or clinically prior to 1 month following completion of therapy unless the patient has been previously irradiated.

Mitomycin, an alkylating antibiotic, has been used in the treatment of gastrointestinal, breast, and lung cancers. More than 30 patients have been reported to have had pulmonary injury associated with its use. In the majority of these cases, additional drugs or radiation therapy had been received.

The approximate incidence of pulmonary toxicity from mitomycin is 3 to 12%, the variance presumably due to concomitant therapy. The total dose associated with pulmonary toxicity ranges from 20 to 200 mg/m^2. Patients who have received previous or concurrent irradiation may develop pulmonary toxicity at a lower dose. Oxygen therapy also may enhance the pulmonary disease.

Two types of syndromes are associated with mitomycin lung toxicity: (1) acute respiratory failure, and (2) insidious cough, dyspnea on exertion and constitutional symptoms. Fever is not a prominent finding. PFTs show a restrictive ventilatory defect and a decrease in DLCO. The diagnosis can be established by lung biopsy. Open lung biopsy provides a larger piece of tissue and may be more advantageous in excluding other etiologies and in diagnosing the drug-induced lung disease.

The chest radiograph usually shows a diffuse reticular pattern with nodularity, acinar pattern, hilar enlargement, and pleural effusions present uncommonly. Lobar or segmental infiltrates have not been reported.

The lung biopsy shows Type II pneumocyte proliferation and atypia, Type I pneumocyte necrosis, endothelial damage and collagen deposition. Alveolar septal edema and mononuclear cell infiltration of the interstitium is seen commonly.

The mortality of mitomycin lung disease is high, especially if the diagnosis is not established early. Corticosteroids can cause dramatic improvement in some patients.

In the present patient, transbronchial lung biopsy showed Type II pneumocyte hyperplasia, intraalveolar accumulation of foamy macrophages, accumulation of blood and fibrin within some airways, prominent endothelial cells, and a chronic mononuclear cell inflammation. The patient had a dramatic improvement with corticosteroid therapy. This most likely represented a case of mitomycin lung toxicity potentiated by radiation therapy. It would be an atypical presentation of radiation pneumonitis, as there was diffuse interstitial disease outside of the radiation port and occurrence of symptoms 2 weeks following cessation of radiation therapy. As has been observed with bleomycin toxicity, radiation therapy or high concentrations of oxygen can either cause or reexacerbate the drug toxicity.

Clinical Pearls

1. Radiation pneumonitis most commonly occurs 2 to 3 months (up to 6 months and rarely prior to 1 month) following radiation therapy and rarely prior to 1 month unless the patient has had previous irradiation.

2. Mitomycin causes pulmonary toxicity in up to 12% of patients with a total dose reported of 20 to 200 mg/m^2. Toxicity occurs at lower doses if there has been prior radiation therapy or the use of high concentrations of oxygen.

3. Steroids may result in dramatic improvement in mitomycin-induced lung disease.

REFERENCES

1. Cooper AD Jr, White DA, Matthay RA. Drug-induced pulmonary disease. Part I: Cytotoxic drugs. Am Rev Respir Dis 1986; 133:321–340.
2. Orwoll ES, Keissling PJ, Patterson JR. Interstitial pneumonia from mitomycin. Ann Intern Med 1978; 89:352–355.
3. Gross NJ. Pulmonary effects of radiation therapy. Ann Intern Med 1977; 86:81–92.

PATIENT 74

A 43-year-old man with a history of diabetes mellitus presenting with cough, chest pain, and upper lobe infiltrate

A 43-year-old man with brittle diabetes was admitted complaining of cough, fever, and left chest pain. He had required admission twice during the previous 4 months for diabetic ketoacidosis.

Physical Examination: Temperature 102°; respirations 22; pulse 110; blood pressure 111/77. Patient coughed frequently, producing scant clear sputum. HEENT normal; scattered rhonchi; cardiac normal.

Laboratory Findings: Hct 34%; WBC 12,200/μl with 95% neutrophils. ABG (room air): pH 7.45, $PaCO_2$ 37 mmHg, PaO_2 72 mmHg. Sputum Gram stain showed numerous neutrophils with a paucity of bacteria; potassium hydroxide and Ziehl-Nielson stains were negative. Chest radiograph revealed a dense infiltrate in the left upper lobe.

The patient received intravenous penicillin without improvement in symptoms or chest radiographic findings after 48 hours.

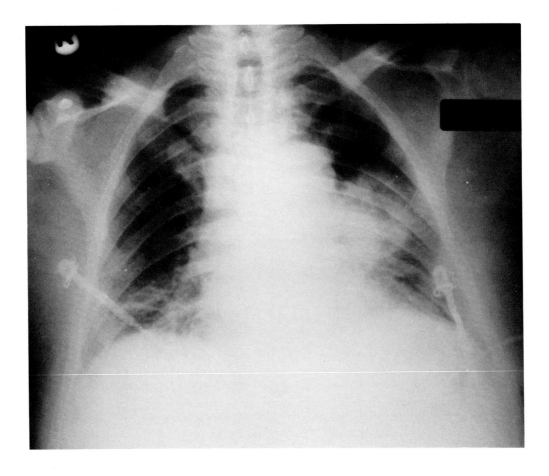

Diagnosis: Pulmonary mucormycosis.

Discussion: Although most patients with community-acquired pneumonia have a limited spectrum of bacterial pathogens that account for the majority of infections and respond adequately to antibiotics, the presence of comorbid disease, such as brittle diabetes, increases the likelihood of unusual or opportunistic pathogens. The presence of immunocompromise warrants more aggressive diagnostic procedures either at the patient's initial presentation or after the patient fails to respond to empiric antibiotics. A number of diagnostic techniques are available to determine the underlying pathogen in complicated pneumonias; the present patient underwent bronchoscopy because of the diagnostic sensitivity of protected catheter brushing and BAL for both bacterial and fungal pathogens.

The presence of hyphae in bronchoscopic specimens compatible with mucor confirmed the diagnosis of pulmonary mucormycosis—an infection caused by fungi belonging to the order mucorales in the class Zygomycetes. These ubiquitous fungi exist in soil and decaying organic material and rarely cause infection in normal hosts because of their low virulence. The presence of underlying severe immunosuppression, as caused by leukemia, lymphoma, profound neutropenia, or steroid and immunosuppressive drugs, markedly increases the pathogenicity of these organisms. Less common underlying disorders associated with mucormycosis include diabetes, renal failure, burns, and, rarely, solid tumors.

Brittle diabetes appears to predispose to mucormycosis beyond the immunosuppressive effects of hyperglycemia alone, since the infection is more common in patients with recent ketoacidosis. Laboratory investigations have supported this clinical observation by demonstrating that animals with drug-induced diabetes do not become easily infected with mucor unless they have associated acidosis. The presence of recurrent diabetic ketoacidosis in the present patient was a clinical clue suggesting the possibility of mucormycosis.

Clinical forms of mucor associated with diabetes include rhinocerebral, pulmonary, cutaneous, gastrointestinal, and widely disseminated infection. The pulmonary form of the disease develops after inhalation of the organism that invades pulmonary vascular walls, causing arteritis, intravascular thrombosis, abscess formation, and pulmonary hemorrhage with ischemic necrosis. Although mucor is one of the most fulminant fungal diseases known, usually demonstrating rapid progression of pulmonary infiltrates, chronic forms of infection occasionally occur. Early symptoms of pulmonary mucormycosis include cough, fever, and variable sputum production that may rapidly progress to pleuritic chest pain, massive pulmonary hemorrhage, and severe systemic toxicity.

The radiographic manifestations of pulmonary mucormycosis are varied. Initial zones of infection appear as patchy or nodular infiltrates that spread to cavitary lobar consolidation, simulating necrotizing bronchopneumonia. Fungus balls containing mucor hyphae may form within the cavities. A miliary pattern and pleural effusions are rare radiographic manifestations, but vascular thrombosis commonly causes distal infarction, thereby creating a wedge-shaped infiltrate.

Diagnosis of pulmonary mucormycosis usually depends on detection of the organism in lung biopsy specimens or airway secretions, since mucor does not grow well in culture. The fungus appears as broad (15-50 μm) nonseptate hyphae with right angle branching, as distinct from Aspergillus species, which are septate with acute angle branching. The presence of the organism in airway secretions is strong evidence of disease, since mucor is rarely a pulmonary saprophyte.

Optimal therapy for pulmonary mucor is uncertain. The underlying cause of immunosuppression should be reversed whenever possible. Rapid initiation of full-dose systemic amphotericin B has resulted in complete cure in diabetics with mucormycosis. Because some patients fail medical therapy with amphotericin B, surgical resection of infected lobes may be indicated in adequate operative candidates who have localized disease.

Because of continued symptoms and the history of diabetes, the present patient underwent bronchoscopy with transbronchial biopsy, bronchoalveolar lavage (BAL), and protected catheter brushing in consideration of an opportunistic or unusual pathogen. The biopsy and BAL specimens demonstrated fungal hyphae with characteristic features of mucor. The patient was treated with intravenous amphotericin B with complete resolution of radiographic and clinical evidence of infection. No recurrence of disease has been noted during a one-year follow-up.

Clinical Pearls

1. Pulmonary mucormycosis should be suspected in a febrile diabetic with recurrent ketoacidosis and a pulmonary infiltrate.

2. Mucor rarely grows in culture, and diagnosis of pulmonary mucormycosis depends on microscopic detection of the organism in lung tissue or secretions.

3. Although the ideal therapy of pulmonary mucor is uncertain, lobectomy should be considered in a surgical candidate with localized disease.

REFERENCES

1. Lehrer RI, Howard DH, Sypherd PS, et al. Mucormycosis. Ann Intern Med 1980; 93:93–108.
2. Bigby TD, Serota ML, Tierney LM, Matthay MA. Clinical spectrum of pulmonary mucormycosis. Chest 1986; 89:435–439.
3. Brown JF, Gottlieb LS, McCormick RA. Pulmonary and Rhinocerebral mucormycosis: successful outcome with amphotericin B and griseofulvin therapy. Arch Intern Med 1977; 137:936–938.

PATIENT 75

A 47-year-old alcoholic woman with a 12-day history of cough, purulent sputum, and right pleuritic chest pain

A 47-year-old alcoholic woman was transferred to our hospital 12 days following the onset of cough, purulent sputum, and right pleuritic chest pain. She was seen by a local physician who diagnosed right lower lobe pneumonia and began a third-generation cephalosporin. She remained intermittently febrile and was noted to have a right pleural effusion 10 days following onset of symptoms. She denied recent heavy alcohol consumption, loss of consciousness, or shaking chills. There was a remote history of intravenous drug abuse and occasional use of marijuana.

Physical Examination: Temperature 102°; pulse 110; respirations 28; no acute distress but appeared toxic; poor dentition and gingivitis. Chest examination: flat percussion note, decreased fremitus, and distant breath sounds on the right.

Laboratory Findings: WBC 29,900/μl, 78% PMNs, 12% lymphocytes, 9% monocytes; Hct 29%. Right thoracentesis under ultrasound guidance: nucleated cells 15,500/μl, 85% PMNs, total protein 5.8 g/dl, LDH 383 IU/L, glucose 10 mg/dl, pH 6.83. Chest radiograph (PA and lateral decubitus): large non-free flowing right pleural density. CT scan: loculated right pleural effusion with thick rind and evidence of right lower lobe necrosis.

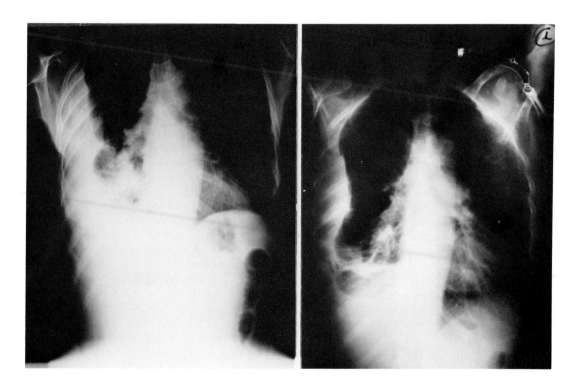

Diagnosis: Anaerobic pleuropulmonary infection.

Discussion: Anaerobic pulmonary infection should be suspected in the appropriate setting when there is impaired consciousness or esophageal disease. The major predisposing conditions are alcoholism, other drug abuse, cerebrovascular accidents, nasogastric tube feeding, seizures, and general anesthesia. Periodontal disease and gingivitis are important background factors, as the quantity of anaerobes is substantially higher with poor oral hygiene than in normal or edentulous patients. Despite aspiration of oropharyngeal contents, most individuals have good clearance mechanisms, as the distal airways and parenchyma are generally sterile. However, in the previously mentioned predisposing conditions, normal pulmonary host defenses are impaired, multiplication of organisms can occur, and pneumonitis is initiated.

Anaerobic pneumonia is most commonly found in dependent segments, the posterior segments of the upper lobes, and the superior segments of the lower lobes. The pneumonia frequently is pleural-based and initially may resemble a pulmonary infarction. Anaerobic pleuropulmonary infection in the absence of predisposing factors should raise the suspicion of pulmonary embolism, endobronchial obstruction by tumor, and extension of infection from below the diaphragm.

The anaerobes most commonly involved in pulmonary infection are Bacteroides, *Fusobacterium nucleatum,* Peptostreptococcus, and microaerophilic streptococcus. Ninety percent of patients with aspiration pneumonia and lung abscess and 75% of postpneumonic empyemas are caused by anaerobes.

The clinical presentation may be that of acute pneumonia with fever, cough, and pleurisy, or be more insidious, with patients having a history of days to weeks of low-grade fever and cough. When tissue necrosis ensues, patients will present with either necrotizing pneumonia, lung abscess, or empyema. Physical examination frequently demonstrates poor oral hygiene, impaired or absent gag reflex, and the ravages of alcoholism.

The chest radiograph shows areas of pneumonia in dependent lung segments, evidence of necrosis, and either lung abscess or loculated pleural effusion.

The sputum Gram stain shows multiple gram-negative bacilli or coccobacillary forms, pale-staining gram-negative cells with tapered ends, and small gram-positive cocci in chains. However, a sputum sample cannot be used for anaerobic culture because it is contaminated by large numbers of indigenous mouth anaerobes. Foul-smelling sputum may suggest anaerobic infection but its absence does not negate the diagnosis. Empyema fluid provides a good source for a specific diagnosis. It is important that the specimen be placed under anaerobic conditions in an appropriate transport tube immediately after being aspirated. Blood cultures are infrequently positive in anaerobic infections, and transtracheal aspirate and fiberoptic bronchoscopy with a protected specimen brush and quantitative cultures could be helpful in certain clinical situations. However, the diagnosis usually can be based on the clinical presentation.

Appropriate prolonged antibiotic therapy to prevent relapse is critical in treatment. Moderate to high dosages of penicillin, clindamycin, and metronidazole are usually satisfactory in the noncritically ill patient. In the seriously ill patient with evidence of necrosis, a combination of clindamycin and penicillin, or metronidazole and penicillin or chloramphenicol may be more advantageous. Drainage of an empyema needs to be instituted as soon as the diagnosis is established. In anaerobic infections, this usually requires a thoracotomy for debridement and decortication, as these patients present late in the course of infection.

The present patient was taken to the operating room where a large amount of partially organized, purulent material was removed from the pleural space, and the lung decorticated. She became afebrile three days following surgery and was discharged on oral penicillin 12 days later.

Clinical Pearls

1. In 90% of patients with aspiration pneumonia and lung abscess and in 75% of patients with postpneumonic empyema, anaerobic bacteria are involved.

2. Anaerobic pleuropulmonary infection should be suspected in the setting of impaired consciousness, particularly in the alcoholic who also has defects in lung defense mechanisms.

3. The patient may present with low-grade fever and constitutional symptoms, have poor oral hygiene, and have evidence of peripheral infiltrates in the dependent portions of the lung.

4. Most patients with anaerobic empyema due to the natural history of the disease will not respond to bedside chest tube drainage and require an empyemectomy and decortication.

REFERENCES

1. Bartlett JG, Finegold SM. Anaerobic infections of the lung and pleural space. Am Rev of Respir Dis 1974; 110:207–226.
2. Bartlett JG, Gorbach SL, Finegold SM. The bacteriology of aspiration pneumonia. Am J Med 1974; 56:202–207.
3. Bartlett JG, Gorbach SL, Thadepalli H, Finegold S. The bacteriology of empyema. Lancet 1974; 1:338–340.

PATIENT 76

A 47-year-old man with subcutaneous nodules, diplopia, and fever of 3 weeks' duration

A 47-year-old man experienced headaches, double vision, mild cough, and fever three weeks before admission. One week later he noted painful subcutaneous nodules on his arms and legs that had a purplish discoloration. He denied additional respiratory symptoms or a history of smoking.

Physical Examination: Temperature 101°. Lymph nodes normal; numerous subcutaneous tender nodules on arms and legs. Chest and abdomen normal.

Laboratory Findings: Hct 39%, WBC 7,300/μl; creatinine 1.1 mg/dl; urinalysis normal. Chest radiograph was normal except for subtle basilar interstitial infiltrates. A CT scan of the head showed several 1.5 cm mass lesions in the occipital cerebral cortex.

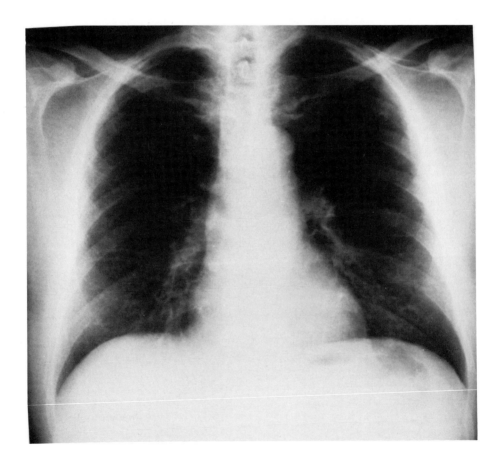

Diagnosis: Lymphomatoid granulomatosis with involvement of the central nervous system and skin.

Discussion: Despite the patient's nonspecific presentation, the subtle pulmonary radiographic abnormality with cerebral mass lesions and fever should suggest the possibility of lymphomatoid granulomatosis. This disorder, first described by Liebow et al. in 1972, is characterized as a form of angiitis and granulomatosis affecting small- and medium-sized blood vessels with an angiocentric and angiodestructive infiltration of mononuclear cells. Although often included in general reviews of systemic vasculitis, lymphomatoid granulomatosis is not a true vasculitis, since vascular inflammatory necrosis is not a feature. Similarly, this condition differs from Wegener's granulomatosis by the absence of a polymorphous inflammatory cell response and the rarity of a true granulomatous tissue reaction. These histopathologic features and the proclivity for development of malignant lymphoma characterize lymphomatoid granulomatosis as a part of the spectrum of malignant lymphoproliferative disorders.

The typical patient presents with fatigue, weakness, weight loss, and fever. More than 60% of patients note chest discomfort, pleuritic chest pain, cough, shortness of breath or dyspnea on exertion in the early phases of the disease, with essentially all patients eventually developing pulmonary manifestations. Skin lesions are the commonest extrapulmonary manifestation of the disease, usually appearing as 1 to 4 cm painful, erythematous nodules that can occasionally erode through the overlying skin. Neurologic involvement occurs in 20% of patients and may be the presenting complaint. Angiodestructive mononuclear cell infiltration of nerve tissue creates a mass lesion effect in either the central or peripheral nervous system. As opposed to most causes of vasculitis, renal involvement usually does not impair renal function, since the interstitium rather than the glomeruli is infiltrated. Although infiltration of the skeletal muscle, mesentery, salivary glands, liver, adrenals, heart, and gastrointestinal tract has been reported, lymphomatoid granulomatosis typically spares the lymph nodes, bone marrow, and spleen.

Lymphomatoid granulomatosis is suspected clinically when a patient with constitutional, respiratory, or neurologic symptoms presents with an abnormal chest radiograph suggestive of the disorder. Most patients have bilateral pulmonary nodules ranging in size from 1 to 9 cm, simulating metastatic disease that may cavitate in 30% of patients or spontaneously clear. Other radiographic features include patchy or diffuse inhomogeneous infiltrates with a lower lobe predominance, fleeting infiltrates, rare pleural effusions, or regions of dense alveolar consolidation. The major clinical point is that almost all patients will have an abnormal chest radiograph, and the subtle abnormalities in the present patient are unusual. The diagnosis is confirmed by open lung biopsy, although some patients without obvious pulmonary disease may undergo biopsy of other organs.

Since the disease is rapidly progressive, with death often resulting from CNS involvement, urgent initiation of therapy is requisite. Aggressive diagnostic evaluations for an underlying lymphoproliferative neoplasm are required, since many patients with lymphomatoid granulomatosis will have an occult malignant lymphoma at presentation. Combination chemotherapy comprising corticosteroids and cyclophosphamide with radiation therapy directed at CNS foci are the initial treatment modalities. Because as many as 13 to 47% of patients develop lymphoma during therapy, a poor response to corticosteroids and cyclophosphamide warrants more aggressive therapy for an occult lymphoma. Once corticosteroids and cyclophosphamide induce a long-term remission in patients with lymphomatoid granulomatosis, lymphoma tends not to develop subsequently.

A skin biopsy specimen revealed the diagnosis in the present patient. He underwent chemotherapy and radiation therapy with a dramatic improvement in symptoms after an initial evaluation did not demonstrate lymphoma. He died suddenly 1 month later of pulmonary emboli, and an autopsy demonstrated residual CNS disease with foci of malignant transformation.

Clinical Pearls

1. Despite its name, lymphomatoid granulomatosis rarely demonstrates true granulomas in biopsy specimens.

2. Lymphomatoid granulomatosis is a lymphoproliferative disorder rather than a vasculitis, since inflammatory necrosis of blood vessels is not found.

3. The incidence of malignant lymphoma in lymphomatoid granulomatosis is so high that patients not responding to chemotherapy should be assumed to have an underlying neoplasm.

REFERENCES

1. Fauci AS, Haynes BF, Costa J, et al. Lymphomatoid granulomatosis: Prospective clinical and therapeutic experience over 10 years. N Engl J Med 1982; 306:68–74.
2. Bone RC, Vernon M, Sobonya RE, Rendon H. Lymphomatoid granulomatosis: Report of a case and review of the literature. Am J Med 1978; 65:709–716.
3. Chandler DB, Fulmer JD. Pulmonary vasculitis. Lung 1985; 163:257–273.
4. Leavitt RY, Fauci AS. Pulmonary vasculitis. Am Rev Respir Dis 1986; 134:149–166.

PATIENT 77

A 63-year-old man with a history of irradiated lung cancer presenting with cough, fever, and a progressive pulmonary cavity

A 63-year-old man noted cough, fever, and weight loss. Nine months earlier, he had undergone radiation therapy for unresectable squamous cell carcinoma of the lung, which presented as a right hilar mass with mediastinal extension. Two months later he developed a right upper lobe paratracheal infiltrate considered to be radiation fibrosis. During the next 7 months of follow-up, the infiltrate enlarged, progressing to pleural thickening and cavity formation despite oral penicillin therapy.

Physical Examination: Temperature 100°. Chronically ill appearing edentulous male with productive cough; right upper lobe consolidation with rales; cardiac normal.

Laboratory Findings: WBC 12,000/μl; Hct 31%. Chest radiograph: left upper lobe cavitary infiltrate with pleural thickening. Sputum Gram stain and acid-fast smears unrevealing.

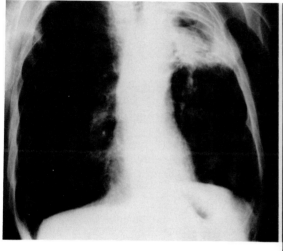
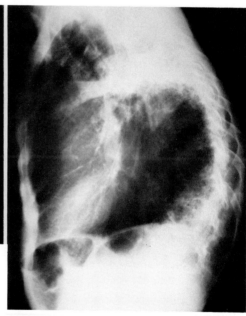

Diagnosis: Chronic necrotizing aspergillosis with intracavitary fungus ball. Additional considerations include anaerobic pneumonitis, progressive lung cancer, tuberculosis, and other fungal infections.

Discussion: Aspergillus species are ubiquitous fungal organisms that are usually innocuous but have the potential to cause a spectrum of pulmonary disorders. Chronic necrotizing aspergillosis is a form of pulmonary disease that has been recently emphasized to be a distinct entity from the more familiar allergic, saprophytic, and rapidly invasive forms of aspergillosis. First described over 50 years ago as chronic granulomatous aspergillosis, this disorder is an indolent, cavitating pulmonary process that results from slowly progressive invasion of tissue by Aspergillus.

Most patients with chronic necrotizing aspergillosis are middle-aged with either underlying lung disease or some condition causing mild immunocompromise, such as insulin-dependent diabetes mellitus or corticosteroid therapy. The history of lung disease may be COPD, pulmonary resection, sarcoidosis, pneumoconiosis, radiation therapy, inactive tuberculosis, or nonspecific lung cysts. These disorders interfere with pulmonary clearance of inhaled fungal spores, allowing initiation of localized infection that slowly extends across a region of the lung. Since Aspergillus species have a proclivity for invading arterioles, tissue necrosis occurs, resulting in thick-walled cavities that contain devitalized tissue and fungal elements. These resultant fungus balls arising in foci of Aspergillus bronchopneumonia differ from simple aspergillomas complicating pre-existing lung cavities because of the absence of fungal tissue invasion in the latter condition.

Patients presenting with chronic necrotizing aspergillosis typically note fever, cough, and sputum production. Weight loss, lassitude, and anorexia almost always occur, and hemoptysis and leukocytosis are variable manifestations. The duration of symptoms are notably prolonged: 76% of patients demonstrate progressive radiographic abnormalities or symptoms from 1 to 6 months, with the remaining 24% from 6 to 24 months. The radiologic manifestations are typically distinctive, revealing a localized infiltrate that progresses to parenchymal necrosis, a characteristic rim of thickened pleura, and cavity formation with or without a fungus ball. The presence of a fungus ball is often associated with a crescent of air within the cavity. The process most often involves the upper lobes or superior segment of the lower lobes, thereby suggesting the differential diagnoses comprising tuberculosis, anaerobic infection, lung cancer, and other fungal infections such as histoplasmosis, coccidioidomycosis, and blastomycosis. The disorder is indolently progressive, with infection capable of extending to the entire lung, contralateral hemithorax, pleural space, chest wall, or mediastinum.

Diagnosis of chronic necrotizing aspergillosis is most certain when lung tissue obtained by transbronchial biopsy, needle aspiration, or open surgical biopsy demonstrates invasive fungal hyphae. The diagnosis may be strongly suspected when expectorated or aspirated airway secretions grow Aspergillus in the absence of other pathogens or pulmonary disorders that can adequately explain the patient's radiographic and clinical features. Positive Aspergillus precipitins are almost always positive and further support the diagnosis.

Many patients respond well to therapy. Although the ideal therapeutic approach is controversial, medical management with systemic amphotericin B with or without 5-fluorocytosine is generally recommended. Patients failing to respond or with contraindications to systemic therapy have been successfully managed with intracavitary instillation of amphotericin B. Pulmonary resection is usually avoided, because most patients have underlying pulmonary disorders that interfere with surgical recovery and cause a greater than 40% postoperative morbidity rate. If patients have localized disease, good pulmonary function, or contraindications to medical therapy, surgical therapy can be considered. Without data to guide us, most physicians recommend a short pre- and postoperative course of amphotericin B to prevent Aspergillus empyemas or stump infections.

The present patient grew *Aspergillus fumigatus* from a sputum specimen, prompting fiberoptic bronchoscopy with transbronchial biopsy of the right upper lobe that demonstrated branching fungal hyphae invading lung tissue. He was started on intravenous amphotericin B but died suddenly. The autopsy confirmed the diagnosis and excluded recurrent neoplasm in the upper lobe.

Clinical Pearls

1. Chronic necrotizing aspergillosis is suspected when a patient with preexisting lung disease develops chronic, necrotizing bronchopneumonia that results in a fungus ball or pleural thickening.

2. Fungus balls resulting from chronic necrotizing aspergillosis differ from simple aspergillomas, which require a preexisting lung cavity and do not invade tissue.

3. In contrast to simple aspergillomas, chronic necrotizing aspergillosis may respond to systemic amphotericin B.

REFERENCES

1. Gefter WB, Weingrad TR, Epstein DM, et al. "Semi-invasive" pulmonary aspergillosis. Diagn Radiol 1981; 140:313–321.
2. Binder RE, Faling J, Pugatch RD, et al. Chronic necrotizing pulmonary aspergillosis: A discrete clinical entity. Medicine 1982; 61:109–124.

PATIENT 78

A 43-year-old man with rheumatoid arthritis, nonpleuritic chest pain, and bilateral pleural effusions

A 43-year-old white male with a 3-year history of rheumatoid arthritis was admitted for evaluation of bilateral pleural effusions. Approximately 15 months prior, the patient was noted to have a right-sided pleural effusion associated with nonpleuritic chest pain. The right effusion never resolved completely and he subsequently developed bilateral pleural effusions with intermittent chest pain and dyspnea on exertion. Articular disease had been active. Current medications included prednisone and a nonsteroidal antiinflammatory agent.

Physical Examination: Temperature 99°, respirations 20; no acute distress; bilateral pleural friction rubs; rheumatoid nodules on the extensor surface of the upper extremities; symmetric synovitis of multiple joints.

Laboratory Findings: WBC 9500/μl, 54% PMNs, 34% lymphocytes; ESR 35 mm/h. Chest radiograph: bilateral pleural effusions with loculation on the right, no evidence of parenchymal rheumatoid disease. Left thoracentesis: yellowish-green fluid, nucleated cells 1584/μl, 7% PMNs, 70% lymphocytes; glucose 3 mg/dl; pH 7.05; protein 6 g/dl; LDH 1065 IU/L; rheumatoid factor 1:320; C3, C4 and total hemolytic complement: all low. Right thoracentesis: milky pleural fluid, nucleated cells 1500/μl, 80% lymphocytes, 15% macrophages, 5% PMNs; pH 7.00; glucose 6 mg/dl; protein 5.5 g/dl; cholesterol 300 mg/dl; triglycerides 25 mg/dl; numerous cholesterol crystals.

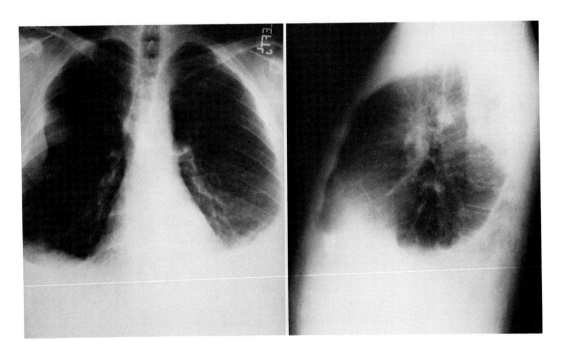

Diagnosis: Bilateral rheumatoid pleural effusions (one-sided cholesterol effusion).

Discussion: Pleural involvement probably is the most common thoracic manifestation of rheumatoid disease. Clinical evidence of rheumatoid pleurisy occurs in approximately 5% of patients with rheumatoid disease; however, based on autopsy findings, clinical disease grossly underestimates the number of patients who have pleural involvement. Grossly, the pleural space may show small areas of visceral pleural fibrosis, numerous visceral pleural nodules, or extensive fibrosis with complete obliteration of the pleural space. The visceral pleural nodules have the characteristic features of fibrinoid necrosis, palisading cells, and lymphocytic or plasma cell infiltration.

Rheumatoid pleurisy has a striking male predominance, the usual patient presenting in the sixth decade approximately 5 years after the onset of rheumatoid disease. However, effusions can develop either before or as late as 20 years following the onset of arthritis. At the time of presentation, patients usually manifest moderate to severe arthritis, subcutaneous nodules, and a high serum rheumatoid factor. They may present with pleuritic chest pain or dyspnea or the disease may be discovered on a routine chest radiograph. Fever is not a frequent manifestation of rheumatoid pleurisy in contrast to lupus pleuritis. The chest radiograph usually shows a small to moderate unilateral pleural effusion without evidence of rheumatoid lung disease; however, this may occur in up to one-third of patients. On thoracentesis, the fluid may have a yellowish-green tint and, occasionally, may be milky due to an increased cholesterol concentration. The fluid may appear to contain debris (due to exfoliation of cells from the rheumatoid nodules). The leukocyte count varies from a few hundred up to 20,000/μl. Cellular predominance depends on the timing of thoracentesis in relation to the active pleural process. The most striking and consistent features are a low pleural fluid glucose (usually < 30 mg/dl), a pH of about 7.00, and an LDH of > 1000 IU/L. However, when first evaluated, approximately 20% of patients with rheumatoid pleurisy will have a normal pleural fluid glucose. If the effusion persists for several weeks, the pleural fluid glucose concentration will decrease to < 50 mg/dl. Other common findings are low pleural fluid total hemolytic and complement components, a high rheumatoid factor ($\geq$ 1:320), and an increased concomitant serum value. Patients who develop severe pleural fibrosis and trapped lung with a chronic pleural effusion commonly have an abundance of cholesterol crystals and high concentrations of cholesterol, which make the fluid appear milky. Triglyceride concentrations will be < 50 mg/dl, cholesterol/triglyceride ratio > 1.0, and lipoprotein electrophoresis will not show chylomicrons, excluding the diagnosis of chylothorax and supporting the diagnosis of a cholesterol or chyliform effusion.

The course of a patient with rheumatoid pleurisy is variable. It is uncommon, however, for resolution to occur in less than 3 to 4 weeks; the effusion will generally resolve over several months. Some patients have a protracted course that lasts years and occasionally progresses to marked pleural thickening, requiring decortication. There are no scientific data available concerning the use of corticosteroids or nonsteroidal antiinflammatory drugs in the treatment of rheumatoid pleurisy. If treatment with antiinflammatory drugs is to be of value, it probably would need to be instituted early and continued until the inflammation ceases. The current patient's prednisone dose was increased to 40 mg daily with some diminution of fluid and improvement in symptoms over a few weeks.

Clinical Pearls

1. Patients with rheumatoid pleurisy may present prior to or as late as 20 years after onset of articular disease.

2. Patients with rheumatoid pleurisy have the classic triad of low pleural fluid pH and glucose and LDH > 1000 IU/L. However, up to 20% of patients initially presenting with rheumatoid pleurisy have a normal pH and glucose and an LDH < 1000 IU/L.

3. Other diagnoses associated with the above triad include empyema and paragonimiasis. Since patients with rheumatoid pleurisy are frequently on corticosteroids and appear to have an increased incidence of empyema, Gram stain and culture of this fluid need to be performed.

REFERENCES

1. Lillington GA, Carr DT, Mayne JG. Rheumatoid pleurisy with effusion. Arch Intern Med 1971; 128:754–768.
2. Walker WC, Wright V. Pulmonary lesions and rheumatoid arthritis. Medicine 1968; 47:501–519.
3. Halla JT, Schronhenloher RE, Volanakis JE. Immune complexes and other laboratory features of pleural effusions. Ann Intern Med 1980; 92:748–752.
4. Jones FL, Blodgett RC. Empyema in rheumatoid pleuropulmonary disease. Ann Intern Med 1971; 74:665–671.
5. Coe JE, Aikawa JK. Cholesterol pleural effusion. Arch Intern Med 1961; 108:163–174.

PATIENT 79

A 24-year-old woman with a history of cystic fibrosis and massive hemoptysis

A 24-year-old woman with cystic fibrosis was admitted with massive hemoptysis. She had required continuous antibiotics and home oxygen for severe respiratory dysfunction during the previous 2 years. Recurrent airway suppuration necessitated 3 hospitalizations within the previous 6 months. Recently she had been feeling well until she suddenly coughed up 500 ml of bright red blood.

Physical Examination: Respirations 22; pulse 100; blood pressure 118/65. Thin-appearing woman with mild respiratory distress; hyperresonant chest with diffuse rales and scattered rhonchi.

Laboratory Findings: CBC normal with adequate platelets. Prothrombin time 12.5/11 sec. ABG (2 L/min): pH 7.43, $PaCO_2$ 35 mmHg, PaO_2 72 mmHg. Chest radiograph: diffuse fibrotic and cystic parenchymal changes consistent with the diagnosis of cystic fibrosis.

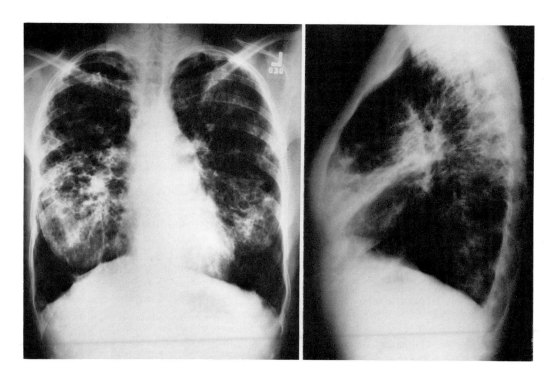

Diagnosis: Massive hemoptysis related to cystic fibrosis.

Discussion: Cystic fibrosis (CF) is the most common lethal genetic disorder among whites in the United States, occurring in approximately 1 of every 2,000 live births. During the last several decades, advances in management along with earlier detection of mild forms of the disease have improved the life expectancy of CF from 2 years to now more than 20 years.

Complications of chronic pulmonary disease are the major sources of morbidity and mortality for the CF patient and represent the most important challenge to the physician. Of several potential complications, massive hemoptysis is the greatest risk for sudden death. The majority of patients with CF experience some degree of mild to moderate hemoptysis that usually responds to antibiotic therapy. Massive hemoptysis, defined as more than 500 ml of blood during a 24-hour period, occurs in 5 to 7% of patients, of whom 11 to 30% may die from uncontrolled hemorrhage and asphyxiation. Most patients with massive hemoptysis have severe pulmonary dysfunction, but occasionally major bleeding occurs in patients with mild CF.

Patients with CF have a proclivity for airway hemorrhage for a number of reasons. Chronic purulent bronchiectasis generates growth of granulation tissue in the endobronchial and peribronchial regions which has a rich vascular supply from the bronchial circulation. Furthermore, bronchial arteries in bronchiectatic sections of airways become tortuous and dilated, forming bronchial-pulmonary artery anastomoses. This vascular supply along with underlying pulmonary hypertension and suppurative tissue necrosis contributes to recurrent hemoptysis. Additionally, long-term antibiotic therapy and pancreatic insufficiency may cause clotting abnormalities further aggravating bleeding.

The approach to the patient with CF and massive hemoptysis is directed to encourage a prompt cessation of hemorrhage. Clotting and intravascular volume abnormalities are corrected, bedrest with mild sedation is initiated, respiratory therapy is temporarily suspended, and antibiotics are employed to treat *Staphylococcus aureus* and *Pseudomonas aeruginosa*.

If major, life-threatening hemorrhage continues despite conservative measures, localization of the site of bleeding is critical to direct further therapeutic efforts. During active hemorrhage, fiberoptic bronchoscopy is successful in more than 90% of patients to identify the segmental or subsegmental source of blood. Bronchial angiography is less sensitive, requiring more active bleeding to demonstrate a radiologic "blush" of contrast agent, but can be employed if bronchoscopy is unavailable.

With localization of the bleeding source, several therapeutic interventions are available. Balloon occlusion of the bleeding segmental bronchus with a Fogarty catheter placed through a bronchoscope may successfully tamponade hemorrhage in most patients. The majority of patients will stop bleeding, although in 22% bleeding will recur during the subsequent weeks to months. The small number of patients with CF treated by Fogarty catheters does not allow this intervention to be considered the preferred form of therapy. Several large studies indicate that bronchial artery embolization with absorbable gelatin sponge successfully arrests hemorrhage in CF in 88% of patients during the initial procedure. If unsuccessful, embolization can be repeated until all potential vessels supplying the region of hemorrhage are embolized. The most frequent complications are low-grade fever and mild thoracic discomfort that lasts 2 to 3 days. Transverse myelitis is a major concern, but most series do not note its occurrence. Unfortunately, 23% of patients eventually redevelop massive hemoptysis.

Thoracotomy is initially avoided in patients with CF and massive hemoptysis. Underlying severe pulmonary dysfunction causes an unacceptably high operative mortality of 18%, which is higher than the mortality of 11% from the bleeding alone. Careful patient selection can reserve thoracotomy with lobectomy for patients most likely to tolerate the procedure and who have demonstrated the greatest need for surgery. Patients with unrelenting, life-threatening hemorrhage despite other interventions (bronchial artery embolization and/or Fogarty catheter placement) with good physical activity levels and an FVC and FEV_1 greater than 50% of predicted may have adequate pulmonary reserve to tolerate thoracotomy.

The present patient underwent bronchoscopy that localized the bleeding to the right upper lobe. After three attempts, bronchial artery embolization successfully controlled the hemorrhage.

Clinical Pearls

1. Massive hemoptysis occurs in 5 to 7% of patients with CF and has a mortality rate of 11 to 30%.

2. If conservative measures fail, the patient should undergo bronchoscopy with bronchial artery embolization or airway Fogarty catheter placement.

3. Thoracotomy in patients with CF and massive hemoptysis has an 18% mortality and is reserved for patients with uncontrollable hemorrhage and adequate pulmonary reserve.

REFERENCES

1. Porter DK, Van Every MJ, Anthracite RF, Mack JW Jr. Massive hemoptysis in cystic fibrosis. Arch Intern Med 1983; 143:287–290.
2. Davis DB. Cystic fibrosis. Semin Respir Med 1985; 6:243–342.
3. Taussig LM. Cystic Fibrosis. New York, Thieme-Stratton, Inc., 1984.

PATIENT 80

A 16-year-old girl with hemoptysis and recurrent pulmonary infiltrates during a 5-year period

A 16-year-old girl was admitted because of rapidly developing shortness of breath and hemoptysis. She had three similar episodes during the previous five years that were treated with antibiotics for "severe, bilateral pneumonia." She denied chronic symptoms other than fatigue during the last two months.

Physical Examination: Pulse 110; respirations 30. Skin normal; bilateral crackles with tubular breath sounds; cardiac normal.

Laboratory Findings: CBC normal except for Hct 31%; urinalysis normal; renal function tests normal. ABG (room air): pH 7.50, PCO_2 30 mmHg; PO_2 52 mmHg. Chest radiograph demonstrated bilateral alveolar infiltrates with consolidation.

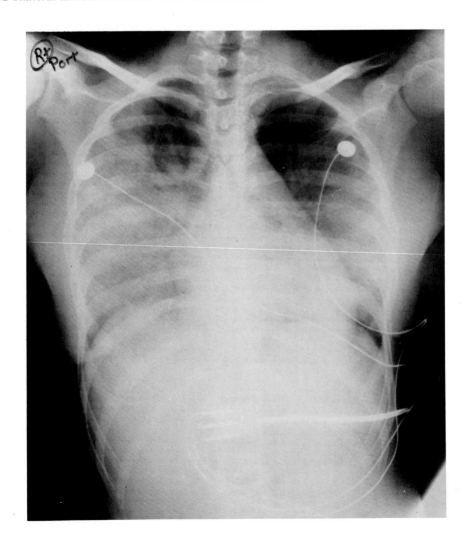

Diagnosis: Idiopathic pulmonary hemosiderosis (IPH).

Discussion: The onset of diffuse alveolar hemorrhage with hemoptysis and hypoxemia is an alarming mode of presentation for patient and physician alike. The patient is often moderately to severely ill, the alveolar hemorrhage may be initially occult in the absence of hemoptysis, and a wide range of disparate disorders may precipitate the clinical condition.

The initial approach to the patient is assisted by recognizing that six diseases are the major causes of most instances of pulmonary hemorrhage: antibasement membrane disease, nonspecific systemic necrotizing vasculitis, Wegener's granulomatosis, lupus, idiopathic rapidly progressive glomerulonephritis, and IPH. To determine which of these conditions underlies an episode of alveolar hemorrhage requires a careful clinical assessment, serologic studies, and biopsy of the kidneys or other extrapulmonary organs when indicated. With the exception of IPH, the major causes of pulmonary hemorrhage are associated with renal insufficiency or preexisting symptoms in other organ systems. Because pulmonary histopathology is nonspecific, sharing similar features with varied diseases associated with alveolar hemorrhage, lung biopsy is not required in the majority of patients.

IPH is a diagnosis of exclusion, since it is defined as a nonimmunologically dependent intraalveolar hemorrhage that occurs unassociated with infection, chemical exposures, bleeding diathesis, hemodynamic abnormalities, glomerulonephritis, or other extrapulmonary disease. The diagnosis is considered in the setting of isolated pulmonary hemorrhage with negative serologic studies for antibasement membrane antibody when cardiovascular abnormalities such as mitral stenosis are excluded. The chest radiograph ranges from patchy to diffuse bilateral acinar or confluent infiltrates; after repeated hemorrhages cause underlying pulmonary fibrosis, a mixed interstitial-alveolar infiltrate may occur. When IPH is strongly suspected, an open lung biopsy is indicated to exclude other unusual disorders and to confirm the presence of typical histopathologic features of IPH, which are intraalveolar hemorrhage, hemosiderin-laden macrophages, and interstitial fibrosis.

The etiology of IPH remains uncertain. Since some patients respond to corticosteroids and others have had coexisting celiac disease, an immunologic pathophysiology has been suggested. This theory is supported by the presence of elevated serum IgA in 50% of patients with IPH and reports of IgA deposition in the renal glomeruli. Many patients, however, do not respond to corticosteroids, and lung biopsy specimens do not detect antibody or immune complex deposition.

Determination of optimal therapy for patients with IPH is difficult because acute hemorrhage may resolve spontaneously and the disease may undergo long remissions. Corticosteroids appear to be of benefit in the acute situation but do not improve the long-term course. Patients with active hemorrhage not responding to corticosteroids may improve with immunosuppressive agents. The pulmonary infiltrates wane within 48 hours and may resolve in two weeks. Patients need to be followed subsequently to exclude the possibility of late development of underlying lupus or a systemic vasculitis. The typical course of IPH is marked by recurrent hemorrhage that may generate pulmonary fibrosis, chronic dyspnea, clubbing, and cor pulmonale.

The clinicians recognized the significance of anemia and hemoptysis occurring in the setting of diffuse alveolar infiltrates, hypoxemia, and recurrent acute respiratory illnesses, and considered the possibility of diffuse alveolar hemorrhage in the present patient. The absence of renal or other extrapulmonary disease suggested IPH, which was later confirmed by open lung biopsy. The patient was managed with intravenous corticosteroids, and her episode of alveolar hemorrhage remitted. She subsequently bled again six months later.

Clinical Pearls

1. IPH is the only major cause of diffuse alveolar hemorrhage unassociated with renal or other extrapulmonary disease.

2. Up to 50% of patients with IPH have elevated serum IgA.

3. Patients with diffuse alveolar hemorrhage benefit from a careful clinical and serologic evaluation occasionally complemented by kidney or other extrapulmonary organ biopsy. Lung biopsies become useful primarily in confirming IPH when other causes of alveolar hemorrhage are excluded.

REFERENCES

1. Leatherman JW. Immune alveolar hemorrhage. Chest 1987; 91:891–897.
2. Leatherman JW, Davies SF, Hoidal JR. Alveolar hemorrhage syndromes: diffuse microvascular lung hemorrhage in immune and idiopathic disorders. Medicine 1984; 63:343–361.

PATIENT 81

A 21-year-old man with an 8-week history of fever, pleurisy, nonproductive cough, weight loss, and hilar and mediastinal adenopathy

A 21-year-old white male college student was well until 8 weeks prior to admission when he noted chest tightness while running. Six weeks previously, he had developed right anterior pleuritic chest pain, nonproductive cough, and fever. There was fatigue, anorexia, and a weight loss of 10 pounds.

Physical Examination: Temperature 100.4°; pulse 84; respirations 20. No acute distress but frequent coughing episodes during examination. Chest examination: no adventitious sounds. Abdomen: no hepatosplenomegaly. Skin: no lesions.

Laboratory Findings: WBC 7600/μl, 76% PMNs, 2% bands, 11% lymphocytes, 7% monocytes, 3% eosinophils; ESR 43 mm/hr; urinalysis normal. ABG (room air): pH 7.40, PCO_2 38 mmHg, PO_2 98 mmHg. Chest radiograph: bilateral hilar and right paratracheal and subcarinal adenopathy with right mid-zone infiltrate. Pulmonary function studies: FVC 4.58 L (82% of predicted), FEV_1 3.56 L (79%), FEV_1/FVC ratio 78%, DL/VA 4.37. Angiotensin converting enzyme 20 U/ml; PPD skin test negative; controls positive; fungal serologies pending. Fiberoptic bronchoscopy and transbronchial lung biopsy (6 specimens) and direct mucosal biopsy (2 specimens) showed minimal inflammatory changes without evidence of granuloma. Fungal and tuberculosis cultures of the lung tissue were plated.

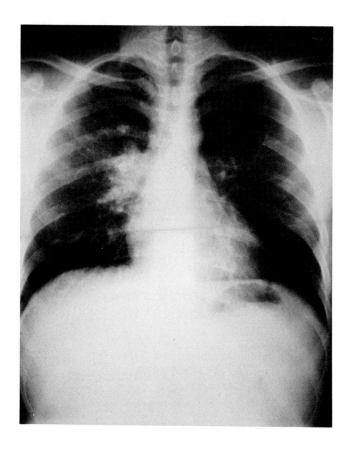

Diagnosis: Symptomatic primary infection with histoplasmosis.

Discussion: *Histoplasma capsulatum,* a dimorphic fungus, is found in the soil in its mycelial form, particularly in the Mississippi and Ohio River Valleys. Man is infected when contaminated soil is disturbed, releasing high concentrations of the spores which may be inhaled and reach the alveoli. Once the spores reach the alveoli, germination begins and primary infection ensues; the sequence is similar to initial tuberculous infection. Prior to the development of cellular immunity, local growth of the organism takes place, with dissemination by the lymphatic and hematogenous routes. Metastatic lesions characteristically involve the liver and spleen. After 2 to 6 weeks, when cellular immunity develops, inflammatory reaction takes place at the initial site of infection, in regional lymph nodes, and metastatic foci, resulting in caseous necrosis and fibrous encapsulation. In adults after 5 or more years, the inflammatory lesions become calcified. Histoplasma calcifications are usually larger than 4 mm in the lung parenchyma and greater than 1 cm in the hilar and mediastinal nodes. "Mulberry" calcifications in the paratracheal nodes, and splenic and hepatic calcifications are highly suggestive of primary histoplasmosis.

The usual primary infection from histoplasma is essentially asymptomatic without clinical sequelae. The rare symptomatic primary infection from minimal inhalation of the fungus is usually seen in infants and young children and is similar to acute symptomatic histoplasmosis resulting from heavy spore inhalation in a previously uninfected adult. Patients frequently have an impressive cough related to the mechanical effect on the tracheobronchial tree of markedly enlarged mediastinal and hilar lymph nodes. Fever usually is present but the degree and duration are variable; fever may persist for several weeks in the more severe cases. The chest radiograph usually shows hilar and mediastinal adenopathy with patchy bronchopneumonia. The disease may disseminate in immunocompromised patients, manifested by hepatosplenomegaly, fungemia, and positive cultures in the urine and on liver biopsy. The lymphadenopathy may persist for months following resolution of constitutional symptoms. These nodes can cause an obstructive pneumonia and rarely may rupture endobronchially producing histoplasma pneumonia.

Acute histoplasmosis or epidemic histoplasmosis is a syndrome that follows heavy spore inhalation, with symptoms proportional to the magnitude of the inhalation. It usually is seen following exposure to a site in which the presence of fowl or bat excrement has favored abundant growth of the organism, when dusty conditions prevail, and with an event that makes the spores airborne. The sweeping of an unused chicken house, bulldozing a starling roost, or exploration of a bat cave are classic examples.

Serologic tests are important diagnostic tools. Most commonly used are the immunodiffusion (ID) tests, which detect M and H bands, and the more sensitive complement fixation (CF) test, performed with yeast and mycelial antigens. A positive M band by ID is relatively specific for histoplasmosis but not very sensitive. Concomitant M and H bands in the same serum is highly specific for current infection but is uncommon, occurring in about 20% of patients. CF is more sensitive than ID but less specific. CF antibodies against the yeast antigen are more frequent and in higher titer than the mycelial antigens. The results of CF to the mycelial antigen are not very useful and the test persists because of tradition. False-positive CF antibodies ($\leq$ 1:16) occur because of cross reactivity with other fungal infections or with tuberculosis. A four-fold increase in titer over a period of observation or a titer of 1:32 or higher on a single determination is suggestive of current infection. About 25% of patients with a positive CF yeast phase have a negative ID, but less than 1% of patients with a positive ID have a negative yeast CF test.

Acute histoplasmosis usually does not require treatment. In adults, prolongation of symptoms beyond 2 weeks raises the question of immunologic compromise, and some have suggested treating the illness persisting greater than 2 to 3 weeks with 1000 mg of amphotericin. Ketoconazole has been used successfully in the therapy of non-life-threatening histoplasmosis in a dose of 200 to 600 mg/day for at least 6 months.

The present patient's CF antibody titer to the yeast antigen was 1:32 and both the H and M bands were positive on ID. By the time we evaluated the patient, he was virtually asymptomatic with the exception of exercise-induced cough; he was observed without therapy. By 6 months, the patient's CF titers had dropped to 1:16 and the ID was negative. Mediastinal and hilar adenopathy had decreased.

Clinical Pearls

1. Symptomatic primary histoplasmosis infection in the adult is a rare occurrence.

2. Cough, fever, and constitutional symptoms with insidious onset in conjunction with hilar and mediastinal adenopathy and patchy parenchymal infiltrates on chest radiograph suggest the diagnosis. Adenopathy often persists for several months following the resolution of constitutional symptoms.

3. Serologic tests are important diagnostic tools. Immunodiffusion is the most specific test for current infection but is not as sensitive as the yeast complement fixation. A four-fold rise in CF titer or titer $\geq$ 1:32 on a single determination is suggestive of current infection.

4. Acute histoplasmosis rarely requires therapy unless symptoms persist for greater than 2 to 3 weeks, raising suspicion of immunocompromise.

REFERENCES

1. Goodwin RA Jr, Desprez RM. Histoplasmosis. Am Rev Respir Dis 1978; 117:929–956.
2. Wheat LJ, Slama TG, Eitzen HA, et al. A large urban outbreak of histoplasmosis: clinical features. Ann Intern Med 1981; 94:331–337.
3. Davies SF. Serodiagnosis of histoplasmosis. Semin Respir Infect 1986; 1:9–15.

PATIENT 82

A 55-year-old woman with bilateral emphysematous bullae

A 55-year-old woman was referred for evaluation of severe dyspnea on exertion. She was a long-time smoker, discontinuing this habit 3 years before. She noted shortness of breath 2 years earlier that progressed to the present severity, limiting her to room ambulation. She had been treated with oral and inhaled bronchodilators without improvement in her condition.

Physical Examination: Normal body habitus; thoracic hyperresonance with generalized decreased breath sounds. Cardiac exam consistent with pulmonary hypertension.

Laboratory Findings: ABG (room air): pH 7.35, PCO_2 42 mmHg, PO_2 68 mmHg. Chest radiograph was remarkable for bilateral upper lung zone lucencies compatible with giant bullae with compression of basilar lung tissue. Pulmonary function tests are shown below. Thoracic surgery consultation was obtained.

TEST	RESULT	% PRED	PREDICTED
FEV_1 (L)	0.84	40	2.09
FVC (L)	1.82	65	2.78
FEV_1/FVC (%)	46	61	75
TLC-Body Box (L)	4.33	102	4.22
TLC-Helium (L)	3.33	71	4.22

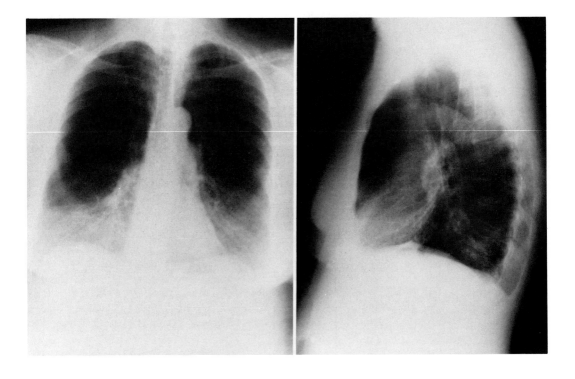

Diagnosis: Surgical candidate for bullectomy.

Discussion: The surgical approach to the management of respiratory symptoms in patients with emphysema is largely limited to excision of space-occupying giant bullae. These parenchymal abnormalities, also termed pneumatoceles or acquired cysts, most commonly occur in the upper lobes and right hemithorax, although bilateral disease, as in this patient, also develops. Bullae become symptomatic as they enlarge and progressively compress adjacent functioning lung tissue.

The goals of surgical therapy are to excise the bullae, thereby allowing reexpansion of relatively normal tissue and improvement in lung function. The key to a successful outcome is careful patient selection to avoid removing a bullus that is not limiting lung function. For instance, patients with "vanishing lungs" have an entire lobe destroyed by a bullus without displacement of neighboring lung tissue and do not benefit from bullectomy. Conversely, resection of a small bullus occupying less than one-third of the hemithorax typically does not improve measurable lung function. Pulmonary hypertension is not a contraindication for surgery, since lung compression results in raised pulmonary vascular resistance, and patients with pulmonary hypertension may have the most striking improvement after surgery. Suppurative bronchitis, however, portends a poor surgical outcome.

The preoperative evaluation is aided by laboratory studies. The chest radiograph often shows evidence of compressed lung tissue around a giant bullus that occupies more than 50% of the hemithorax, thereby suggesting a suitable operative candidate. If expiratory chest views indicate that the bullus does not decrease in size but neighboring lung zones are further compressed, a positive surgical outcome is more likely. Additional studies assist difficult decisions in borderline patients. A perfusion lung scan will quantitate the degree of function of the lung region planned for resection. A pulmonary angiogram may show crowding of vasculature to the adjacent compressed lung, suggesting the potential for improvable function after reexpansion.

Pulmonary function tests may further support an operative decision. Most surgical candidates are nearly normoxic because lung perfusion and ventilation are matched in affected lung regions; the presence of profound hypoxemia or hypercarbia indicates that the emphysema is diffuse and the patient may not improve after surgery. The classical spirometry and lung volume finding in these patients is a proportional decrease in FEV_1 and FVC that results in a normal $FEV_1/FVC\%$ compatible with a restrictive defect and occurs because the bullae do not communicate with the airways. A low FEV_1/FVC ratio, as found in this patient, indicates either considerable obstructive airways in the remaining lung or partial communication of the bullae with the airways. Since helium wash-in and wash-out are slow in the bullae, the difference between TLC measured by helium compared to body plethysmography (body box) approximates the volume of the bullae.

Surgical bullectomy has a low mortality rate (less than 2%) but is complicated by persistent air leak or pleuropulmonary infection in 14 to 45% of patients. Preservation of lung tissue is an important consideration and the surgeon should avoid a lobectomy whenever possible, removing the bullae by wedge excision and plication. Results of surgery depend on the degree of lung compression preoperatively. Patients with the largest bullae tend to have the greatest improvement in lung function. Often functional improvement is striking and persists for several years after surgery. Although recurrent bullae do not develop, a decline in lung function may occur 5 to 7 years after bullectomy, and patients may return to preoperative status after 12 to 15 years. Even a temporary improvement in functional capacity and quality of life, however, more than warrants surgery.

An expiratory chest radiograph in the present patient showed no change in bullae size but marked compression of adjacent lung tissue. A lung scan detected no perfusion of the bullae, and a pulmonary angiogram demonstrated crowding of adjacent pulmonary vasculature. The patient underwent bilateral bullectomies through a median sternotomy incision and noted marked improvement in pulmonary function almost immediately after surgery.

Clinical Pearls

1. Giant bullae occupying less than 30% of the hemithorax do not adversely affect pulmonary function.

2. Patients with pulmonary hypertension may have the greatest degree of improvement after bullectomy.

REFERENCES

1. Gaensler EA, Cugell DW, Knudson RJ, FitzGerald MX. Surgical management of emphysema. Clin Chest Med 1983; 4:443–463.
2. Laros CD, Gelissen HJ, Berstein PGM, et al. Bullectomy for giant bullae in emphysema. J Thorac Cardiovasc Surg 1986; 91:63–70.

PATIENT 83

A 19-year-old male recruit with sore throat, cough, dyspnea, chest pain, and subcutaneous emphysema

A 19-year-old Marine recruit was transferred because of progressive dyspnea, chest pain, and subcutaneous emphysema. He was well until 24 hours prior when he had developed a sore throat, rhinitis, and productive cough.

Physical Examination: Temperature 98.6°; respirations 28; pulse 92; moderate respiratory distress; uncomfortable due to substernal chest pain; bilateral wheezes and rhonci; subcutaneous air palpated in the neck.

Laboratory Findings: WBC 14,800/μl, 87% PMNs, 2% bands. ABG (40% face mask): pH 7.45, PCO_2 30 mmHg, and PO_2 86 mmHg. Sputum Gram stain: PMNs without a predominant organism. Chest radiograph: subcutaneous and mediastinal air, elevated left hemidiaphragm, atelectasis on left.

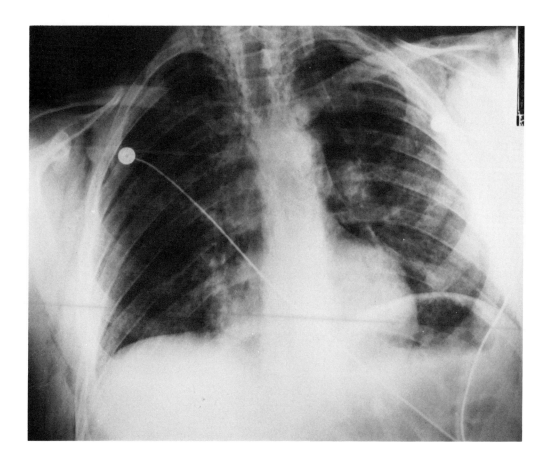

Diagnosis: Viral bronchitis and bronchiolitis with pneumomediastinum.

Discussion: When air is found in the neck, mediastinum, subcutaneous tissue, pulmonary interstitium, or retroperitoneum area, the etiology needs to be addressed, as this is not a normal finding. Subcutaneous emphysema may occur: (1) following trauma (esophageal rupture, tracheobronchial rupture), as air is introduced directly into the mediastinum; (2) from gas-forming organisms; (3) spontaneously, as the alveolar-interstitial space gradient increases to cause alveolar rupture; and (4) following surgery, as in thyroidectomy and tracheotomy. In the present case, it was postulated that airways obstruction due to viral bronchitis and bronchiolitis resulted in marginal alveolar rupture and mediastinal and subcutaneous emphysema.

Over 40 years ago, Macklin and Macklin postulated the mechanisms involved in mediastinal and subcutaneous emphysema. They provided experimental data that when overinflated alveoli rupture, the gas moves into the surrounding interstitium. The interstitial air is almost never visualized on the chest radiograph, as there is an air-air interface. Alveoli are more likely to rupture when there is airways obstruction, such as in status asthmaticus or inflammatory bronchiolitis. When intraalveolar pressure increases or perivascular interstitial pressure decreases, a gradient is created and alveoli may rupture, resulting in air entry into the interstitium of the lung. As the pressure in the lung periphery exceeds mediastinal pressure, air will tend to move toward the mediastinum along the bronchovascular sheaths. Mediastinal air accumulates until it reaches a critical pressure and then decompresses into the area of least resistance (cervical and subcutaneous tissues, retroperitoneum). If decompression is not adequate or mediastinal pressure rises abruptly, the mediastinal pleura will rupture, resulting in pneumothorax. Besides airway inflammation, pneumomediastinum has been associated with other conditions generally having in common abdominal, diaphragmatic, and thoracic muscular contraction against a closed glottis. This may occur with parturition, coughing, vomiting, or weight lifting. Spontaneous pneumomediastinum has also been reported in patients with diabetic ketoacidosis.

The most common symptom is a nonlocalized anterior chest pain, probably resulting from pressure in the interstitial soft tissues due to dissection of air. With careful examination, subcutaneous air can be documented in the neck, either by auscultation or palpation. Hamman's sign, a crunching noise synchronous with the cardiac cycle, may be heard over the sternum in over 50% of patients with pneumomediastinum. The radiologist frequently alerts the clinician to the diagnosis of pneumomediastinum. The chest radiograph will demonstrate air in the tissue planes of the neck and the pectoral muscle. Air in the mediastinum is documented by finding a thin radiolucent line, usually best appreciated along the left cardiac border, that represents the displaced mediastinal pleura. Lateral radiograph will show retrosternal air or air outlining the aorta or other structures in the mediastinum. The key is early diagnosis so that reassurance and observation of the patient can be initiated without the necessity of further diagnostic testing.

Treatment of nontraumatic causes of subcutaneous and mediastinal emphysema is conservative. Reduction in airways resistance should be accomplished with bronchodilator therapy and removal of bronchial secretions. Prophylactic chest tubes should be avoided as they are of no value and will result in risk and discomfort for the patient.

The present patient was treated with inhaled bronchodilators, chest physiotherapy, and erythromycin with a good clinical response. Cold agglutinins were positive but acute and convalescent mycoplasma CF titers were negative.

Clinical Pearls

1. Consider pneumomediastinum as a diagnostic possibility in a young individual who presents with diffuse anterior chest pain and has been involved in an activity associated with abdominal or thoracic muscle contraction against a closed glottis.

2. A lateral chest radiograph should always be performed in the patient with suspected pneumomediastinum, as a PA view alone may result in misdiagnosis.

3. The initial management of spontaneous pneumomediastinum should be conservative.

REFERENCES

1. Macklin MT, Macklin CC. Malignant interstitial emphysema of the lungs and mediastinum as an important occult complication in many respiratory diseases and other conditions: an interpretation of the clinical literature in light of laboratory experiments. Medicine 1944; 23:281–352.
2. Wohl MEB, Chernick V. Bronchiolitis. Am Rev Resp Dis 1978; 118:759–781.
3. Maunder RJ, Pierson DJ, Hudson LD. Subcutaneous and mediastinal emphysema: pathophysiology, diagnosis, and management. Arch Intern Med 1984; 144:1447–1453.

PATIENT 84

A 48-year-old man with massive hemoptysis

A 48-year-old man was admitted for management of hemoptysis. He had been followed by another physician for pulmonary sarcoidosis that was stable on low-dose prednisone. One year earlier, he had two episodes of mild hemoptysis that were not investigated. Blood-streaked sputum developed 1 day before admission, followed through the night by "coughing up handfuls of blood." While giving the history, the patient coughed up several tablespoons of bright red blood.

Physical Examination: Temperature 99°; pulse 100; blood pressure 120/89. Chest diffuse rhonchi; cardiac normal.

Laboratory Findings: Hct 33%; WBC 7,900/μl; platelet count normal; prothrombin time 12.0 sec; electrolytes and renal function tests normal. Chest radiograph demonstrates a left upper lobe cavity with an intracavitary mass and overlying pleural reaction. Mediastinal adenopathy and upper lobe interstitial infiltrates are also present.

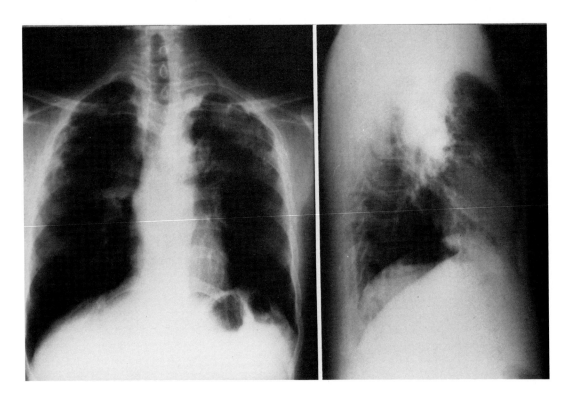

Diagnosis: Pulmonary sarcoidosis with hemoptysis secondary to an intracavitary aspergilloma.

Discussion: Aspergillomas are common complications of cavitary lung disease, occurring in up to 10 to 15% of patients with cavitary tuberculosis. Although middle-aged patients are most frequently affected, aspergillomas may develop in any age group. Since hemoptysis is the most common manifestation of the disease, an aspergilloma should be considered in any patient presenting with hemoptysis and a radiographic cavity.

Although Aspergillus species are also capable of causing pulmonary disorders by invasive and immunologic mechanisms, aspergillomas are examples of saprophytic disease. The organism initially establishes colonization in pulmonary cavities resulting from underlying lung disease such as sarcoidosis, tuberculosis, bronchial cysts, pulmonary fibrosis, and lung abscess. Occasionally, the aspergilloma develops in a cavity created by pulmonary infection from underlying invasive or chronic necrotizing aspergillosis or in bronchiectatic airways of patients with allergic bronchopulmonary aspergillosis. As the fungus grows, it creates a mass of fungal mycelia intertwined with inflammatory cells, fibrin, mucus, and amorphous debris that forms the fungus ball that may be freely mobile or attached to the cavity wall by granulation tissue.

Most patients with aspergillomas have either pulmonary or constitutional symptoms. Hemoptysis occurs in 50 to 80% of patients; cough, dyspnea, malaise, and weight loss present less frequently. The etiology of the hemoptysis is unknown, but mechanical effects of the fungoma, fungal toxins and enzymes, and an inflammatory response probably contribute to localized injury to the cavity wall. The diagnosis is usually confirmed radiographically, since the chest radiograph is often diagnostic. The cavity is usually 3 to 5 cm in diameter with thickened walls. Thickening of the overlying pleura is a characteristic feature that is invariably present. The fungoma may fill the cavity, creating a surrounding crescent of air between the fungoma and cavity wall. If the fungoma is not apparent on routine chest radiographs, its presence can be confirmed by either tomography or CT scan. Sputum cultures for Aspergillus are positive in only 50 to 60% of patients, since the cavity may not communicate with the bronchi. Aspergillus precipitins are almost always positive.

Patients with aspergillomas present management difficulties when hemoptysis develops. The initial approach is bronchoscopy to confirm the segmental location of the bleeding site, since patients usually have diffuse underlying lung disease with several potential sources of hemorrhage. Bedrest and antitussive agents are then employed, since most initial episodes of hemorrhage are not major and 10% of aspergillomas may eventually spontaneously lyse. After several episodes of hemorrhage, however, bleeding may become life-threatening and more difficult to control. Therapeutic options include thoracotomy with lobectomy for patients with adequate pulmonary function or bronchial artery embolization for patients who are not surgical candidates. An important clinical consideration affecting therapeutic decisions is that most patients with aspergillomas and hemoptysis do not die of bleeding but rather have a limited prognosis because of the severity of the underlying pulmonary disease. In this regard, patients with sarcoidosis and aspergillomas do not live as long as patients with aspergillomas complicating more localized disease, such as tuberculosis.

The present patient underwent urgent fiberoptic bronchoscopy, confirming the segmental source of blood loss. Tomography of the upper lobes confirmed a fungus ball within a pulmonary cavity. Aspergillus precipitins were subsequently positive. After several days of bed rest and antitussive agents, the patient was discharged without further hemoptysis.

Clinical Pearls

1. Although an intracavitary crescent of air around a fungoma is the classic radiographic feature of aspergilloma, adjacent pleural thickening is invariably present and serves as a reliable radiographic finding.

2. Most patients with hemoptysis from an aspergilloma do not die of hemorrhage.

3. The survival in patients with aspergillomas correlates with the severity of the underlying pulmonary disease.

REFERENCES

1. Butz RO, Zvetina JR, Leininger BJ. Ten-year experience with mycetomas in patients with pulmonary tuberculosis. Chest 1985; 87:356–358.
2. Daly RC, Pairolero PC, Piehler JM, et al. Pulmonary aspergilloma. J Thorac Cardiovasc Surg 1986; 92:981–988.
3. Wollschlager C, Khan F. Aspergillomas complicating sarcoidosis. A prospective study in 100 patients. Chest 1984; 86:585–588.
4. Glimp A, Bayer AS. Pulmonary aspergilloma. Diagnostic and therapeutic considerations. Arch Intern Med 1983; 143:303–308.
5. Tomlinson JR, Sahn SA. Aspergilloma in sarcoid and tuberculosis. Chest 1987; 92:505–508.

PATIENT 85

A 63-year-old man with increasing ascites, pleural effusions, and dyspnea at rest after diagnosis of carcinoma of the colon metastatic to the peritoneum and pleura

A 63-year-old man with carcinoma of the colon metastatic to the peritoneum and pleura was referred for chemical pleurodesis. He was diagnosed 4 months prior and had documented malignant ascites and right pleural effusion. He had progressive dyspnea on exertion, which was now present at rest. Over the previous several weeks he had noted increased abdominal girth and a "very tense belly." He had less than 10 pack-years of cigarette smoking and had quit years ago. There was no history of prior or current pneumonia, heart failure, or thromboembolic disease.

Physical Examination: Temperature 98.2°; pulse 100; respirations 36. A chronically ill appearing male in minimal respiratory distress at rest with a markedly protuberant abdomen. Chest examination: decreased breath sounds in the bases with minimal basilar rales. Cardiac: neck veins flat at 45°, regular tachycardia without gallops or murmurs. Abdomen: tense, protuberant with fluid wave; 1+ peripheral edema.

Laboratory Findings: WBC 6400/μl with normal differential, Hct 33%, alkaline phosphatase 385 IU/L; BUN, creatinine, electrolytes, calcium and phosphorus: normal. Chest radiograph: small lung volumes, increased haziness of the upper abdomen, small right pleural effusion. Pulmonary function tests: FVC 2.45 (51% of predicted), FEV, 1.96 L (57%), FEV$_1$/FVC 80%, MVV 93 L/min (72%), TLC 4.90 L (67%), FRC 2.17 L (53%), RV 2.13 L (86%), ERV 0.04 L (2%). ABG: (room air): pH 7.45, PCO$_2$ 33 mmHg, PO$_2$ 72 mmHg. A procedure was recommended.

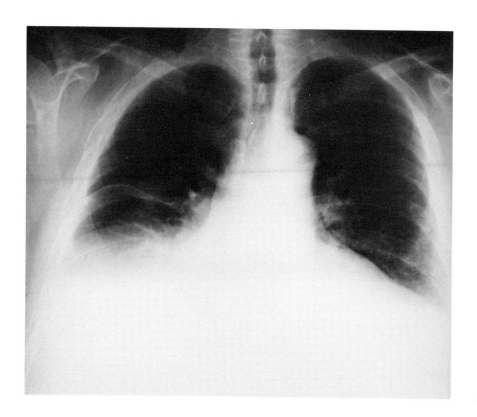

Diagnosis: Dyspnea due to massive ascites.

Discussion: Ascites, pneumoperitoneum, and pregnancy all increase intraperitoneal pressure and have been shown to reduce ventilatory capacity. Patients with massive ascites have a breathing pattern characterized by rapid and shallow breathing. Following therapeutic paracentesis, the tidal volume increases and the respiratory rate decreases, with minute ventilation remaining unchanged. Fluoroscopy has documented elevation and decreased maximal excursion of the diaphragm with massive ascites. These changes result in a reduction of all lung volume compartments. The reduced vital capacity is caused by a decrease in both of its components, the inspiratory capacity and the expiratory reserve volume. The residual volume tends to be reduced somewhat less but, in conjunction with a decreased expiratory reserve volume, results in a decreased functional residual capacity. The changes in lung volume in massive ascites have been attributed to an increase in peritoneal pressure which is transmitted to the pleural space, resulting in an increase in intrapleural pressure. It has been shown experimentally that as abdominal pressure increases, respiratory rate increases, a response probably mediated by the Hering-Breuer reflex. Massive ascites also results in distention and increased rigidity of the abdominal wall and relative fixation of the diaphragm. Thus, this part of the functional thoracic cage, the diaphragm and abdominal wall, become less compliant and therefore the overall elasticity of the thoracic cage is affected. This in turn requires additional amounts of energy for thoracic cage movement and an increased work of breathing. At rest, the work of breathing is small; however, during exercise, the work of breathing increases considerably and probably is the major cause of the increase in oxygen consumption associated with ascites. The decreased maximum voluntary ventilation (MVV) with ascites is due not only to the severe restrictive defect but also to the increased stiffness of the diaphragm and abdominal wall; this is supported by the fact that in patients with restrictive defects, the MVV is not affected until the vital capacity becomes severely reduced.

Following therapeutic paracentesis, there is an increase in all lung volume components but they usually do not return to normal. This observation probably can be explained by decreased tone of the abdominal wall, discomfort at the paracentesis site, residual ascites, and the presence of cardiopulmonary disease. Nevertheless, pulmonary function may show progressive improvement several days after paracentesis. In massive ascites, there is marked reduction in both inspiratory capacity and total lung capacity, in contrast to pneumoperitoneum and pregnancy where reduction of the functional residual capacity is offset by an increase in inspiratory capacity, with the total lung capacity remaining unchanged. This difference is probably explained by the relatively greater increase in intraabdominal pressure by massive ascites.

To explain dyspnea in patients with massive ascites, other cardiopulmonary disease, whether or not related to the primary process, must be considered; this includes pleural effusions, COPD, pneumonia, or congestive heart failure. Factors related to dyspnea without ascites include reduction of ventilatory capacity, increased work of breathing, and increased stimulus to respiration. These patients also are at increased risk for pulmonary infection secondary to impaired cough and atelectasis. The failure of therapeutic paracentesis to relieve dyspnea suggests that other cardiopulmonary factors, either related or unrelated to the primary disease, are contributory.

The present patient underwent therapeutic paracentesis with removal 3500 cc of fluid; prompt improvement in dyspnea was accompanied by an increase in all components of the lung volume and a decrease in respiratory rate. Manipulation of the pleural space was not indicated.

Clinical Pearls

1. Massive ascites results in a restrictive ventilatory defect characterized by a reduced total lung capacity and its components and a decrease in MVV.

2. Dyspnea from massive ascites probably is due to a combination of restrictive ventilatory defect, stiffness of the abdominal wall and fixation of the diaphragm, resulting in increased work of breathing and compensatory reflexes resulting in hyperventilation.

3. Therapeutic paracentesis results in immediate relief of dyspnea with an improvement of all lung volumes if ascites is the major factor responsible for the dyspnea.

REFERENCES

1. Abelmann WH, Frank NR, Gaensler EA, Cugell DW. The effects of abdominal distention by ascites on lung volume in ventilation. Arch Intern Med 1954; 93:528–540.
2. Prinzmetal M, Kountz WB. Intrapleural pressure in health and disease and its influence on body function. Medicine 1935; 14:457–498.
3. Patton WE, Abelmann WH, Frank NR, et al. Pulmonary function in pregnancy. II. Comparison of the effects of pneumoperitoneum and pregnancy in young women with functionally normal lungs and serial observations during pregnancy and postpartum pneumoperitoneum. Am Rev Tuberc 1953; 67:755–778.
4. Richards DW Jr. The nature of cardiac and pulmonary dyspnea. Circulation 1953; 7:15–29.

PATIENT 86

A 76-year-old man with carcinoma of the pancreas, percutaneous biliary drainage, and a right pleural effusion

A 76-year-old male presented with abdominal pain, jaundice, and orthostasis. There had been weight loss and vague constitutional symptoms.

Physical Examination: Temperature 99.5°, pulse 100, blood pressure 100/65; ill appearing male in no acute distress; scleral icterus; hepatomegaly without tenderness; chest examination: unremarkable.

Laboratory Findings: WBC 12,300/μl, 82% PMNs, 2% bands, 12% lymphocytes; Hct 31%, alkaline phosphatase 485 IU/L; total bilirubin 7.8 mg/dl. Ultrasound: dilated biliary tree; endoscopic retrograde cholangiopancreatography (ERCP) was unsuccessful. Percutaneous biliary drainage was established with a 6 F catheter. During the cholangiogram an overzealous injection of contrast dye was noted to fill and dilate the subcapsular hepatic space. Percutaneous needle aspiration of the pancreas: adenocarcinoma. Seven days following percutaneous biliary drainage, the patient had a decrease in biliary drainage, a three-fold increase in serum bilirubin, and a new large, right-sided pleural effusion. Thoracentesis: serosanguinous; WBC 9280/μl, 82% PMNs, 12% macrophages, 6% lymphocytes, total protein 3.5 g/dl, LDH 332 IU/L, glucose 163 mg/dl, pH 7.80, amylase 279 IU/L, total bilirubin 2.1 mg/dl; serum bilirubin 1.5 mg/dl.

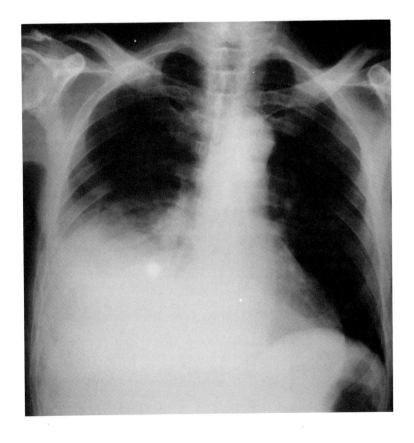

Diagnosis: Biliopleural fistula as a complication of percutaneous biliary drainage.

Discussion: Blunt or penetrating thoracoabdominal trauma is the most common cause of biliopleural fistula in the Western world. Biliopleural fistula from disease of the biliary tree is extremely uncommon. Worldwide, hepatic disease with echinococcus and entamoeba probably is the most common etiology. Postoperative stricture of the bile ducts predisposes to biliopleural fistula, especially when associated with subphrenic abscess.

Percutaneous drainage of an obstructed biliary system has been a useful adjunct to definitive surgical therapy of obstructive jaundice. When technical placement of an internal biliary stent is not feasible, patients with unresectable malignant disease can obtain palliation from complications of obstructive jaundice by percutaneous biliary drainage. Percutaneous biliary drainage, however, is not without inherent complications, which include cholangitis and catheter dislodgement, obstruction, and leaking; peritonitis, hemobilia, arteriovenous malformation, hemorrhage, and subphrenic abscess also have been reported. Pleural complications appear to be uncommon despite documented transgression of the pleural sulcus using the intercostal approach. Hemothorax, pneumothorax, empyema, rib erosion, and malignant pleural seeding, in addition to biliopleural fistula, have been reported.

Features that appear to be common to the development of biliopleural fistula include complete biliary obstruction, catheter placement between the 9th and 10th ribs in the midaxillary line, and prolonged drainage (one week to several weeks). It is possible that prolonged drainage permits the formation of a well-defined fistulous tract and that biliopleural fistula requires dysfunction of the percutaneous biliary drainage catheter; biliopleural fistula has been reported following inadvertent catheter removal. With catheter dislodgement rates up to 20%, catheters should be secured effectively and patients should be educated concerning taping changes.

Empyema appears to be a frequent accompaniment of biliopleural fistula. Reasons for empyema could be a direct tract from the skin to the pleura with seeding without adequate pleural drainage or as a complication of cholangitis, a frequent occurrence when the biliary tract is completely obstructed, leading to a peritoneal or subdiaphragmatic collection of bile.

The diagnosis of biliopleural fistula should be suspected when a patient with a percutaneous biliary drainage catheter develops a right pleural effusion. Confirmation is obtained on thoracentesis when greenish-yellow fluid is aspirated that has a pleural fluid total bilirubin/serum bilirubin ratio of >1.0. Experimentally, it has been shown that bilirubin is cleared rapidly following entry into the pleural space. An early finding in biliopleural fistula is a high pleural fluid LDH value that decreases rapidly following cessation of bile entry. Thus, thoracentesis performed late in the course of biliopleural fistula, after the leak has ceased, may be nondiagnostic.

Early institution of another form of biliary drainage appears to be the single most important factor in successful management. This concept is supported by surgical experience with traumatic biliopleural fistula. Establishing percutaneous biliary drainage can be difficult in the setting of biliary decompression into the chest. The relative amount of ongoing biliary drainage, reactive exudate effusions, and suppurative complications determines the presentation.

The present patient underwent repeat ERCP, which did establish definitive internal drainage. The right pleural effusion resolved rapidly following removal of the percutaneous biliary drainage catheter.

Clinical Pearls

1. Biliopleural fistula as a complication of percutaneous biliary drainage may be more likely to occur when there is complete biliary obstruction, catheter placement between the 9th and 10th ribs in the midaxillary line, and prolonged drainage (one to several weeks).

2. Biliopleural fistula usually requires a well-defined fistulous tract that results from prolonged drainage and dysfunction of the percutaneous biliary drainage catheter.

3. The diagnosis should be suspected when a patient with a percutaneous biliary drainage catheter develops a right pleural effusion and is confirmed by obtaining greenish-yellow fluid at thoracentesis that has a pleural fluid total bilirubin/serum total bilirubin ratio of >1.0.

REFERENCES

1. Boyd BP. Bronchobiliary and bronchopleural fistulas. Ann Thorac Surg 1977; 24:481–487.
2. Mueller PR, van Sonnenberg E, Ferrucci JT. Percutaneous biliary drainage: technical and catheter related problems in 200 procedures. AJR 1982; 138:17–23.
3. Hanlin JA, Friedman M, Stein MG, Bray J. Percutaneous biliary drainage: complications of 118 consecutive catheterizations. Radiology 1986; 158:199–202.
4. Strange C, Allen ML, Freidland P, Cunningham J, Sahn SA. Biliopleural fistula with the complication of percutaneous biliary drainage: experimental evidence for pleural inflammation. Am Rev Respir Dis 1988; 137:959–961.

PATIENT 87

A 64-year-old man with the insidious onset of chest pain and a pleural effusion

A 64-year-old male security guard had the insidious onset of right chest pain; the pain was nonpleuritic, aching, and at times referred to the shoulder. He had worked at his present job for the past 25 years. When he was in his early 20's, he worked for several years as a construction worker.

Physical Examination: Vital signs normal; no acute distress; patient did not appear chronically ill. Flat percussion note; decreased fremitus; absent breath sounds at right base.

Laboratory Findings: WBC 10,000/μl, normal differential; Hct 35%; ESR 30 mm/h. Chest radiograph: lobulated pleural density and small pleural effusion without contralateral mediastinal shift. Thoracentesis: serosanguinous fluid, nucleated cells 4500/μl, 40% mononuclear cells, 30% lymphocytes, 20% PMNs, glucose 35 mg/dl, pH 7.11. Cytology: suspicious for malignancy; pleural biopsy: suspicious for malignancy; bronchoscopy: no endobronchial lesions; bronchial washings: negative on cytologic examination. A thoracotomy was performed.

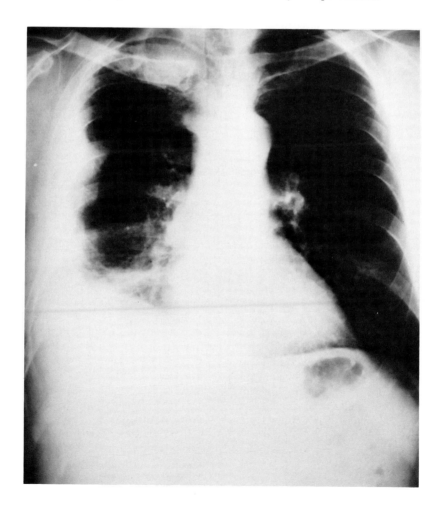

Diagnosis: Malignant mesothelioma.

Discussion: In 1960, Wagner and colleagues reported on the association between asbestos exposure and malignant mesothelioma. Since that time, additional studies have clearly implicated asbestos exposure in both pleural and peritoneal malignant mesotheliomas in miners, insulation workers, and other trades. The association, however, does not apply to the solitary or localized (benign) mesothelioma. The incidence of mesothelioma ranges from one per million per year in populations not directly exposed to asbestos to rates 2 to 5 times higher in industrialized countries and 20-fold higher among insulation workers and asbestos factory workers. The risk of mesothelioma is highest with crocidolite, found both occupationally and environmentally, which has a very high length-diameter ratio. Chrysolite, which represents 90% of the commercially used asbestos, has a relatively low potential for causing mesotheliomas due to its short fibers.

The latency period from the time of exposure to asbestos to the appearance of the tumor is, on the average, 30 to 45 years. There seems to be a linear dose-response curve. Smoking does not increase the risk for development of mesothelioma.

Malignant mesotheliomas are more commonly found in males in the 50 to 70 year age group. The onset is usually insidious, with chest pain or dyspnea on exertion. In contrast to patients with adenocarcinoma of the pleura, it is distinctly unusual for patients with mesothelioma to be diagnosed when they are asymptomatic. Pleural effusion usually is present at the time the patient is first seen and can range from small to massive in volume. Absence of contralateral mediastinal shift with a large pleural effusion should suggest mesothelioma as a diagnostic possibility. This finding usually is observed at a later stage of the disease when the tumor has grown along the mediastinum and prevents shift from occurring. In this situation, dyspnea may not be as prominent and is less likely to be relieved by thoracentesis. A lobulated appearance of the "pleural fluid meniscus" is suggestive of the diagnosis. Pleural fluid may be serous to bloody and viscous, and is exudative with a low number of nucleated cells. Approximately 70% of patients with malignant mesothelioma have a low pleural fluid glucose and pH. This is due to the abnormal pleura, which is composed of tumor and fibrosis, inhibiting glucose transport into the pleural space and efflux of hydrogen ions, the end product of glucose metabolism.

The diagnosis of malignancy generally is not difficult but differentiating adenocarcinoma of the pleura from mesothelioma may be a diagnostic dilemma. Exfoliative cytology is of uncertain value in diagnosis, as it may be impossible to distinguish between reactive mesothelial cells and tumor cells or impossible to distinguish between metastatic tumor and primary pleural malignancy. A high level of hyaluronic acid in pleural fluid is more common with mesothelioma than other pleural exudates; however, the test is not specific, as high levels have been found in inflammatory exudates and with metastatic malignancy. Large pieces of pleural tissue usually are required for the diagnosis. Pleural biopsy usually does not provide sufficient tissue. Thoracoscopy has been recommended, although thoracotomy often is required. There appears to be a relatively high incidence of tumor invasion of surgical scars and some recommend giving prophylactic radiation therapy postoperatively. Electron microscopy may be of value in differentiating adenocarcinoma from mesothelioma. With a combination of special stains, new immunologic techniques, and electron microscopy, the diagnosis usually can be established antemortem.

The survival following diagnosis is dependent mainly upon the stage of the disease at presentation. Those presenting with chest pain appear to have a worse prognosis than those presenting with dyspnea only. When tumor is confined to the ipsilateral pleura and lung, median survival is 16 months; when tumor involves the chest wall, mediastinum and pericardium or contralateral pleura, median survival is 9 months; and when tumor involves both thorax and abdomen or lymph nodes outside the chest, median survival is 5 months.

No modality of treatment is curative; however, pleurectomy may be palliative in some patients. Radiotherapy has been found to reduce pleural fluid and sometimes relieve pain; combination chemotherapy has reduced tumor burden in individual cases but its effectiveness requires confirmation in a large series with randomization.

The present patient was diagnosed at thoracotomy as having the epithelial variety of mesothelioma. Following thoracotomy, he developed tumor metastasis in the surgical scar and required radiation therapy for relief of pain. The patient continued with moderate to severe chest pain and died 10 months following diagnosis.

Clinical Pearls

1. Patients with mesothelioma are usually males in the 50 to 70 year age group who have had initial exposure to asbestos 30 to 45 years previously. There is no association between ciagarette smoking and mesothelioma.

2. Almost all patients presenting with a malignant mesothelioma have symptoms, the most common being chest pain and dyspnea. Therefore, in a patient with a pleural effusion who is asymptomatic, it is unlikely that the cause is malignant mesothelioma.

3. Approximately 70% of patients with malignant mesothelioma have a low pH, low glucose pleural effusion; this is in contrast to the 30% incidence of this pleural fluid profile in carcinoma metastatic to the pleura.

REFERENCES

1. Wagner JC, Sleggs CA, Marchand P. Diffuse pleural mesothelioma and asbestos exposure in the Northwestern Cape Province. Br J Indust Med 1960; 17:260–271.
2. Taryle DA, Lakshminarayan S, Sahn SA. Pleural mesotheliomas. An analysis of 18 cases and review of the literature. Medicine 1976; 55:153–162.
3. Antman KH. Malignant mesothelioma. N Engl J Med 1980; 303:200–202.
4. Hillerdal G. Malignant mesothelioma 1982: review of 4710 published cases. Br J Dis Chest 1983; 77:321–343.

PATIENT 88

A 78-year-old man with decreased sensorium and pulmonary edema 12 hours after evacuation from a house fire

A 78-year-old man was transferred 12 hours following evacuation from a housefire. When seen at the local emergency room, his pants were smoldering. He was noted to have thermal burns to the lower extremities below the knees (approximately 15% total body surface). In the local emergency room the patient was said to be stable without evidence of inhalation injury. He was given IV fluids and transferred. On arrival to the burn unit, the patient had decreased sensorium and pulmonary edema with expectoration of carbonaceous sputum. He was intubated and placed on a mechanical ventilator.

Physical Examination: Temperature 97°; pulse 110 regular; respirations 32. Lethargic and in moderate respiratory distress; no evidence of singed nasal hairs or soot on the face; diffuse rhonchi and wheezes bilaterally; tachycardia without gallops or murmurs; second and third degree burns to lower extremities below the knees.

Laboratory Findings: WBC 8000/μl; Hct 37%; serum HCO_3 19 mEq/L. ABG (40% face mask): pH 7.13, PCO_2 50 mmHg, PO_2 50 mmHg; carboxyhemoglobin level 3.7%. Chest radiograph: bilateral perihilar and predominantly upper zone alveolar infiltrates; normal cardiac silhouette; small right pleural effusion. An endotracheal tube, a central venous line and a nasogastric tube are in place.

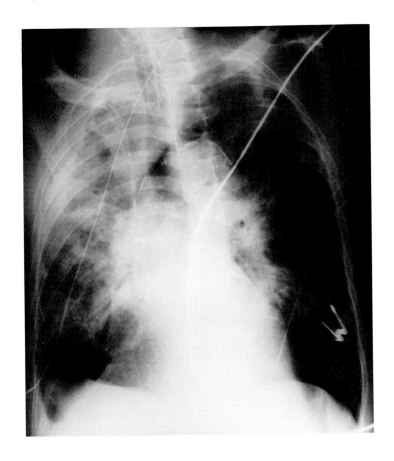

Diagnosis: Pulmonary edema secondary to smoke inhalation.

Discussion: Respiratory failure resulting from inhalation of hot air and smoke is the major cause of death from fire. Understanding the pathophysiology of smoke inhalation injury is important in early diagnosis and therapy, and the only chance of improving survival in these individuals. There are three components of this injury: (1) carbon monoxide poisoning and, to a lesser extent, cyanide toxicity leading to impaired tissue oxygen delivery; (2) heat injury to the upper airway leading to upper airway edema, increased work of breathing, and hypoventilation; and (3) chemical injury to the lower airways from potent acids and aldehydes.

Carbon monoxide poisoning is an early manifestation of smoke inhalation with the patient presenting with subtle symptoms such as headache, confusion, nausea, and dizziness (carboxyhemoglobin levels 20 to 40%). Severe intoxication (40 to 50% carboxyhemoglobin) may produce a semicomatose state as a result of decreased oxygen delivery to the brain. Carboxyhemoglobin levels greater than 60% are generally fatal. Although the oxygen content of blood is decreased, the PaO_2 remains normal and the patient may not be tachypneic, as carotid body chemosensors are responsive to oxygen tensions rather than oxygen content. Auscultation of the chest and the chest radiograph usually are normal.

Heat injury to the upper airway generally results in clinical symptoms 12–24 hours following exposure. The patient may complain of dyspnea and be tachypneic and cyanotic. Examination of the chest may reveal stridor and expiratory upper airway sounds. Upper airway edema leads to an increased work of breathing and, at times, hypoventilation. The diagnosis of heat injury to the upper airways is made by history and direct laryngoscopy or fiberoptic bronchoscopy demonstrating erythema and edema at the level of the larynx. Flame exposure sufficient to produce a facial burn and singed nasal hairs often is associated with temperatures sufficiently high to produce mucosal damage. Concomitant burns to the face can result in massive facial and oropharyngeal swelling, impairing the ability to manage oral secretions and possibly leading to tracheal compression.

The chemical injury from smoke inhalation is of more serious consequence than the thermal injury. Toxic gases, as well as carbon particles, coated with aldehydes and organic acids can result in injury to both the upper and lower airways, the location depending upon the duration of exposure, size of the particles, and gas solubility. The unconscious patient loses the protective mechanisms of breathholding and laryngospasm, which may lead to increased inhalation of the toxic gases. Water-soluble gases such as ammonia, sulfur dioxide, and chlorine from burning plastics or rubber lead to irritation, bronchospasm, mucous membrane ulceration, and edema. Polyvinylchloride, the most commonly used plastic, decomposes into a hydrogen chloride gas when heated and causes severe irritation of the mucous membranes. Upon reaching the lower airways, bronchiolitis and alveolitis may ensue. The oxides of nitrogen (liberated from wallpaper and lacquered wood) and aldehydes (from wood and cotton) are lipid-soluble and can alter the cellular membrane lipid fraction and lead to rapidly fatal pulmonary edema. Ciliary activity is severely impaired in the larger airways, decreasing clearance of mucous and debris. In the first several hours, the response to chemical injury may be absent or similar to that from gastric acid aspiration—bronchoconstriction and bronchorrhea. Fiberoptic bronchoscopy will reveal erythematous and, at times, ulcerated mucosa, which indicates the presence but not the severity of the injury. With severe chemical injury, capillary permeability and pulmonary edema may occur, resulting in the adult respiratory distress syndrome. Sloughing of airway mucosa, leading to distal airways obstruction in conjunction with alveolar edema, will lead to increased work of breathing resulting in hypercapnic as well as hypoxic respiratory failure.

Treatment for carbon monoxide poisoning is 100% oxygen; the concentration of carboxyhemoglobin is reduced by 50% after 30 to 40 minutes of breathing 100% oxygen. One hundred percent oxygen should be used until the carboxyhemoglobin level is below 10% and metabolic acidosis has resolved. Treatment of heat injury to the upper airways is supportive if upper airway obstruction is not likely, with maintenance in the semi-erect position and assistance in removing oropharyngeal secretions. Endotracheal intubation is indicated in the patient with a high risk for obstruction, particularly if there are deep burns to the face and neck.

Treatment of chemical injury to the airways includes prevention of atelectasis, maintenance of small airway patency, and removal of mucopurulent secretions. Inhaled bronchodilators, chest physiotherapy, and monitored fluid administration, preserving a euvolemic state, may be effective in mild cases. With more severe injury, endotracheal intubation with mechanical ventilation and PEEP usually is necessary. Steroids and prophylactic antibiotics are not indicated, with the former associated with increased mortality due to infection. Injury to the mucosa of the tracheobronchial tree with impaired mucociliary activity greatly increases the risk of bronchiolitis and pneumonia as the source for sepsis 1 to 2 weeks following smoke inhalation.

The present patient developed capillary permeability pulmonary edema 12 hours following inhalation injury and initially responded to endotracheal intubation, mechanical ventilation, and PEEP. However, 2 weeks later he developed bilateral pneumonia with marked hypoxemia, leading to an acute myocardial infarction and death.

Clinical Pearls

1. The three components of smoke inhalation injury are carbon monoxide poisoning, thermal injury, and chemical injury.

2. The chemical injury of smoke inhalation usually occurs from 24 to 72 hours (but may occur within hours) following the inhalation and may present with both airways and parenchymal manifestations that include wheezing, rhonchi, and pulmonary edema.

3. Corticosteroids are contraindicated, as they have no proven efficacy and have been found to increase mortality in patients with a combined inhalation injury and cutaneous burn due to pulmonary infection.

REFERENCES

1. Cahalane M, Demling RH. Early respiratory abnormalities from smoke inhalation. JAMA 1984; 251:771–773.
2. Teixidor HS, Rubin E, Novick GS, Alonso DR. Smoke inhalation: radiologic manifestations. Radiology 1983; 149:383–387.
3. Thorning DR, Howard ML, Hudson LD, Schumacher RL. Pulmonary responses to smoke inhalation: morphologic changes in rabbits exposed to pinewood smoke. Hum Pathol 1982; 13:355–364.

PATIENT 89

A 68-year-old man with adenocarcinoma of the lung and swelling of the left arm

A 68-year-old man with adenocarcinoma of the lung, diagnosed 4 months earlier, was admitted with swelling of the left arm. There were episodes of acute dyspnea several times over the previous two months and a weight loss of 15 pounds.

Physical Examination: Temperature 100°; pulse 100 and regular; respirations 24. Cachectic; no acute distress. Chest examination: bilateral rhonchi without consolidation; no peripheral lymphadenopathy; enlarged left arm with 2+ edema and increase in warmth without erythema or pain on palpation.

Laboratory Findings: WBC 7800/μl with a normal differential; Hct 30%; platelet count 575,000/μl. Partial thromboplastin time 20 sec, prothrombin time 9 sec, fibrinogen 480 mg/dl. Chest radiograph: widened superior mediastinum, large right upper lobe lesion and several smaller nodules in both lungs. Venogram: left axillary vein thrombosis with extensive collateral circulation; ventilation-perfusion lung scan: high probability of pulmonary embolism.

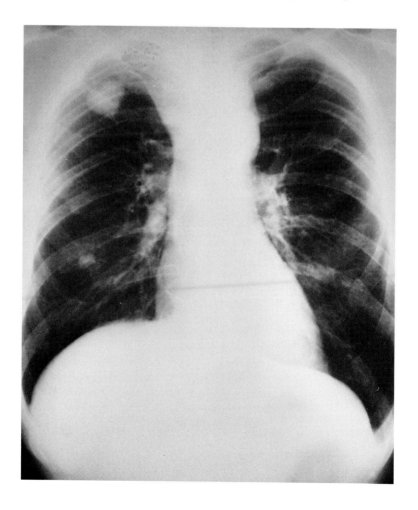

Diagnosis: Hypercoagulability in a patient with carcinoma of the lung with axillary vein thrombosis and pulmonary embolism.

Discussion: Over 100 years ago, Trousseau described the hypercoagulable state of malignancy. Over 50 years ago, the first large study of patients with malignancy revealed accelerated bleeding time in over 60%. Since then elevated clotting factors I, V, VIII, IX, and XI and shortened partial thromboplastin times, prothrombin times, and accelerated clotting times have been documented. Although these parameters are indicative of a hypercoagulable state, there is not a good correlation between these abnormalities and clinical thrombosis. Furthermore, a low-grade intravascular coagulopathy probably is ongoing in these patients, as evidenced by increased fibrinogen turnover and decreased platelet survival, high levels of fibrin degradation products, cryofibrinogens, and fibrin monomers. A shortened survival of fibrinogen and platelets and other coagulation proteins is associated with an over-compensatory increase in coagulation factors and fibrinolytic enzymes. In addition, decreases in the major coagulation inhibitor, antithrombin III, occur. These changes affect the homeostasis between clotting, lysis and clot inhibition, making the patient with malignancy highly sensitive to minor perturbations in the hemostatic system, predisposing to localized intravascular coagulation (thrombosis) or disseminated intravascular coagulation (hemorrhage). Thrombosis is a more common problem and may approach 50% in patients with carcinoma. In some patients, coagulation abnormalities have been correlated directly to tumor bulk and inversely to patient survival. Following surgery, radiation therapy, or chemotherapy, there may be improvement in the coagulopathy. Some malignant tissues produce thromboplastin-like activity, and presumably the amount released is decisive in whether localized intravascular coagulation (thrombosis) or DIC (hemorrhage) occurs. Low antithrombin III levels allow this process to be initiated more readily and proceed without inhibition once started.

Mucinous adenocarcinomas are most commonly associated with thrombosis. The sialic acid moiety of the mucin is capable of initiating clotting by the nonenzymatic activation of factor X. The carcinomas most commonly associated with thrombosis are those affecting the pancreas, stomach, lung, colon, ovary, and gallbladder. In pancreatic carcinoma, the release of trypsin may be the clotting trigger. Carcinoma of the body and tail of the pancreas is more commonly associated with thrombosis; since in carcinoma of the head of the pancreas with duct obstruction, there is minimal trypsin released.

The overall incidence of thrombosis in malignancy is about 15% but is higher with tumors such as pancreatic carcinoma where it exceeds 50%. The postoperative state results in a major risk period for thrombosis for the cancer patient, and thromboembolic disease is one of the major causes of death. A corollary is that persons having thromboembolic phenomena of unknown etiology frequently are found at follow-up to have carcinoma.

Platelet abnormalities may be responsible or contribute to the hypercoagulable state of the patient with carcinoma; these patients have increased numbers, abnormal morphology, and increased platelet adhesiveness.

Anti-tumor therapy, anticoagulants, and antiplatelet drugs have been associated with some correction of the coagulopathy; however, these patients are notoriously resistant to anticoagulants, often with persistent thrombosis. Furthermore, anticoagulants have been associated with significant bleeding that is closely related to tumor necrosis. Patients with decreased antithrombin III levels have a suboptimal heparin response. Aspirin or dipyridamole may be effective for the immediate treatment of thrombus extension as well as for long-term prophylaxis of recurrent thromboses. With adequate levels of antithrombin III, minidose heparin has been found to be as effective as full-dose heparin, with a decreased incidence of bleeding.

The present patient was placed on minidose heparin and dipyridamole, with prevention of recurrent thromboses and resolution of the episodes of dyspnea.

Clinical Pearls

1. Mucinous adenocarcinomas are most frequently associated with thrombosis; thrombosis has been reported to exceed 50% in tumors of the body and tail of the pancreas.

2. Presumably procoagulant substances secreted from carcinoma cells result in activation of the coagulation system; platelet abnormalities may participate in the coagulopathy.

3. Thromboembolism is one of the major causes of death in cancer patients; in thromboembolic disease of unknown cause, follow-up frequently discovers carcinoma.

4. With normal antithrombin III levels, minidose heparin appears to be equally as effective as full-dose heparin in preventing subsequent thromboses with a decreased risk of hemorrhage from tumor necrosis.

REFERENCES

1. Gore JM, Applebaum JS, Greene HL, et al. Occult cancer in patients with acute pulmonary embolism. Ann Intern Med 1982; 96:556–560.
2. Sack GH Jr, Levin J, Bell WR. Trousseau's syndrome and other manifestations of chronic disseminating coagulopathy in patients with neoplasms: clinical, pathophysiologic, and therapeutic features. Medicine 1977; 56:1–37.
3. Rickles FR, Edwards RL. Activation of blood coagulation in cancer. Trousseau's syndrome revisited. Blood 1983; 62:14–31.

PATIENT 90

A 24-year-old woman with a 1-month history of facial and hand swelling with a right paratracheal mass

A 24-year-old woman from Missouri noted the gradual onset of swelling in her face and hands over the previous month. She denied weight loss, recent trauma, or a smoking history, but she had experienced a mild cough and decreased exercise tolerance.

Physical Examination: Vital signs normal. Swelling of the neck, face and both arms with distended neck veins. The remainder of the examination was normal.

Laboratory Findings: CBC and electrolytes normal. Chest radiograph showed clear lung fields with a right paratracheal mass. VDRL negative.

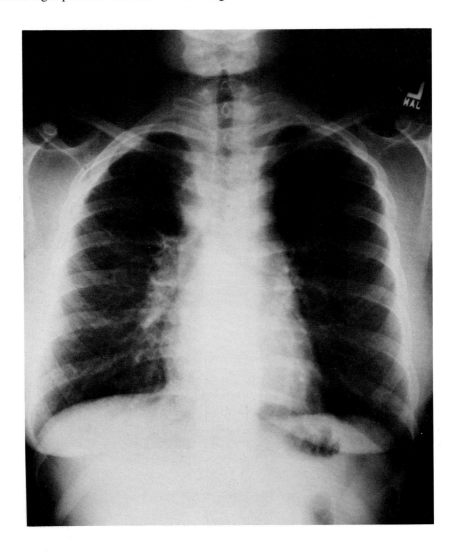

Diagnosis: Fibrosing mediastinitis with superior vena cava syndrome from *Histoplasma capsulatum.*

Discussion: The onset of the superior vena cava syndrome in a previously healthy patient is a dramatic clinical event that usually portends serious underlying disease. The differential diagnosis includes several malignant and benign conditions. Bronchogenic carcinoma is the most common cause of SVC syndrome, accounting for 75% of instances, with lymphoma or metastatic carcinoma underlying an additional 22%. Benign conditions are less common and result either from vascular thrombosis or compression of vascular structures by enlarging tumors or inflammatory masses. Although mediastinal involvement with *H. capsulatum* is an uncommon cause of SVC syndrome, it was recognized as a clinical entity in the mid-19th century and was discussed by Osler in 1903.

Histoplasma involvement of the mediastinum results in either granulomatous enlargement of lymph nodes or fibrosing mediastinitis. Enlarged lymph nodes contain caseous material and become matted together, forming a single encapsulated mass ranging in size from 3–10 cm. Although the masses are typically asymptomatic, being noted incidentally on chest radiographs, occasionally an enlarging mediastinal granuloma will compress mediastinal structures, causing SVC syndrome or bronchial and esophageal dysfunction.

The vast majority of instances of fibrosing mediastinitis are caused by mediastinal infection with *H. capsulatum.* The pathogenesis of the exuberant proliferation of collagen within the mediastinal compartment is uncertain. Immunologic material leaking from a caseous focus may possibly initiate an intense fibrotic reaction. Alternatively, an abnormal host response to granulomatous inflammation may initiate ongoing collagen deposition that persists despite adequate walling off of the fungal organisms. In any event, the end result is dense fibrosis with focal areas of calcification and fibrocaseous material infiltrating the mediastinum and extending into adjacent mediastinal structures.

The course of patients with mediastinal fibrosis is variable. If the fibrosis does not involve mediastinal structures, the patient may remain asymptomatic. If symptoms do occur, the nature of the patient's presentation is dictated by the location of the fibrotic inflammatory reaction. Subcarinal involvement affects the major bronchi and pulmonary veins, resulting in airway symptoms and veno-occlusive manifestations. If the pulmonary vein obstruction is extensive, pulmonary hypertension simulating idiopathic veno-occlusive disease or chronic pulmonary thromboemboli may develop. A hilar location of fibrosis typically affects the bronchi or the pulmonary arteries. Paratracheal fibrosis has the greatest potential to obstruct the SVC, thereby causing the SVC syndrome.

Diagnosis in patients with SVC syndrome from Histoplasma fibrosing mediastinitis requires documentation of organisms in biopsy specimens or exclusion of alternative diagnoses in a clinical situation suggestive of histoplasmosis supported by positive serologic studies. Although the organisms in mediastinal lymph nodes are no longer viable and tissue culture is usually unrevealing, fungi may be detected with special stains. Specific therapy for fibrosing mediastinitis is lacking. Antifungal agents such as amphotericin B or ketoconazole are ineffective, since the organisms are nonviable or inactive. Corticosteroids have been used to suppress the inflammatory response with variable results. Surgery is ineffective because of the extensive fibrosis, except in instances in which a large mediastinal granuloma is compressing the SVC early in the disease course. Fortunately, many patients with SVC symptoms gradually improve as collateral circulation is established.

The present patient underwent a CT scan of the chest that demonstrated enlarged, calcified mediastinal masses that were biopsied at thoracotomy, revealing *H. capsulatum* organisms. After surgery, gradual improvement of symptoms over several weeks was observed.

Clinical Pearls

1. Infection with *H. capsulatum* is the commonest cause of fibrosing mediastinitis.

2. Obstruction of the pulmonary veins may induce pulmonary hypertension, simulating chronic pulmonary thromboemboli or idiopathic veno-occlusive disease.

3. Despite the lack of specific therapy, many patients with SVC syndrome and fibrosing mediastinitis symptomatically improve as collateral circulation develops.

REFERENCES

1. Scully RE, Galdabini JJ, McNeely BU. Case records of the Massachusetts General Hospital. N Engl J Med 1976; 295:381–388.
2. Berry DF, Buccigrossi D, Peabody J, et al. Pulmonary vascular occlusion and fibrosing mediastinitis. Chest 1986; 89:296–301.
3. Goodwin RA, Nickell JA, Des Prez RM. Mediastinal fibrosis complicating healed primary histoplasmosis and tuberculosis. Medicine 1972; 51:227–246.
4. Goodwin RA, Loyd FE, Des Prez RM. Histoplasmosis in normal hosts. Medicine 1981; 60:231–262.

PATIENT 91

A 65-year-old man with severe emphysema developing restlessness, tachycardia, and muscle twitching

A 65-year-old man with severe emphysema was admitted for wheezing and shortness of breath. He smoked cigarettes and took nifedipine as his only medication.

Physical Examination: Moderate breathing difficulties with hyperexpanded thorax and diffuse wheezes; normal cardiac examination.

Laboratory Findings: CBC, liver and renal function tests, and electrolytes normal. Chest radiograph revealed hyperexpanded lung fields without acute infiltrates.

The patient received an inhaled bronchodilator, intravenous corticosteroids, ampicillin, and an intravenous loading dose of 350 mg of aminophylline with a maintenance infusion of 45 mg/min. His respiratory function gradually improved. One day after admission, a theophylline level was 19 μg/ml. On the third hospital day, the patient became restless, experiencing tachycardia and muscle twitching. A serum theophylline level was 30 μg/ml and calcium was 11.9 mg/dl.

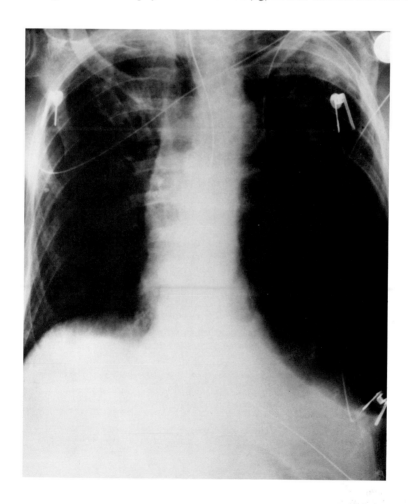

Diagnosis: Theophylline toxicity with theophylline-induced hypercalcemia.

Discussion: Despite widespread usage, theophylline toxicity continues as a major clinical problem for many patients hospitalized with respiratory disorders. The source of these difficulties lies in the variable pharmacokinetics of the drug and the potential for multiple drug interactions in acutely ill patients. Several associated disorders such as liver disease, heart failure, and smoking, in addition to advanced age and high carbohydrate diets, affect theophylline clearance. Commonly prescribed medications in patients with lung disease that either increase or decrease theophylline clearance include macrolide antibiotics, cimetidine, phenobarbital, phenytoin, allopurinol, oral contraceptives, caffeine, verapamil, and nifedipine. The latter drug may have been a factor in the toxicity of the present patient.

An important aspect in the management of patients with pulmonary disease is the wide intrasubject variability of theophylline clearance in the presence of an acute illness. During the first 4 days of respiratory failure, drug elimination may vary up to 300% in an individual patient. Furthermore, drug clearance is dose-dependent: elimination deviates from first order kinetics at high plasma concentrations, causing a large increase in the serum level after a small increment in dose. These combined factors of theophylline pharmacokinetics mandate consideration of the patient's clinical features supplemented by frequent measurements of serum theophylline levels to reliably adjust drug dosages.

Cardiovascular and neurologic complications are the most serious manifestations of theophylline toxicity. Potentially lethal cardiac arrhythmias and hypotension may occur suddenly without warning. Seizures can occur in patients with drug levels as low as 25 μg/ml, often appear as the initial manifestation of theophylline toxicity, and may result in death or neurologic sequelae in 50% of instances. Hypercalcemia, as occurred in the present patient, is an interesting result of theophylline toxicity. Theophylline promotes tissue accumulation of cyclic adenosine monophosphate, which also mediates the calcemic and phosphaturic effects of parathyroid hormone. Nearly 20% of patients with theophylline levels greater than 20 μg/ml have some degree of hypercalcemia.

The presence of theophylline toxicity warrants aggressive therapy to decrease the drug serum level. Hemoperfusion across resin or activated charcoal is an effective means of rapidly increasing theophylline clearance up to five-fold. The procedure is not prevented by nausea and vomiting, which are common symptoms in the presence of theophylline toxicity. Drawbacks include the need for an experienced team, lack of availability in many institutions, and the potential for thrombocytopenia, anemia, and hypotension. Although not as rapid as hemoperfusion, conventional hemodialysis also effectively increases the rate of theophylline elimination.

Because theophylline freely diffuses across the gut membrane and has a small volume of distribution, the oral administration of activated charcoal effectively decreases the serum theophylline level. Activated charcoal has a surface area of 950 m^2/g with tremendous absorptive properties. Superactivated charcoal has even a larger surface area (3,000 m^2/g), and, when administered orally, increases theophylline clearance four-fold. Giving the agent in small doses frequently (30 g of charcoal every two hours) is most effective, suggesting the importance of a constant presence of charcoal in the gut. If severe vomiting is a manifestation of the theophylline toxicity, charcoal can be administered after ranitidine and droperidol control emesis.

The choice of therapy in an individual patient is controversial. Previous guidelines recommend oral charcoal in patients with mild to moderate drug levels, and hemoperfusion for patients with critical toxicity defined by drug levels greater than 60 μg/ml, advanced age, and associated conditions limiting drug elimination. More recent studies, however, demonstrate no correlation of symptom severity with theophylline serum levels, patient age, or underlying clinical condition. These investigations support the use of oral charcoal in the absence of major complications of toxicity such as loss of consciousness, aspiration, seizure, or ventricular arrhythmias.

The present patient received oral charcoal, resulting in a rapid fall in serum theophylline level and improved symptoms.

Clinical Pearls

1. Oral charcoal rapidly lowers serum theophylline levels in patients receiving both oral or parenteral theophylline.

2. Hypercalcemia is a common associated finding in patients with theophylline toxicity.

3. Complications of theophylline toxicity are not correlated with patient age, underlying clinical conditions, or serum drug level.

REFERENCES

1. Aitken ML, Martin TR. Life-threatening theophylline toxicity is not predictable by serum levels. Chest 1987; 91:10–14.
2. McPherson ML, Prince SR, Atamer ER, et al. Theophylline-induced hypercalcemia. Ann Intern Med 1986; 105:52–54.
3. Amikai Y, Yeung AC, Moye J, Lovejoy FH. Repetitive oral activated charcoal and control of emesis in severe theophylline toxicity. Ann Intern Med 1986; 105:386–387.
4. Bukowskyj M, Nakatsu K, Munt PW. Theophylline reassessed. Ann Intern Med 1984; 101:63–73.

PATIENT 92

A 58-year-old man with ankylosing spondylitis and fever, purulent sputum, hemoptysis, and weight loss of several weeks' duration

A 58-year-old white male with a 37-year history of ankylosing spondylitis presented with intermittent fevers, chronic purulent sputum with blood streaking, and weight loss. Three years prior to admission the patient was noted to have left upper lobe fibrosis and cavitation. All diagnostic studies in pursuit of an etiologic diagnosis of the left upper lobe disease were negative. Over the subsequent 2 years, he developed similar disease in the right upper lobe.

Physical Examination: Temperature 99°; respirations 20. A chronically ill appearing male in no acute distress; decreased range of motion of the neck; bronchial breath sounds in both apices; no clubbing; neurologic examination intact.

Laboratory Findings: WBC 13,200/μl, 92% PMNs; Hct 31%; ESR 137 mm/h. Electrocardiogram normal. Chest radiograph: bilateral upper lobe fibrocavitary disease with an air/fluid level on the left. Sputum AFB stain: 4+ positive; sputum culture: plated for AFB.

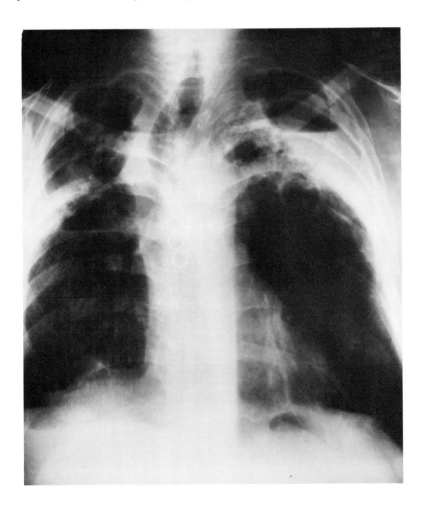

Diagnosis: Ankylosing spondylitis with bilateral fibrocavitary upper lobe disease and *Mycobacterium fortuitum* infection.

Discussion: In 1949, Hamilton provided the first report of ankylosing spondylitis and upper lobe fibrosis which mimicked tuberculosis. Since this initial report, over 60 patients have been described. It does not appear that the etiology of the lung disease is specific pulmonary infection such as tuberculosis or fungal diseases. However, it is postulated that impaired mechanics and altered mucociliary clearance might predispose some patients to repeated low-grade infection of the upper lobes.

Early chest roentgenographic findings are small nodules or linear densities in the apices. Coalescence and progression occur and cavitation may develop. The disease may be unilateral at onset but most often becomes bilateral; however, asymmetry may persist. Aspergillomas can develop in these cavities, and infection with group IV mycobacteria also have been cited as secondary invaders.

The rapidly growing mycobacteria are rare pathogens; only *M. fortuitum* and *M. chelonei* have been found to be pathogenic in man. These organisms have worldwide distribution and are common inhabitants of the soil. Numerous reports have documented the consistent recovery of *M. fortuitum* from the sputum of patients with chronic pulmonary disease, clinically indistinguishable from tuberculosis, and in patients with malignancy. The clinical problem is to determine whether *M. fortuitum* is a colonizer or tissue invader. Chest radiographs and routine laboratory studies usually are not helpful in identifying characteristics of invasive disease. Patients with disease due to *M. fortuitum* usually have symptoms of productive cough with hemoptysis and weight loss. The association of rheumatoid disease and ankylosing spondylitis with *M. fortuitum* infection has been well documented.

A number of problems arise when the diagnosis of *M. fortuitum* is pursued: (1) if cultures for AFB are not requested specifically, the organism probably will not be isolated; (2) *M. fortuitum* resembles diphtheroids on blood agar and may be mistaken for them on Gram stain unless AFB stains are done; (3) it may take from 7 to 12 weeks for the mycobacterial culture to become positive on primary isolation; this may be due to the toxic effect of chemical digestion before plating or the inhibitory effect of other antimicrobials that the patient may be taking. Furthermore, chemical digestion prior to inoculation onto culture media has been shown to decrease the viability of *M. fortuitum*.

M. fortuitum may be isolated repeatedly from the sputum in patients with normal chest radiographs; this is indicative either of colonization or bronchitis. A definitive diagnosis of *M. fortuitum* infection requires demonstration of the organism in lung tissue with a reaction to the organism or isolation of *M. fortuitum* from pleural fluid or blood in a patient with pulmonary disease compatible with mycobacteriosis. The usual pathologic change is a granulomatous reaction, usually with AFB positivity.

The assessment of therapy for pulmonary disease due to *M. fortuitum* is difficult to interpret because of the unknown natural history. *M. fortuitum* is resistant in vitro to all first-line and most second-line antituberculous drugs. In vitro sensitivity to the tetracyclines, vancomycin, erythromycin, amikacin, and kanamycin has been reported. There are anecdotal reports of both failure and success with surgical resection and chemotherapy. Treatment of pulmonary disease should be guided by in vitro susceptibility testing using the least toxic agent with safely attainable serum levels. Appropriate duration of therapy is unknown and should be guided by clinical response and evidence of drug toxicity. It is not clear whether multiple drug therapy is more effective than single drug therapy.

The present patient's sputum culture grew *M. fortuitum*. BAL was positive on AFB smear and grew *M. fortuitum* on culture; transbronchial biopsy demonstrated *M. fortuitum* in tissue with granulomatous reaction. The patient was treated with amikacin for eight weeks and then switched to doxycycline and demonstrated partial improvement of symptoms.

Clinical Pearls

1. *Mycobacterium fortuitum* has been documented to cause pulmonary infection in patients with chronic lung disease, including ankylosing spondylitis.

2. Diagnosis can only be established with certainty by demonstrating the organism in tissue with a compatible inflammatory reaction or in isolation from the blood or pleural fluid with compatible pulmonary disease.

3. *M. fortuitum* is resistant in vitro to all first-line and most second-line antituberculous drugs. In vitro sensitivity to amikacin, doxycycline, vancomycin, and erythromycin have been reported.

4. Therapy should be guided by in vitro sensitivities using the least toxic drug to obtain safe serum levels.

REFERENCES

1. Gacad G, Massaro B. Pulmonary fibrosis in Group IV mycobacterial infection of the lungs and ankylosing spondylitis. Am Rev Respir Dis 1974; 109:274–278.
2. Dreisin RB, Scoggin C, Davidson PT. The pathogenicity of *Mycobacterium fortuitum* and *Mycobacterium chelonei* in man: report of 7 cases. Tubercle 1976; 57:49–57.
3. Dalovisio JR, Pankey GA. Problems in diagnosis and therapy of *Mycobacterium fortuitum* infections. Am Rev Respir Dis 1978; 117:625–630.

PATIENT 93

A 62-year-old woman with a 3-month history of cough, dyspnea, malaise, and an upper lobe infiltrate

A 62-year-old woman was referred for pulmonary consultation. Three months earlier, she had noted a prolonged flu-like illness followed by cough, dyspnea, and malaise. Her physicians detected a left lower lobe alveolar infiltrate and hospitalized her for pneumonia. The infiltrate failed to improve with two weeks of antibiotics, and, after an extensive negative medical evaluation, she underwent a nondiagnostic bronchoscopy followed by an open lung biopsy. The lung specimen demonstrated "organizing pneumonia." One month after discharge, the patient's symptoms continued and a chest radiograph revealed a right upper lobe infiltrate.

Physical Examination: Temperature 100°. Chest: basilar rales.

Laboratory Findings: CBC and electrolytes normal; erythrocyte sedimentation rate 100 mm/hr. Chest radiograph showed a right upper lobe infiltrate with air bronchograms and left-sided pleural reaction.

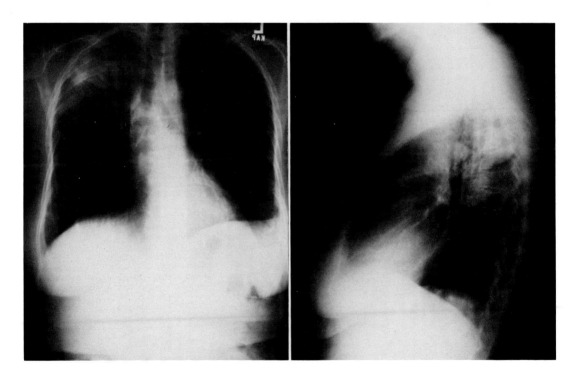

Diagnosis: Idiopathic bronchiolitis obliterans with organizing pneumonia (BOOP).

Discussion: Bronchiolitis obliterans is characterized pathologically by injury to small conducting airways that become plugged with granulation tissue during the reparative process, resulting in obliterative bronchiolar scarring. Extension of the granulation tissue into alveolar ducts is termed organizing pneumonia and completes the nomenclature of BOOP. Although first described in 1901, bronchiolitis obliterans has received renewed attention recently because of the clinical recognition of the unique idiopathic form of the disorder.

Causes of bronchiolitis obliterans include various respiratory infections, drug reactions, toxic fume inhalations, connective tissue diseases, and localized lesions such as bronchiectasis, cancer, or airway obstruction. The idiopathic form of the disease occurs in the absence of an apparent etiologic factor and differs sufficiently in clinical manifestations and prognosis to warrant its consideration as a separate entity.

The clinical presentation of idiopathic BOOP often suggests the diagnosis. A 40- to 60-year-old patient typically presents with a prolonged flu-like illness or slowly resolving viral pneumonia. A persistent, nonproductive cough develops associated with fever, sore throat, malaise, and mild dyspnea that is unresponsive to general therapy for several weeks or months. The physical examination detects basilar rales and rarely wheezes.

The chest radiograph is characteristic with bilateral, patchy "ground glass" or alveolar opacities without a particular lobar predominance. Infiltrates may start as a focal lesion and eventually spread bilaterally or remit in one location to appear in another. Although the appearance of the chest radiograph may simulate that of pneumonia, BOOP should be suspected in the presence of nonpurulent sputum, a prolonged course, and no response to antibiotic therapy. As opposed to idiopathic pulmonary fibrosis, diffuse infiltrates of a reticular or nodular quality seldom occur and volume loss is not a radiographic finding. Pulmonary function tests demonstrate reduced lung volumes and impaired gas exchange.

The timely diagnosis of BOOP depends on an awareness of the typical clinical and radiographic features of the disease. Confirmation of clinical suspicions, however, requires lung biopsy. Since bronchoscopic specimens are too small to adequately exclude associated conditions such as cancer or infection, open lung biopsy is the preferred biopsy procedure. Despite adequacy of tissue specimens, idiopathic pulmonary fibrosis is a common pathologic misdiagnosis, particularly when extensive organizing pneumonia in BOOP results in a component of interstitial scarring. BOOP can be recognized by emphasizing the histologic hallmarks of the disease that include a uniformity of temporal maturation of the granulation plugs across the specimen, a patchy distribution of the reaction, and preservation of background lung architecture.

Idiopathic BOOP generally has a favorable prognosis in contrast to bronchiolitis obliterans related to collagen vascular diseases. Although the disease occasionally remits spontaneously, prednisone is the preferred therapy, since it results in rapid and dramatic symptomatic and radiographic improvement. Once initiated, prednisone is tapered after several months and continued for one year to avoid clinical relapses.

The present patient's open lung biopsy specimen demonstrated the characteristic histopathologic features of BOOP. The patient denied a history of exposure to toxic fumes and did not have any of the underlying conditions commonly associated with the disorder. She was treated with prednisone with a prompt improvement in symptoms and clearing of the chest radiograph.

Clinical Pearls

1. A prolonged "viral" illness with a persistent radiographic infiltrate compatible with "pneumonia" should prompt a clinical evaluation for BOOP.

2. The chest radiograph in BOOP is characterized by patchy infiltrates without evidence of volume loss.

3. When interstitial fibrosis is present, BOOP may histologically simulate idiopathic pulmonary fibrosis unless the distinctive airway granulation plugs are recognized.

REFERENCES

1. Chandler PW, Shin MS, Friedman SE, et al. Radiographic manifestations of bronchiolitis obliterans with organizing pneumonia vs usual interstitial pneumonia. AJR 1986; 147:899–906.
2. Epler GR, Colby TV, McLoud TC, et al. Bronchiolitis obliterans organizing pneumonia. N Engl J Med 1985; 312:152–158.
3. McLoud TC, Epler GR, Colby TV, et al. Bronchiolitis obliterans. Radiology 1986; 159:1–8.

PATIENT 94

A 58-year-old woman with alcoholic cirrhosis and a left pleural effusion

A 58-year-old woman with a diagnosis of alcoholic cirrhosis of the liver was transferred to our hospital with increasing dyspnea on exertion, nonproductive cough, and an increase in abdominal girth over several weeks. She had been drinking heavily.

Physical Examination: Temperature 99.1°; pulse 96; respirations 24; blood pressure 130/64 without orthostasis; numerous spider angiomata; icteric sclera; flat percussion note, decreased fremitus and breath sounds over the majority of the left posterior chest; no jugular venous distention; marked abdominal distention with a fluid wave; liver 12 cm; 2+ pretibial edema; stool was brown and positive for occult blood.

Laboratory Findings: WBC 11,500; Hct 30%; prothrombin time 19.5 sec. ABG (room air): pH 7.52, PCO_2 35 mmHg; PO_2 74 mmHg. Chest radiograph: a large pleural effusion on the left; increased radiodensity of the abdomen suggested ascites. Total bilirubin 8.1 mg/dl; protein 7.1 g/dl; LDH 260 IU/L; SGOT 143 IU/L. Thoracentesis: bloody fluid; 75,000 RBCs (75% crenated); nucleated cells 5300, 80% PMNs, 10% macrophages, 4% lymphocytes, 3% mesothelials; total protein 2.5 g/dl; glucose 128 mg/dl; pH 7.44; amylase 35 IU/L; cytology negative. Simultaneous paracentesis: serous fluid; 396 RBCs/μl; 120 nucleated cells/μl, 60% macrophages, 20% PMNs, 15% lymphocytes, 3% mesothelial cells; total protein 1.1 g/dl; glucose 152 mg/dl; amylase 19 IU/L; LDH 41 IU/L; pleural fluid LDH 124 IU/L; cytology negative.

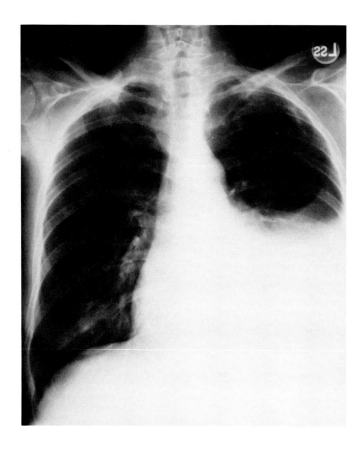

Diagnosis: Cirrhosis with ascites and left pleural effusion due to pleuroperitoneal communication.

Discussion: Pleural effusions occur in approximately 6% of patients with cirrhosis of the liver and clinical ascites. Pleural fluid results from movement of ascitic fluid through diaphragmatic defects or via diaphragmatic lymphatics. Defects have been noted as blebs on the diaphragmatic pleural surface, and movement of air from the peritoneal to pleural space has been observed through these defects at thoracoscopy. The defects are usually small (< 1 cm in diameter) and often can be overlooked even at postmortem examination without use of dyes or air bubble techniques. Blebs form because of defects in the muscle and collagen bundle structure at their base. Under the influence of increased abdominal pressure, the peritoneum may herniate through the defect and form a bleb. Sudden rupture may give rise to pleural effusion at various times after the development of ascites.

A patient with a pleural effusion due to liver disease usually has physical stigmata of cirrhosis and clinically apparent ascites. With a large to massive effusion, the patient may present with acute dyspnea but with a smaller pleural effusion may only manifest dyspnea on exertion or come to attention because of a routine radiographic finding. When clinical ascites is not evident in a patient with cirrhosis with a large to massive effusion, a large diaphragmatic defect should be suspected. An acute hydrothorax has been described in association with a simultaneous decrease in ascitic fluid.

The usual chest radiograph shows a normal cardiac silhouette and a right-sided pleural effusion (70%) that varies from small to massive (< 1%); effusions may be isolated to the left pleural space (15%) or be bilateral (15%). Thoracentesis usually shows a serous transudate but occasionally the fluid is serosanguinous or frankly bloody; the hemorrhagic fluid usually has no clinical importance and is due to the patient's coagulopathy. The leukocyte count is generally low (< 1500/μl) but, on occasion, has been reported up to 10,000 cells/μl without evidence of an acute infectious process. There usually is a mononuclear predominance but, infrequently, there may be a predominance of PMNs. The glucose is similar to serum, the pH is > 7.40, and the amylase is normal.

The diagnosis is established by demonstrating transudative effusions in both the peritoneal and pleural space that have similar biochemical findings. However, the protein and LDH are usually slightly higher in the pleural fluid. This may be due to portal hypertension, which prevents reabsorption of nonprotein containing fluid by the peritoneum. If there is any question concerning the diagnosis, injection of technetium sulfur colloid into the ascitic fluid with imaging up to 1 hour demonstrates passage of the radiolabel into the appropriate hemithorax.

The finding of an isolated left pleural effusion in cirrhosis is unusual enough to warrant a careful evaluation of the etiology of the effusion. The finding of a bloody effusion, exudate, or marked inflammation manifested by a high leukocyte count with predominance of PMNs should increase the index of suspicion for an alternative diagnosis and lead to appropriate diagnostic tests.

The treatment of hepatic hydrothorax is directed at the ascites, with sodium restriction and diuresis. The pleural effusion frequently persists unchanged until all the ascites has been mobilized clinically. Patients refractory to therapy who remain symptomatic can be treated effectively with chemical pleurodesis.

The present patient had a technetium sulfur colloid scan. Images at 15 minutes revealed diffuse activity throughout the peritoneal cavity and in the left pleural space. This activity progressively increased through 60 minutes, at which time activity also was noted in lymph nodes in the left hemithorax. Repeat pleural fluid cytology was negative, as were cultures for tuberculosis, fungal disease, and bacteria. With salt restriction, diuretics, and spironolactone, the ascites and pleural effusion diminished in size and symptoms improved.

Clinical Pearls

1. Approximately 15% of patients with cirrhosis and clinical ascites present with an isolated left-sided pleural effusion.

2. A rare patient may have a pleural effusion due to cirrhosis without clinically demonstrable ascites. Such a patient usually has a large diaphragmatic defect, resulting in rapid movement of fluid from the peritoneal to pleural space.

3. On occasion, an hepatic hydrothorax may be grossly bloody and have a PMN predominance.

4. The following findings in the setting of a pleural effusion and ascites warrant further investigation: (1) an isolated left effusion; (2) a hemorrhagic effusion; (3) an exudate; or (4) a large number of leukocytes with PMN predominance.

REFERENCES

1. Lieberman FL, Hidemura R, Peters RL, Reynolds TB. Pathogenesis and treatment of hydrothorax complicating cirrhosis with ascites. Ann Intern Med 1966; 64:341–351.
2. Johnston RF, Loo RB. Hepatic hydrothorax: studies to determine the source of the fluid and report of 13 cases. Ann Intern Med 1964; 61:385–401.
3. Mirouze D, Juttner H-U, Reynolds TB. Left pleural effusion in patients with chronic liver disease and ascites. Prospective study of 22 cases. Dig Dis Sci 1981; 26:984–988.
4. Hartz RS, Bomalaski J, LoCicero J, Murphy RL. Pleural ascites without abdominal fluid: surgical considerations. J Thorac Cardiovasc Surg 1984; 87:141–143.

PATIENT 95

A 47-year-old man with insidious onset of fever, pleurisy, cough, dyspnea, and hemoptysis

A 47-year-old white male smoker was admitted with the insidious onset of right, pleuritic chest pain, cough, hemoptysis, dyspnea, fever, and constitutional symptoms. He had been well prior to the development of symptoms, which persisted despite antibiotic therapy for the 10 days prior to admission. He was from rural South Carolina but worked indoors.

Physical Examination: Temperature 100°; pulse 100; respirations 24; minimal discomfort due to right posterior chest pain; diminished breath sounds and rales in the right base without evidence of consolidation; abdominal examination unremarkable; absence of peripheral edema, erythema, or pain on compression of the lower extremities; clubbing absent.

Laboratory Findings: WBC 10,000/μl with a normal differential; urinalysis and routine chemistries normal. Chest radiograph: volume loss on the right with an elevated hemidiaphragm, blunting of the right costophrenic angle and small peripheral right lower zone infiltrate. ABG (room air): pH 7.44, PCO_2 35 mmHg, PO_2 75 mmHg. Thoracentesis: serosanguinous fluid, nucleated cells 6000, 65% lymphocytes, 20% PMNs, 10% macrophages, total protein 3.8 g/dl, LDH 210 IU/L, cytology negative; Gram stain and culture negative; tuberculosis and fungal cultures negative; VQ scan: low probability; impedance plethysmography normal.

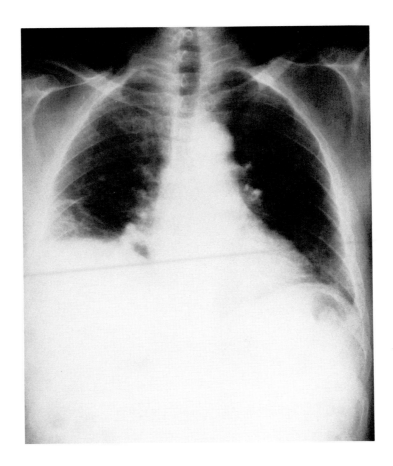

Diagnosis: Pulmonary cryptococcosis with pleural involvement.

Discussion: Cryptococcus neoformans, a yeast-like organism ubiquitous in soil enriched by pigeon excrement, is a relatively rare cause of infection in man suggesting that, in the normal host, defense mechanisms antagonize tissue invasion. Cryptococcal infection of the lungs is usually self-limited; however, dissemination occurs particularly in individuals with impaired cell-mediated immunity, such as those with lymphoproliferative malignancies, AIDS, or sarcoidosis, or those being treated with corticosteroid or cytotoxic agents. It has now been established that saprophytic colonization of the respiratory tract can occur without tissue invasion; this is most likely to occur in the setting of pre-existing chronic lung disease or lung cancer. Furthermore, the presence or absence of anticryptococcal antibodies does not distinguish between tissue invasion and colonization. Even when pulmonary tissue invasion occurs, the patient is often asymptomatic and the diagnosis is suspected when a routine chest radiograph is obtained.

Chest pain is the most common presenting symptom; however, cough, mucoid sputum production, fever, and malaise also occur frequently. The course of patients with pulmonary cryptococcosis is most commonly subacute or chronic. There is a poor correlation between the patient's symptoms and disease activity assessed either radiographically or pathologically.

There are no characteristic radiographic features of pulmonary cryptococcosis. The following patterns have been described: (1) cryptococcomas, (2) segmental consolidation, (3) poorly defined masses, and (4) mass-like infiltrates. Fibrosis, calcification, and evidence of substantial volume loss are distinctly unusual. Hilar adenopathy may be present, and cavitation occurs in up to 10% of patients. There is no predilection for lung zones. It has been suggested that diffuse pulmonary cryptococcosis is most often associated with dissemination. In contrast, focal patchy infiltrates or nodules are more likely to reflect localized pulmonary infection.

The pleura becomes involved when the infected focus extends to the adjacent pleural surface. Cryptococcal pleural effusions occur with equal frequency with pulmonary and disseminated cryptococcus, with no apparent predisposing factors associated with localized disease. Patients with cryptococcal pleural disease do not appear to have distinguishing features.

Up to 1980, only 30 cases of cryptococcal pleural effusions were reported in the literature. The effusions are usually unilateral, minimal to massive in size, and are almost always associated with accompanying parenchymal lesions. Half of the time they are serosanguinous or frankly bloody. Cell counts range from a few hundred to $12,000/\mu l$ with a predominance of lymphocytes. Effusions are exudates with cultures of the fluid being positive in about 40% of cases. Cryptococcal antigen has been demonstrated in pleural fluid.

The diagnosis of isolated pulmonary cryptococcosis is difficult, as there are no specific clinical features; however, the chest radiograph appears worse than the patient's symptoms. The diagnosis should be considered when a patient not in a high risk group for lung cancer or an immunocompromised host presents with a mass-like lesion on chest radiograph. When *C. neoformans* is isolated from the sputum, bronchial washings, or BAL in a patient with a new radiographic infiltrate, spinal fluid, blood, urine, and bone marrow should be examined and cultured. If the aforementioned tests are negative, tissue should be obtained by transbronchial biopsy. The finding of cryptococcal antigen in serum, cerebrospinal fluid, or pleural fluid is conclusive proof of active cryptococcosis.

Immunocompromised hosts with documented pulmonary cryptococcosis should be treated with amphotericin B and flucytosine. Normal hosts with isolated pulmonary disease do not need to be treated. The latter patients need a thorough examination for evidence of extrapulmonary disease and should be followed closely for several years.

The present patient had fiberoptic bronchoscopy with transbronchial biopsy and bronchoalveolar lavage. The airways were normal; cryptococcus was cultured from the BAL and from lung tissue but was negative in pleural fluid. Blood, urine, CSF and bone marrow were negative on culture and cryptococcal antigen could not be demonstrated. The patient has been followed closely with serum cryptococcal antigens and has done well clinically.

Clinical Pearls

1. *Cryptococcus neoformans* can colonize the lower respiratory tract without tissue invasion, most commonly with pre-existing chronic pulmonary disease or lung cancer.

2. Patients with isolated pulmonary cryptococcosis may be asymptomatic or present with a subacute or chronic history of chest pain, productive cough, and constitutional symptoms.

3. Pleural effusions are probably more common than previously appreciated and have been found equally between those with localized and disseminated disease.

4. Patients with documented pulmonary cryptococcosis (isolation from lung tissue or pleural fluid) should be examined for evidence of dissemination (culture of blood, urine, CSF, and bone marrow). If dissemination is diagnosed or the patient is a compromised host, treatment with amphotericin B and flucytosine needs to be instituted. In the normal host without evidence of dissemination, the patient should be followed closely clinically and with serum cryptococcal antigen studies.

REFERENCES

1. Kerkering TM, Dumar RJ, Shadomy S. The evolution of pulmonary cryptococcosis. Ann Intern Med 1981; 94:611–616.
2. Young EJ, Hirsh DD, Fainstein B, Williams TW. Pleural effusion due to *Cryptococcus neoformans:* a review of the literature and report of two cases with cryptococcal antigen determinations. Am Rev Respir Dis 1980; 121:143–147.
3. Hammerman KG, Powell KE, Christianson CS, Huggin PM, et al. Pulmonary cryptococcosis: clinical forms and treatment. Am Rev Respir Dis 1973; 108:1116–1123.

PATIENT 96

A 64-year-old man with hemoptysis and an upper lobe cavity

A 64-year-old white man from Texas noted progressive, mild cough with recent streaky hemoptysis. He had smoked cigarettes for 40 years and enjoyed good health with the exception of dyspnea on exertion related to chronic obstructive pulmonary disease.

Physical Examination: Temperature 98°. No lymphadenopathy; decreased breath sounds throughout with increased tympany.

Laboratory Findings: Chest radiograph revealed hyperlucent lung fields with left upper lobe cavitary and fibronodular infiltrates. Three of three sputum specimens were positive on smear for acid-fast organisms that were identified as *Mycobacterium avium* complex by Bactec methods 10 days later.

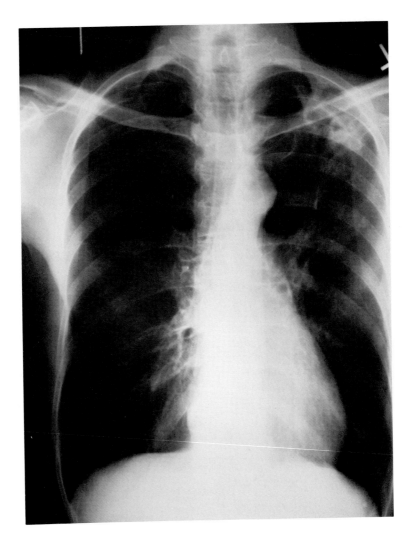

Diagnosis: Pulmonary *M. avium* complex infection.

Discussion: During each of the last several decades, the prevalence of pulmonary tuberculosis has progressively declined, whereas occurrences of nontuberculous mycobacterial (NTM) pulmonary infections have either remained stable or increased in frequency. Presently, a patient with pulmonary infiltrates and positive sputum smears for acid-fast organisms in certain regions of the southeastern United States may be just as likely to have a nontuberculous as a tuberculous mycobacterial infection. The majority of these clinical isolates of NTM prove to be *M. avium* complex with the remainder comprising *M. kansasii, M. fortuitum, M. scrofulaceum,* and *M. chelonei.* Although organisms of the *M. avium* complex are commonly isolated from water and soil, the source of human infection is largely unknown, and person-to-person transmission does not occur.

The typical patient with pulmonary infection from *M. avium* complex has underlying chronic obstructive pulmonary disease, which appears to predispose to disease because of impaired clearance of airway secretions. Previously, the disease was most prevalent in white males in southeastern rural areas, but recent epidemiologic data suggest an equal sex ratio, an increasing prevalence in urban areas, and a racial distribution approximating that of the general population. Patients usually present with mild, nonspecific symptoms such as dyspnea, malaise, weight loss, cough, or hemoptysis, and the chest radiograph shows upper lobe disease with cavities or patchy, nodular infiltrates. Although the cavities have been described as thin-walled in contrast to those found in *M. tuberculosis,* no radiographic features can confidently separate the two diseases in an individual patient.

Diagnosis of pulmonary infection remains a major clinical problem in approaching patients with positive sputum cultures for *M. avium* complex. Since the organism is a common saprophyte in diseased airways and most occurrences of infection develop in patients with underlying lung disease, separating mycobacterial infection from airway colonization is often difficult. Clinical data suggest that most patients with simple airway colonization in contrast to active infection can convert their sputum to negative after short periods of chemotherapy or regimens to improve their sputum airway clearance, such as bronchial hygiene. Based on these findings, the following criteria for infection have been proposed: (1) unexplained cavitary lung disease with positive sputum cultures after 2 weeks of appropriate antimycobacterial therapy, (2) noncavitary pulmonary infiltrates without a decline in sputum colony counts after 2 to 4 months of aggressive bronchial hygiene, or (3) detection of organisms in biopsy specimens with evidence of granulomatous inflammation.

Once diagnosis is confirmed, therapy is complicated by the resistance of *M. avium* complex organisms to most antituberculous drug regimens and a poor correlation between in vitro sensitivity testing and clinical results. Although no prospective, controlled therapeutic trials have ever been performed, most investigators consider prolonged therapy with multiple agents to be necessary to arrest the disease. Recent results have been encouraging utilizing isoniazid, ethambutol, and rifampin for 18 to 24 months supplemented with streptomycin biweekly for the first 6 months, which has resulted in a 91% sputum conversion rate.

Because of the marked drug resistance and the need for prolonged therapy, some clinicians approach infection with *M. avium* complex as a surgical lesion. Although controlled studies have not been performed, lobectomy may be recommended for patients with localized disease and adequate pulmonary reserve if the sputum cultures convert to negative after 4 to 5 months of chemotherapy.

The present patient was considered to have pulmonary infection with *M. avium* complex and was started on chemotherapy with isoniazid, ethambutol, rifampin, and streptomycin. Because his FEV_1 was 1.1 L, he was not evaluated for surgical removal of the infected left upper lobe.

Clinical Pearls

1. Previously considered a disease of middle-aged white males from rural areas, pulmonary infection from *M. avium* complex now commonly occurs in urban settings with an equal sex ratio and racial distribution approximating the general population.

2. No radiographic findings accurately differentiate between tuberculous and non-tuberculous mycobacterial infection.

3. Parenchymal infection can be confirmed in patients with positive sputum cultures for *M. avium* complex organisms by monitoring sputum conversion after appropriate chemotherapy or aggressive bronchial hygiene with inhaled hypertonic saline.

REFERENCES

1. Ahn CH, Ahn SS, Anderson RA, et al. A four-drug regimen for initial treatment of cavitary disease caused by *Mycobacterium avium* complex. Am Rev Respir Dis 1986; 134:438–441.
2. O'Brien RJ, Geiter LJ, Snider DE Jr. The epidemiology of nontuberculous mycobacterial diseases in the United States. Am Rev Respir Dis 1987; 135:1007–1014.
3. Ahn CH, McLarty JW, Ahn SS, et al. Diagnostic criteria for pulmonary disease caused by *Mycobacterium kansasii* and *Mycobacterium intracellulare*. Am Rev Respir Dis 1982; 125:388–391.

PATIENT 97

A 48-year-old man with a history of intravenous drug addiction presenting with mediastinal lymphadenopathy and lymphopenia

A 48-year-old black man with a history of intravenous drug addiction developed low-grade fevers, weight loss, sore throat, and malaise. He denied pulmonary symptoms.

Physical Examination: Temperature 99.9°. Palpable lymph nodes in both axillae and a single 1-cm lymph node in the left supraclavicular fossa; erythematous throat with white exudates; chest and cardiac examinations normal.

Laboratory Findings: CBC normal except for lymphopenia. Chest radiograph revealed mediastinal lymphadenopathy in the right paratracheal region. PPD was negative.

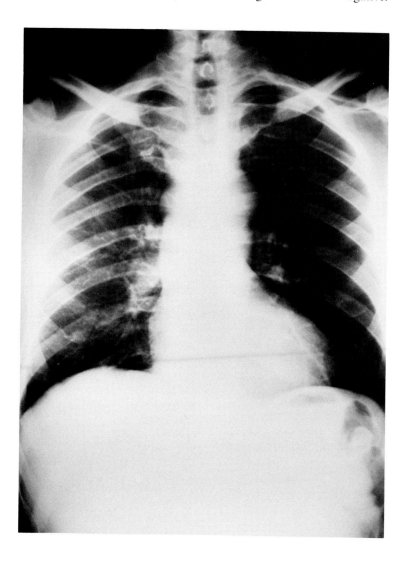

Diagnosis: Acquired immune deficiency syndrome (AIDS) with tuberculosis.

Discussion: The number of tuberculosis cases in the United States reported to the Centers for Disease Control has declined annually by 5 to 7% until 1985 when reported cases were only 0.2% less than the previous year. This diminished decline in tuberculosis morbidity has been attributed to the increasing numbers of persons with AIDS who are infected with the tubercle bacillus. The problem of AIDS and tuberculosis was first recognized in Haitian immigrants with AIDS who have a greater than 60% incidence of tuberculosis. Subsequent studies indicate that up to 10% of non-Haitians with AIDS have active tuberculosis in certain regions of the country. Considering that 10 million people in the United States are infected with tuberculosis, the AIDS epidemic poses a major potential threat to tuberculosis control.

The diagnosis of tuberculosis in patients with AIDS requires a high clinical suspicion, since the infection presents in atypical fashions and may be the presenting manifestation of the underlying immunodeficiency. Pulmonary manifestations differ from non-AIDS tuberculosis in their radiographic appearance. Most patients do not have an upper lung zone predominance of infiltrates, and lung cavities are unusual. Radiographic infiltrates are most commonly localized, involving the middle or lower lung zones, but diffuse miliary and interstitial linear infiltrates also occur. The presence of mediastinal and/or hilar lymphadenopathy is a notable feature of tuberculosis in patients with AIDS, occurring in up to 60% of patients. As demonstrated by the present patient, 20% of patients may have hilar or mediastinal lymphadenopathy without accompanying pulmonary infiltrates, thereby suggesting fungal and Kaposi's sarcoma related lymphadenopathy as additional diagnostic possibilities.

In addition to an atypical radiographic presentation, AIDS-related tuberculosis disseminates to extrapulmonary foci in 60 to 70% of patients compared to 16% of patients without AIDS. This dissemination can involve essentially any organ system, including the skin, pleura, bone marrow, central nervous system, lymph nodes, bowels, and bloodstream. It is clinically important to recognize that dissemination may be far advanced, even though the patient may have a normal chest radiograph, negative tuberculin skin test, and no other clinical features to suggest the diagnosis of tuberculosis.

Confirmation of the diagnosis may require examination of specimens from multiple sites. Sputum smears are often negative, and transbronchial lung biopsies do not show histopathologic features of tuberculosis inflammation, since granulomas are usually absent in patients with AIDS. The organism can be isolated from the urine, skin lesions, lymph nodes, bone marrow, blood, cerebrospinal fluid, or stools, thereby warranting an aggressive evaluation of patients with AIDS considered at risk for tuberculosis. Absence of tuberculous organisms or granulomatous inflammation from any combination of biopsy specimens does not absolutely exclude the diagnosis.

Patients with tuberculosis and underlying AIDS appear to respond well to antituberculous therapy. Although no therapeutic trials with differing drug regimens have been performed, short series report successful outcomes with isoniazid and rifampin. Because of a lack of extensive clinical and bacteriologic data on the response to therapy and the efficacy of short-course chemotherapy, however, the American Thoracic Society presently recommends isoniazid and rifampin plus pyrazinamide supplemented for the first 2 months of therapy. Ethambutol should be added if central nervous system or disseminated disease is present. Therapy should continue for at least 9 months or a minimum of 6 months after sputum conversion.

The present patient's constitutional symptoms, oral thrush, and drug addiction suggested the possibility of acquired immune deficiency syndrome (AIDS) or AIDS-related complex. Serum antibodies to human immunodeficiency virus (HIV) were positive. The mediastinal lymphadenopathy was compatible with early Kaposi's sarcoma, tuberculosis, fungal infections, such as cryptococcus, and persistent diffuse lymphadenopathy related to AIDS. Sputum smears were unrevealing, but biopsy of the palpable left supraclavicular node demonstrated acid-fast organisms without granulomatous inflammation that grew *Mycobacterium tuberculosis* on culture. He was started on antituberculous therapy, with an improvement in symptoms and a resolution of the mediastinal lymphadenopathy. He succumbed 5 months later, however, of pneumonia from *Pneumocystis carinii*.

Clinical Pearls

1. AIDS-related tuberculosis is disseminated in 60 to 70% of patients.
2. Mediastinal and/or hilar lymphadenopathy may be the only radiographic finding in AIDS patients with tuberculosis.
3. As many as 60% of Haitians and 10% of non-Haitians with AIDS have active tuberculosis.

REFERENCES

1. Rieder HL, Snider DE Jr. Tuberculosis and the acquired immunodeficiency syndrome. Chest 1986; 90:469–470.
2. Pitchenik AE, Cole C, Russell BW, et al. Tuberculosis, atypical mycobacteriosis, and the acquired immunodeficiency syndrome among Haitian and non-Haitian patients in South Florida. Ann Intern Med 1984; 101:641–645.
3. Louie E, Rice LB, Holzman RS. Tuberculosis in non-Haitian patients with acquired immunodeficiency syndrome. Chest 1986; 90:542–544.
4. Pitchenik AE, Rubinson HA. The radiographic appearance of tuberculosis in patients with the acquired immune deficiency syndrome (AIDS) and pre-AIDS. Am Rev Respir Dis 1985; 131:393–396.

PATIENT 98

A 62-year-old woman with a suprasternal mass and tracheal deviation

A 62-year-old woman was admitted because of an upper gastrointestinal hemorrhage and was noted to have marked tracheal deviation. She denied shortness of breath or dysphagia.

Physical Examination: Pulse 120; blood pressure 120/70; temperature 37°. Tarry stools; a smooth, hemispheric mass occupied the suprasternal notch. The trachea was not palpable.

Laboratory Findings: CBC, electrolytes, calcium, phosphorus, and thyroid function tests were normal. A portable chest radiograph showed rightward deviation of the trachea and a nasogastric tube.

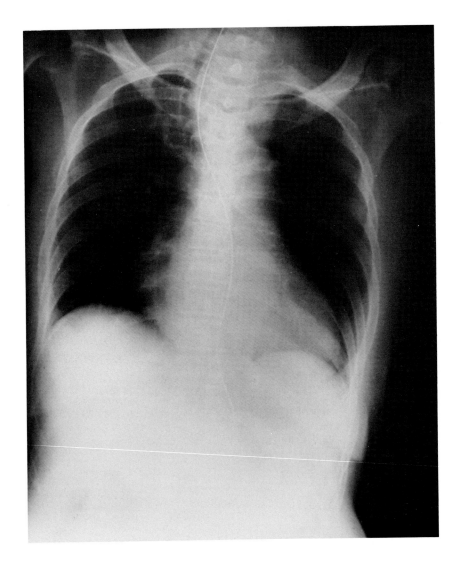

Diagnosis: Tracheal deviation from a substernal euthyroid goiter.

Discussion: Marked tracheal deviation, as noted in this patient, can result either from upper lobe volume loss that pulls or a mediastinal mass that pushes the trachea aside. The normal appearance of the right upper lobe in this patient excluded volume loss and suggested the presence of a mediastinal mass. A mass in the upper mediastinum presents a differential diagnosis that includes several neoplastic and vascular abnormalities. Two of this patient's clinical features, however, indicated a high probability that she had a substernal goiter. First, marked tracheal deviation in an asymptomatic patient with a normal-appearing aortic arch most commonly results from a goiter. Second, a palpable mass in the suprasternal notch that obscures the trachea in the region of the thyroid is invariably noted with a substernal goiter and less commonly found with other causes of upper mediastinal masses.

Enlarged thyroid glands occur most commonly in women older than 30 years but can develop in any age group. Most patients are euthyroid and are typically obese. The major clinical significance of a goiter is the potential for upper airway obstruction that results from external compression of the trachea, which may be associated with both substernal or cervical goiters. The incidence of upper airway obstruction from enlarged thyroids is unknown; however, small patient groups carefully evaluated with spirometry and cervical radiographs suggest that up to 80% of patients with euthyroid goiters will have some degree of tracheal stenosis.

Tracheal narrowing from goiters occurs so insidiously that patients often do not note the onset of respiratory symptoms. When carefully interviewed, however, most patients with euthyroid goiters will admit to varying degrees of dyspnea on exertion, choking sensations, dysphagia, and other sensations that include cough, throat tightness, chest fullness, or dyspnea that worsens in the supine position. The combination of unobtrusive symptoms and an 80% incidence of airway obstruction warrants careful evaluation of any patient with a goiter for tracheal stenosis.

All patients with a goiter should undergo pulmonary function testing with forced inspiratory and expiratory flow-volume loops to assess the presence and degree of tracheal narrowing. Characteristic findings are the diminished peak flow rates and the obstructive flow volume loops noted in both inspiration and expiration. Since spirometry may underestimate the degree of tracheal obstruction, normal results should be supplemented by soft tissue views of the neck in anterior-posterior, lateral, and oblique projections. The presence of moderately severe chronic obstructive pulmonary disease in a patient with a goiter may obscure the spirometric features of upper airway obstruction and may require endoscopy to exclude clinically significant tracheal stenosis.

Upper airway obstruction from a goiter may improve if the gland decreases in size after a period of suppressive therapy with synthetic thyroid hormone. Severe instances of tracheal stenosis with markedly enlarged thyroid glands, however, may fail to respond. If these patients have clinically significant airway obstruction, they should be evaluated for surgical removal of the goiter. Unfortunately, some patients with long-term tracheal compression develop chondromalacia, requiring tracheal resection and reanastomosis or placement of a stent.

The course of patients with goiter and tracheal stenosis is variable. Patients with mild or moderate obstruction may be relatively asymptomatic until they develop upper respiratory tract infections, when obstructive symptoms worsen markedly. Most patients respond favorably to suppressive hormone therapy, with improvement of symptoms and a decrease or stabilization of gland size. Occasionally, however, patients adequately replaced with thyroid hormone have progressive tracheal stenosis, resulting in eventual severe upper airway obstruction. Patients with euthyroid goiters, therefore, should be periodically evaluated with spirometry for worsening airway obstruction despite adequate hormonal replacement.

The present patient had an I[131] thyroid scan that documented a large substernal thyroid that corresponded to the curvature of the deviated trachea. She had 50% narrowing of the trachea demonstrated by cervical radiographs, with mild inspiratory flow limitation. Synthetic thyroid hormone therapy was started with progressive improvement of the tracheal stenosis.

Clinical Pearls

1. Tracheal deviation with a suprasternal mass is highly suggestive of a substernal goiter.

2. Up to 80% of patients with a goiter may have some degree of tracheal narrowing.

3. Most patients with euthyroid goiters have respiratory symptoms, although the insidious progression of airway obstruction may go unnoticed by the patient.

4. Tracheal stenosis from a euthyroid goiter may progress despite adequate replacement therapy.

REFERENCES

1. Jauregui R, Lilker ES, Bayley A. Upper airway obstruction in euthyroid goiter. JAMA 1977; 238:2163–2166.
2. Canham EM, Sahn SA. Recurrent "suppressed" goiter causing upper airway obstruction. Am Rev Respir Dis 1982; 125:757–758.

PATIENT 99

A 58-year-old man with respiratory distress and an abnormal chest radiograph 3 days following subclavian vein catheterization

A 58-year-old white male was transferred following a 24-hour history of headaches and seizures. CT of the head revealed a right temporal subdural hematoma, subarachnoid hemorrhage, and a frontal intracerebral hematoma. Cerebral angiogram showed aneurysms of the left anterior and middle cerebral arteries. A craniotomy was planned to evacuate the subdural hematoma and clip the aneurysms. In preparation for surgery, a right subclavian catheter was inserted by the neurosurgical team without difficulty. The immediate post subclavian line placement radiograph showed the tip of the catheter to overlie the region of the sternoclavicular joint but was otherwise unremarkable. A chest radiograph 3 days later showed a large, right paratracheal soft tissue density, and a supine chest radiograph 1 day later showed the right paratracheal density and increased opacification of the right hemithorax.

Physical Examination: Temperature 103.6°; respirations 32; lethargic; respiratory distress.

Laboratory Findings: Right thoracentesis: sanguinous fluid, nucleated cells 375/μl, 94% PMNs, RBC count 40,000 (100% fresh), pH 7.46, glucose 107 mg/dl, total protein 2.3 g/dl, LDH 85 IU/L.

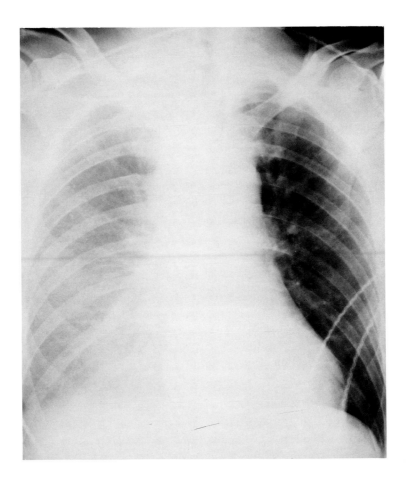

Diagnosis: Mediastinal migration of central venous catheter with infusion of fluid into the mediastinum and right pleural cavity.

Discussion: Numerous complications have been reported with catheterizations of the great intrathoracic veins. Complications of the subclavian vein approach include pneumothorax, hemothorax, hydrothorax, chylothorax, brachial plexus injury, perforation of a vein or the heart, sepsis, thrombophlebitis, air embolism, and hydromediastinum. A malpositioned catheter can result in spurious central venous pressure readings but also can be a clue to other more serious complications.

In a study of over 500 subclavian vein catheterizations, 71% were placed properly, with the tip in the superior vena cava or innominate vein on the initial post-procedure radiograph. Left-sided catheters were more properly positioned than right-sided catheters; right atrial placement was more common with right-sided catheters. The tip of the catheter was curled on itself in 4% of placements. The incidence of complications related to initial catheter placement was 1.6%, with pneumothorax being the only complication associated with successful catheter placement. There were 20 unsuccessful catheterization attempts associated with two complications: hemopneumothorax and a sheered catheter in the infraclavicular soft tissues.

Malposition of a catheter upon placement should be suspected if there is absence of blood return or questionable central venous pressure (CVP) measurements. Evaluation of the immediate post-procedure chest radiograph will confirm proper catheter placement. If the catheter is not in the appropriate vessel, phlebitis, perforation of a vein or the heart, or instillation of fluid into the pleural space or mediastinum may occur. Positioning of the catheter in a vein smaller than the superior vena cava or the innominate veins is more likely to cause intimal injury, which can lead to thrombosis. The catheter tip in the left side of the mediastinum could be in the internal mammary vein, which would necessitate repositioning. A catheter tip in the right mediastinum could be in the superior vena cava or the right internal mammary vein, which overlies the superior vena cava; a lateral chest radiograph may determine catheter position. Injection of contrast into the catheter will verify its position.

In the alert patient, acute infusion of intravenous fluid into the mediastinum frequently results in new-onset chest discomfort and dyspnea. Depending on the rapidity and volume introduced into the mediastinum, tachypnea, worsening respiratory status, and cardiac tamponade may ensue. The classic chest radiograph shows the catheter tip in an abnormal position, a widened mediastinum, and evidence of unilateral or bilateral pleural effusions.

Although extravascular migration of a central venous catheter has been associated with all sites of insertion, it appears to be more common with placement in the external jugular vein. The higher incidence with placement in the left external jugular vein probably is related to the perpendicular position of the catheter tip to the venous wall at the junction of the left external jugular vein with the left subclavian vein, and left innominate vein with the right innominate vein, which leads to easier perforation by the catheter tip. It has been suggested that using 20-cm catheters in adults places the catheter tip in the superior vena cava beyond the union of the innominate veins to prevent extravascular migration. However, this complication has been reported using 20-cm catheters. Unless catheters are fixed securely at the site of insertion, extravascular migration can occur even with 20-cm catheters if head and neck movement are not minimized and traction on the catheter site is not avoided. It is possible that with the use of external jugular venous catheters, catheter movement is more likely to occur.

Proper fluctuation in the central venous pressure during the respiratory cycle and free flow of fluid may not be reliable indicators of intravascular placement. This is probably due to the fact that intrathoracic pressure changes are transmitted to the mediastinum and thus the venous pressure catheter. Aspiration of blood or retrograde flow of blood when the catheter is lowered below the patient's heart level should confirm intravascular catheter placement. If blood cannot be aspirated and the infusate is aspirated instead, extravascular migration is assured. The CVP catheter should be removed. If there is a small effusion, observation is warranted. If the effusion is large, causing respiratory distress, or a hemothorax is discovered, thoracentesis or tube thoracostomy should be performed.

The present patient could not complain of chest pain or respiratory distress due to his underlying mental status but did have evidence of mild hypotension and tachypnea, which were relieved following removal of the catheter and therapeutic thoracentesis.

Clinical Pearls

1. Although extravascular migration of central venous catheters has been associated with all sites of insertion, it is more common with placement using the external jugular vein.

2. Fluctuations in central venous pressure during the respiratory cycle and free flow of infusate are not reliable indicators of intravascular placement; aspiration of blood or retrograde flow of blood when the infusate is below the heart confirms intravascular position.

3. Patients who complain of chest pain or dyspnea following central venous catheter placement should be suspected of having extravascular migration. A chest radiograph showing an abnormal position of the catheter tip, a widening of the mediastinum, and pleural effusion confirms the diagnosis.

REFERENCES

1. Conces DJ Jr, Holden RW. Aberrant locations and complications in initial placement of subclavian vein catheters. Arch Surg 1984; 119:293–295.
2. Moorthy SS, McCammon RL, Deschner WP, Fishel C. Diagnosis and management of mediastinal migration of central venous pressure catheters. Heart and Lung 1985; 14:80–83.
3. Feliciano DV, Mattox KL, Graham JM, et al. Major complications of percutaneous subclavian vein catheters. Am J Surg 1979; 138:869–874.

PATIENT 100

**A 62-year-old woman with insidious dyspnea on exertion
occurring 18 years after diagnosis of carcinoma of the breast**

A 62-year-old woman was referred to our hospital for evaluation for dysphagia. She had a 3-year history of hiatal hernia with progressive esophageal reflux. At presentation she complained of inability to eat solid foods, weight loss, fatigue, and increasing dyspnea on exertion. Carcinoma of the left breast had been diagnosed 18 years previously. She was treated with left radical mastectomy and postoperative radiation therapy; two lymph nodes were found to be positive at the time of surgery. The patient was asymptomatic, except for reflux esophagitis, until the above symptoms occurred.

Physical Examination: Temperature 99°; pulse 120; respirations 20. Cachectic, in no acute distress; left mastectomy scar and skin changes secondary to radiation; decreased bilateral expansion, decreased fremitus, and diminished breath sounds in the bases; neck veins flat at 45°, heart sounds distant without gallops or murmurs.

Laboratory Findings: WBC 9700/μl, 82% PMNs, 9% lymphocytes, Hct 37%. Chest radiograph: absence of left breast, enlarged cardiac silhouette, bilateral pleural effusions. CT scan: thickening of esophageal wall in middle and distal thirds; large pericardial effusion and bilateral pleural effusions. Right thoracentesis: serous fluid, nucleated cells 244/μl, 94% lymphocytes, total protein 3.1 g/dl, LDH 67 IU/L, pleural fluid/serum protein ratio 0.47, pleural fluid/serum LDH ratio 0.38, glucose 95 mg/dl, pH 7.40; Gram stain and AFB stain negative; cytology pending. Left thoracentesis: serous fluid, nucleated cells 820/μl, 78% lymphocytes, 21% PMNs, total protein 3.3 g/dl, pleural fluid/serum protein ratio 0.5, LDH 237 IU/L, pleural fluid/serum LDH ratio 1.3, glucose 75 mg/dl, pH 7.31, cytology pending. Pericardiocentesis: bloody fluid, cytology pending.

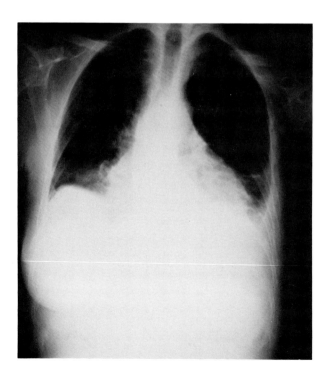

Diagnosis: Breast carcinoma metastatic to mediastinum, left pleura, and pericardium.

Discussion: Malignant pleural effusions are frequently the first manifestation and diagnostic source of the malignancy, signal incurability of lung cancer, represent the initial manifestation of recurrence, and portend a poor prognosis. Malignant effusions signify tumor invasion of the pleura; the diagnosis is established by the finding of malignant cells in either the fluid or in pleural tissue.

Virtually all carcinomas have been reported to metastasize to the pleura. Lung cancer is the most common because of its proximity to the pleural surface and its propensity to invade the pulmonary vasculature and embolize to the visceral pleura. Metastatic breast cancer to the pleura may exceed lung cancer in some series because of its high prevalence; however, on a per tumor basis, lung cancer predominates as a cause of pleural metastasis. Lymphoma accounts for approximately 10% of all malignant effusions and is the most common cause of chylothorax. Ovarian and gastric cancer represent less than 5% of malignant pleural effusions, and approximately 7% of patients have an unknown primary site at the time of initial diagnosis of the malignant effusion.

Obstruction of the lymphatic system draining the pleural space is the predominant mechanism for pleural fluid accumulation in malignancy. Pleural metastasis can be present without clinically demonstrable pleural fluid.

A common presentation of patients with a malignant pleural effusion is dyspnea on exertion. The mechanism of dyspnea is not due solely to a direct plombage effect on the lung. In addition, displacement of the thoracic cage, which results in the inspiratory muscles operating on a disadvantageous portion of their length-tension curve, and neurogenic factors in the lung appear to be contributory. Pleurisy is distinctly unusual and its presence should suggest another cause of the pleural effusion such as pneumonia or pulmonary embolism. Pleural effusion usually can be detected on physical examination since, in most instances, it is greater than 500 ml in volume. Approximately 10% of patients with malignant pleural effusion have massive effusions (occupying the entire hemithorax). When a patient presents with a massive pleural effusion, the most likely diagnosis is malignancy. The finding of bilateral pleural effusions with a normal heart size also is suggestive of malignancy.

The pleural fluid usually is an exudate with a protein concentration of about 4 g/dl. However, 5 to 10% of patients with malignant effusions have transudates. Transudative malignant effusions are due to (1) early stages of mediastinal node involvement; (2) atelectasis from bronchial obstruction; or (3) concomitant congestive heart failure. When the fluid qualifies as an exudate by LDH criteria only, malignancy should be suspected.

Approximately one-third of patients with malignant effusions have a low pleural fluid pH ($<$ 7.30) and a low glucose concentration ($<$ 60 mg/dl). Low pH, low glucose malignant effusions usually are chronic and associated with a large tumor burden and fibrosis of the pleura. These patients have a worse survival, a higher yield on pleural fluid cytologic examination, and a poorer response to tetracycline pleurodesis than those patients with normal pH, normal glucose malignant effusions.

In the patient with breast cancer, the clinician must always be cognizant of recurrence, as this cancer has a propensity to recur years following a "disease free" interval. The finding of bilateral pleural effusions and pericardial effusion without congestive heart failure suggests malignancy. A malignant pericardial effusion, most commonly seen with lung cancer, can occur with any metastatic tumor and can result in pleural effusions on the basis of increased hydrostatic pressure. In other instances, both the pericardium and pleura can be involved directly with the malignant process. Radiation therapy can cause subacute or chronic pleural effusions. Radiation pleuritis occurs over the same time course as radiation pneumonitis, 6 weeks to 6 months following radiation therapy, and results in a unilateral pleural effusion, usually in association with radiation pneumonitis, that may persist for months to years. Radiation therapy also can result in pleural effusions unrelated to pleuritis; these effusions tend to occur 1 to 2 years following radiation therapy and are due to constrictive pericarditis with or without tamponade, superior vena cava obstruction, or mediastinal lymphatic obstruction resulting from fibrosis.

The present patient had evidence of metastatic breast cancer to the pericardium, left pleura, and mediastinum. The effusion on the right was a transudate secondary to impaired lymphatic drainage of the pleural space. The patient had benign esophageal stricture. She underwent esophageal dilatation, a pericardial window, and bilateral chemical pleurodesis, with improvement in oral intake and symptoms. She survived for an additional 11 months with an improved quality of life.

Clinical Pearls

1. Carcinoma of the breast can recur years following an apparent cure and manifest in the thorax as pleural effusion, solitary or multiple nodules, lymphangitic spread, pericardial effusion, or endobronchial metastasis.

2. The major pathogenic mechanism for malignant pleural effusion is impaired lymphatic drainage due to blockage in the lymphatic system anywhere from the pleural surface to the mediastinal lymph nodes.

3. A malignant pleural effusion is most commonly a mononuclear predominant, hemorrhagic exudate but in up to 10% of patients is a serous transudate.

4. A low pH, low glucose malignant effusion implies a short survival time, a high diagnostic yield on cytologic examination, and a poor response to tetracycline pleurodesis.

REFERENCES

1. Chernow B, Sahn SA. Carcinomatous involvement of the pleura. An analysis of 96 patients. Am J Med 1977; 63:695–702.
2. Fentiman IS, Millis R, Sexton S, Hayward JL. Pleural effusion in breast cancer: a review of 105 cases. Cancer 1981; 47:2087–2092.
3. Sahn SA, Good JT Jr. Pleural fluid pH in malignant effusions: diagnostic, prognostic, and therapeutic implications. Ann Intern Med, 1988; 108:345–349.

INDEX